AF851163

Risk Factors for Cardiovascular Disease

Edited by Johnny Chahine

Published in London, United Kingdom

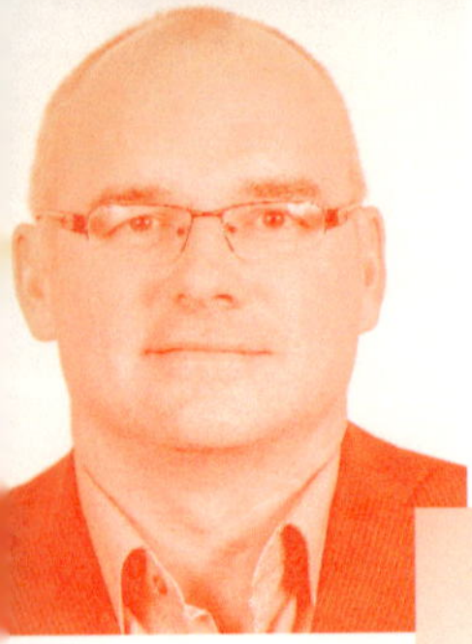
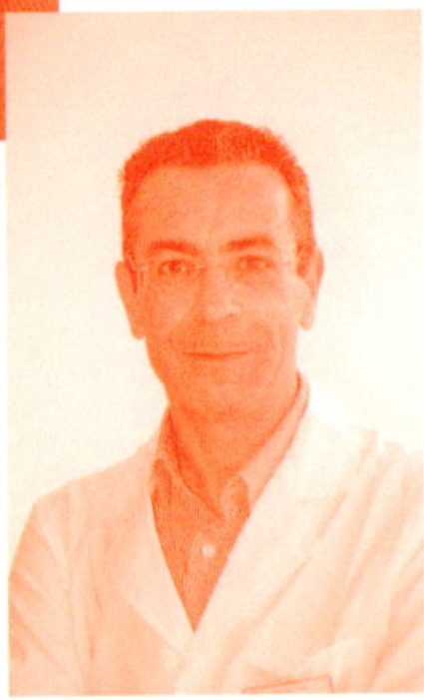
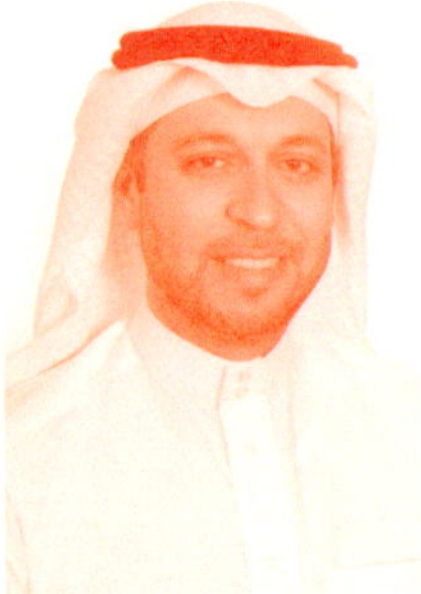
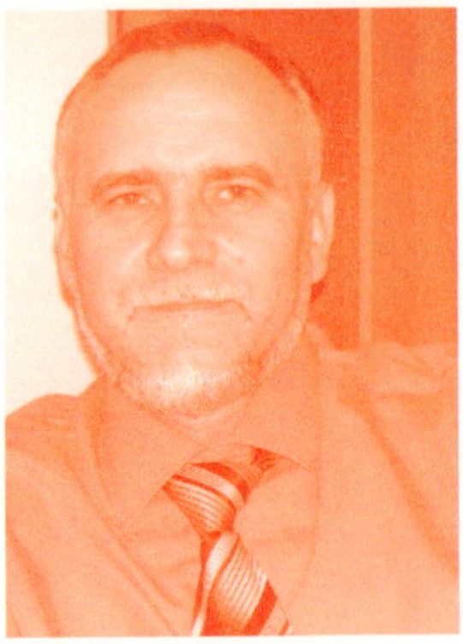
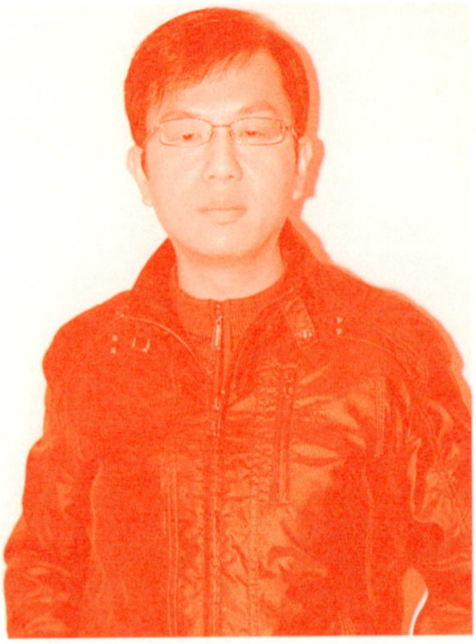
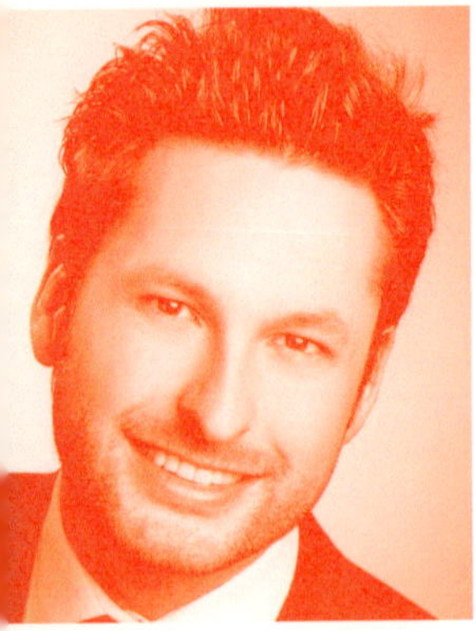
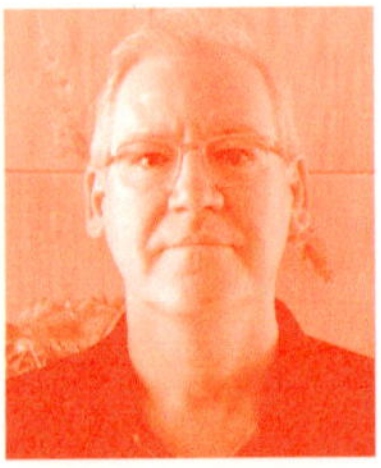

IntechOpen

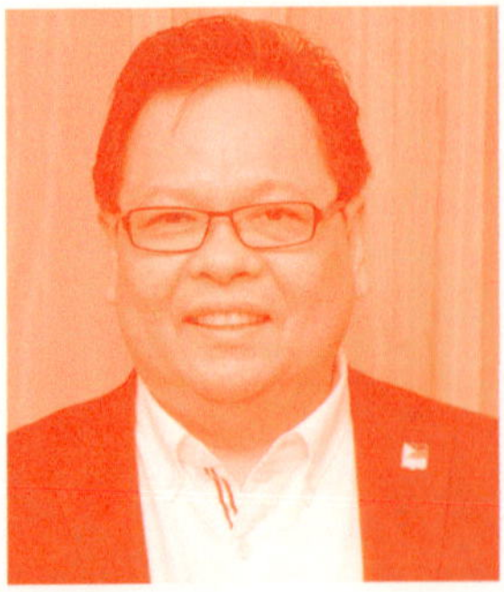
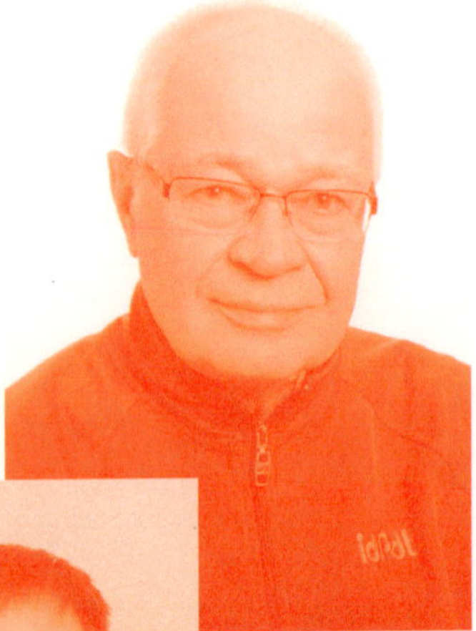
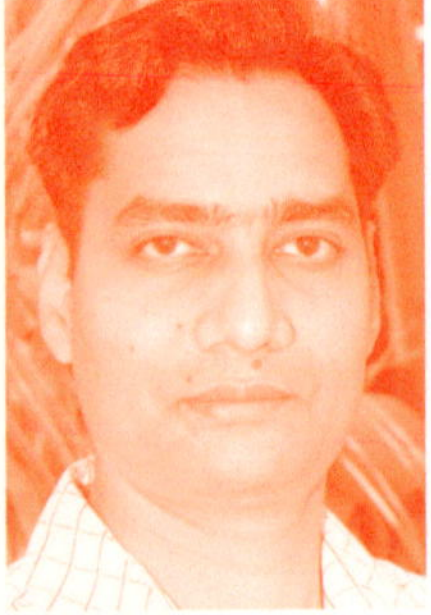
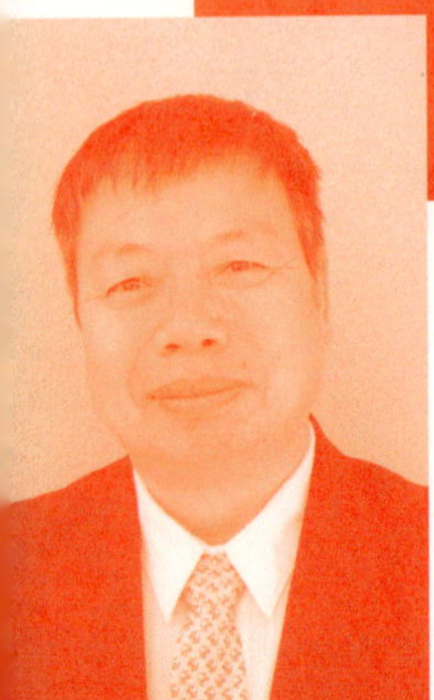
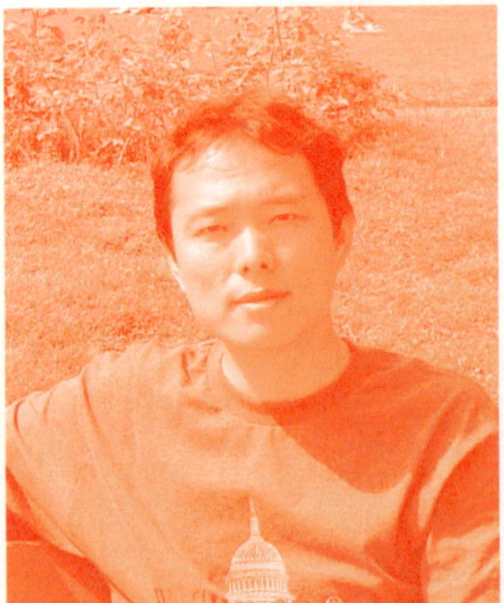
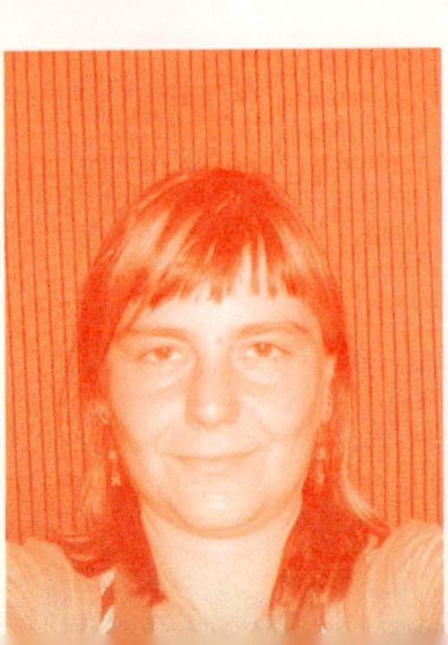

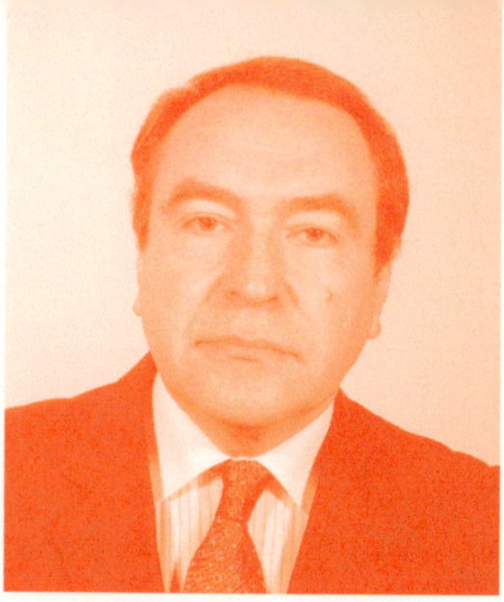
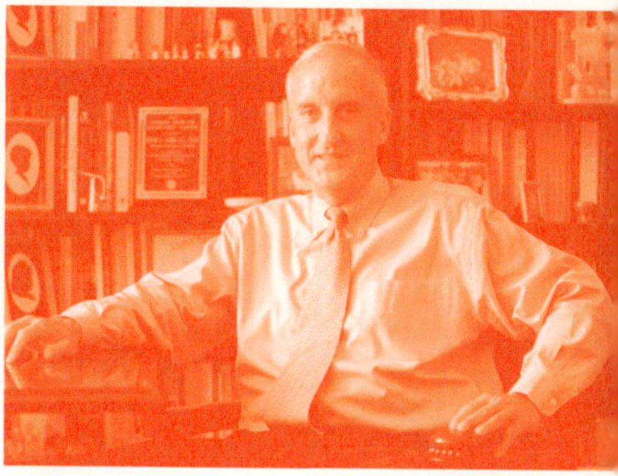
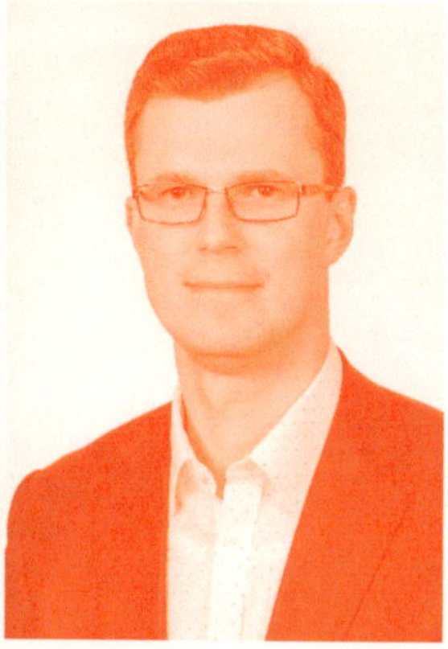
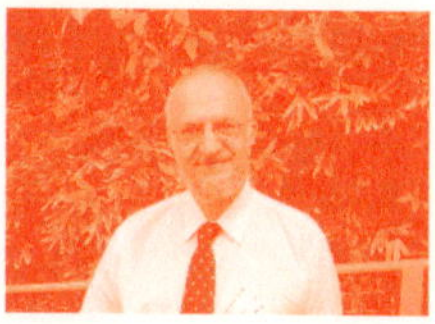
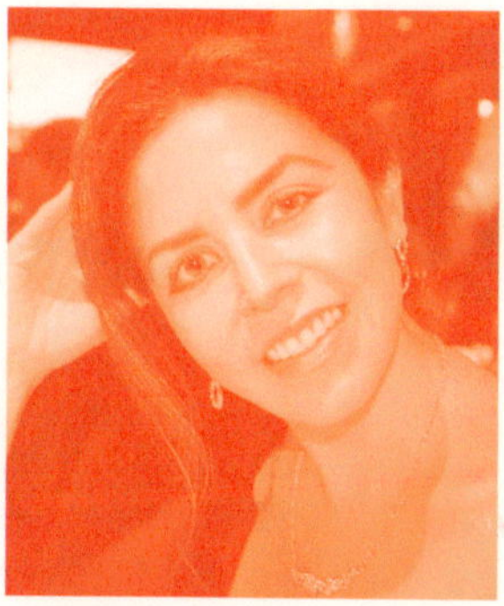

Supporting open minds since 2005

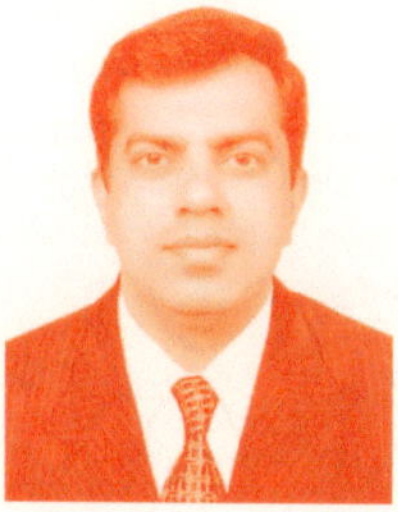
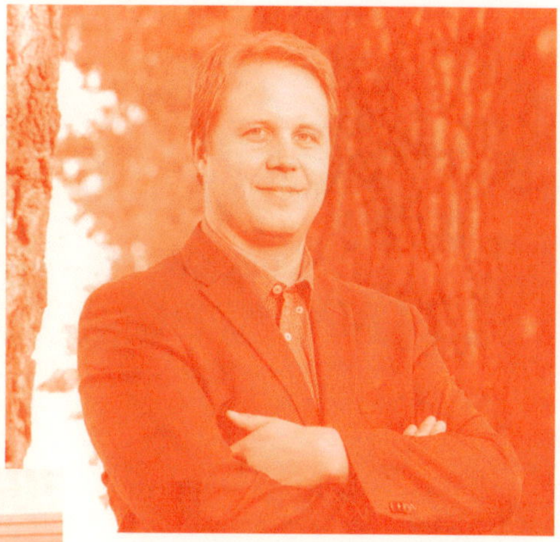
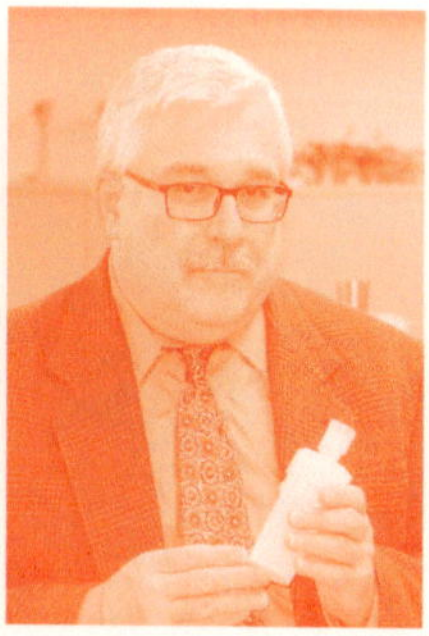
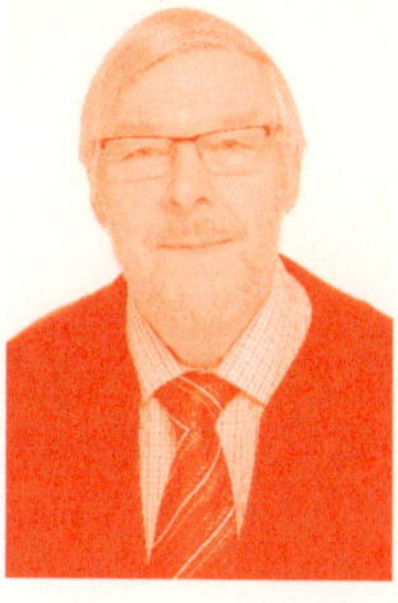
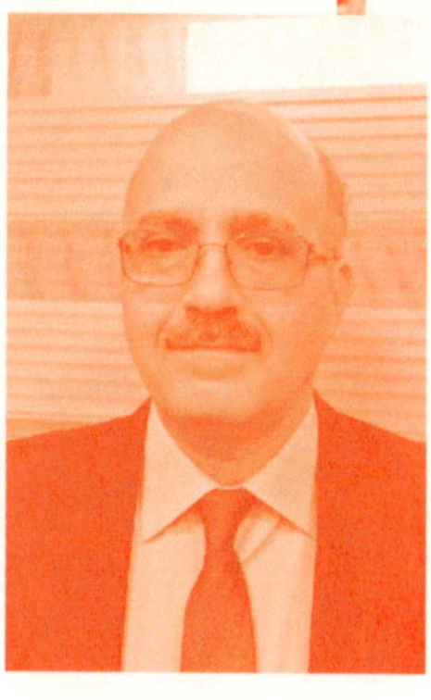
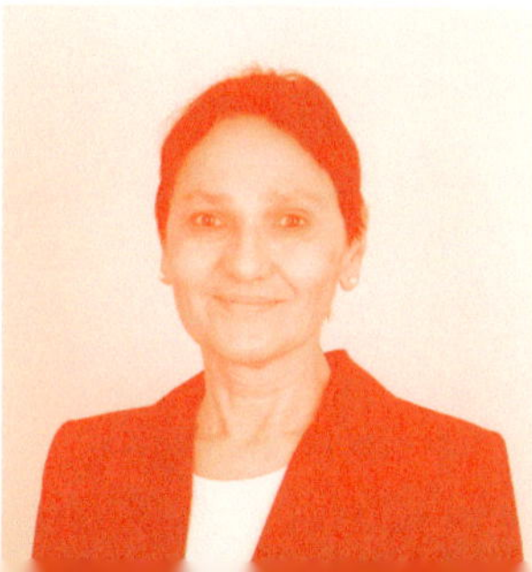
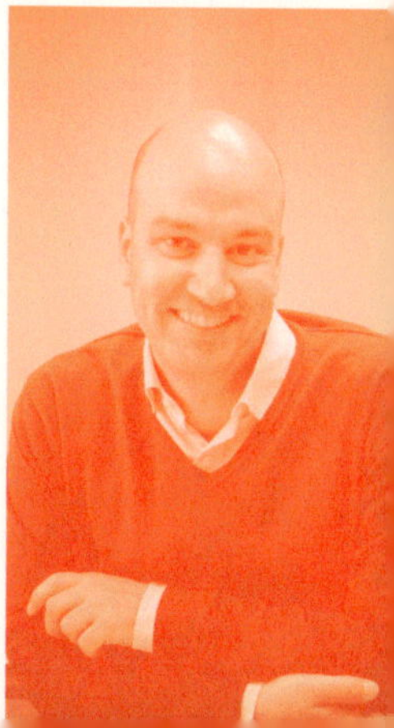

Risk Factors for Cardiovascular Disease
http://dx.doi.org/10.5772/intechopen.94673
Edited by Johnny Chahine

Contributors
Thomas K. Day, Christa Grobler, Wilna Oldewage-Theron, Joseph Musonda Chalwe, Erik Froyen, Mirjam Močnik, Nataša Marčun Varda, Ina Shaw, Brandon S. Shaw, Gregory A. Brown, Valery V. Gafarov, Dmitriy O. Panov, Elena A. Gromova, Eldar A. Krymov, Igor V. Gagulin, Almira V. Gafarova, Ana Paula Andrade da Silva, Roberto Calças Marques, Eduarda Castanheiro Esteves Carias, Nathan B. Buila, Jean René M'Buyamba-Kabangu, Jean-Marc B. Bantu, Elysée M-C. Munyoka, Gilbert K. Kabanda, Van Si Nguyen, Xuan Truong Tran, Thanh Duy Vo, Quang Truong Quang Le, Oytun Erbas, Özge Çağlar, Elif Özyilmaz, Ece Sarı, İlayda Üzümcü, Kaan Erbakan, İlknur Altuntaş

© The Editor(s) and the Author(s) 2022
The rights of the editor(s) and the author(s) have been asserted in accordance with the Copyright, Designs and Patents Act 1988. All rights to the book as a whole are reserved by INTECHOPEN LIMITED. The book as a whole (compilation) cannot be reproduced, distributed or used for commercial or non-commercial purposes without INTECHOPEN LIMITED's written permission. Enquiries concerning the use of the book should be directed to INTECHOPEN LIMITED rights and permissions department (permissions@intechopen.com).
Violations are liable to prosecution under the governing Copyright Law.

CC BY

Individual chapters of this publication are distributed under the terms of the Creative Commons Attribution 3.0 Unported License which permits commercial use, distribution and reproduction of the individual chapters, provided the original author(s) and source publication are appropriately acknowledged. If so indicated, certain images may not be included under the Creative Commons license. In such cases users will need to obtain permission from the license holder to reproduce the material. More details and guidelines concerning content reuse and adaptation can be found at http://www.intechopen.com/copyright-policy.html.

Notice
Statements and opinions expressed in the chapters are these of the individual contributors and not necessarily those of the editors or publisher. No responsibility is accepted for the accuracy of information contained in the published chapters. The publisher assumes no responsibility for any damage or injury to persons or property arising out of the use of any materials, instructions, methods or ideas contained in the book.

First published in London, United Kingdom, 2022 by IntechOpen
IntechOpen is the global imprint of INTECHOPEN LIMITED, registered in England and Wales, registration number: 11086078, 5 Princes Gate Court, London, SW7 2QJ, United Kingdom
Printed in Croatia

British Library Cataloguing-in-Publication Data
A catalogue record for this book is available from the British Library

Additional hard and PDF copies can be obtained from orders@intechopen.com

Risk Factors for Cardiovascular Disease
Edited by Johnny Chahine
p. cm.
Print ISBN 978-1-83968-708-2
Online ISBN 978-1-83968-709-9
eBook (PDF) ISBN 978-1-83968-710-5

For EU product safety concerns:
IN TECH d.o.o., Prolaz Marije Krucifikse Kozulić 3, 51000 Rijeka, Croatia, info@intechopen.com or visit our website at intechopen.com.

We are IntechOpen, the world's leading publisher of Open Access books

Built by scientists, for scientists

5,700+
Open access books available

141,000+
International authors and editors

180M+
Downloads

156
Countries delivered to

Our authors are among the
Top 1%
most cited scientists

12.2%
Contributors from top 500 universities

WEB OF SCIENCE™

Selection of our books indexed in the Book Citation Index (BKCI)
in Web of Science Core Collection™

Interested in publishing with us?
Contact book.department@intechopen.com

Numbers displayed above are based on latest data collected.
For more information visit www.intechopen.com

Meet the editor

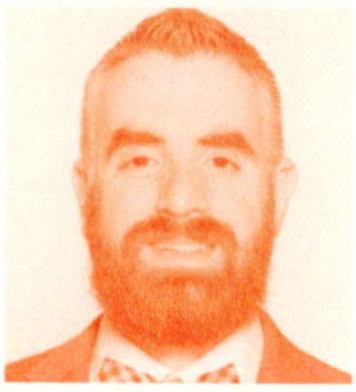

Dr. Chahine graduated from medical school in Lebanon in 2016 and moved to Cleveland, USA for his Internal Medicine residency in 2017. He is currently a cardiology fellow at the University of Minnesota, USA. He is well-published in high-impact journals. Dr. Chahine strives for excellence in his medical knowledge and a friendly environment for his colleagues and patients.

Contents

Preface

With an increasingly aging patient population and changing diets, cardiovascular risk factors are becoming more and more relevant in today's world.

Cardiovascular mortality remains the number one cause of death worldwide, and every attempt should be made to educate the public about the prevention and modification of the various cardiovascular risk factors.

Cardiovascular risk factors are generally divided into those that are modifiable and those that are not. Non-modifiable factors include age, gender, family history, diabetes mellitus (type 1 or 2), hypertension, hyperlipidemia, chronic kidney disease, and various chronic inflammatory diseases. Modifiable risk factors are those that can be addressed through lifestyle modification. These include diet (low fiber, high fat, and high carbohydrate), sedentary lifestyle, smoking, alcohol, obesity, and psychosocial factors. Some factors that are listed as non-modifiable can be largely influenced by lifestyle modification, especially in the early stages of the disease, like the impact of obesity and diet on hypertension and diabetes.

This book highlights the importance of addressing cardiovascular risk factors prior to any cardiovascular event (i.e., primary prevention), as controlling those risk factors as part of secondary prevention is important but not as impactful.

It is crucial to recognize that specific work settings can also predispose people to cardiovascular disease, through traditional or work-specific risk factors. In this book, we address the various cardiovascular risk factors that affect aircrew as an example. Addressing risk factors early on in life is very important, and this book describes cardiovascular risk factors in children and the importance of modifying those risk factors in the initial phases before significant atherosclerotic disease occurs.

I hope this book inspires further research on early recognition and prevention of cardiovascular risk factors.

Johnny Chahine, MD
University of Minnesota,
Minneapolis, MN, USA

Section 1

Cardiovascular Risk Factors in Different Patient Population

Chapter 1

Sex Differences in Long-Term Trends of Psychosocial Factors and Gender Effect on Risk of Cardiovascular Diseases: Arterial Hypertension, Myocardial Infarction and Stroke

Valery V. Gafarov, Dmitriy O. Panov, Elena A. Gromova, Igor V. Gagulin, Almira V. Gafarova and Eldar A. Krymov

Abstract

Introduction: The study aimed to determine gender differences in the prevalence and dynamics of affective states over a long period, i.e., 23 years, and to establish their effect on the risk of cardiovascular diseases (CVD), i.e., arterial hypertension (AH), myocardial infarction (MI), and stroke among the population aged 25–64 in Russia / Siberia. Methods: Between 1994 and 2017, we conducted 4 screening surveys of representative samples (totalling 4,815 people) under the international programs MONICA and HAPIEE in Russia / Siberia. To determine the sex differences in cardiovascular risk from 1994 to 2010, we observed cohorts formed from the screened individuals without CVD and diabetes mellitus (DM). Results: High levels of affective states in the period from 1994 to 2003, especially in women, were replaced by a downward trend in 2013. At the same time, there was a reduction in the gender gap in terms of frequency of depression lower 1%, and men in the younger age groups reported higher levels of personal anxiety (49.3% vs 46.1% in adults aged 35-44y) and vital exhaustion (16.9% vs 15.6%) than women in 2017. We found that men with unfavourable levels of affective states have a 3–5 fold higher risk of hypertension and stroke, while women have a higher risk of myocardial infarction (p for all < 0.05). Hostility in men is associated with a negative risk of myocardial infarction and stroke (HR=0.3 and HR=0.29, respectively; p for all < 0.05). However, this was levelled out by unfavourable social characteristics. Conclusions: The downward trends in prevalence of psychosocial factors were unstable and associated with reduced gender gap for affective states. It had a significant impact on the gender magnitude of cardiovascular risk.

Keywords: anxiety, depression, vital exhaustion, hostility, social support, population, risk, sex differences, arterial hypertension, myocardial infarction, stroke, marital status, education, occupational status

1. Introduction

The widespread and widely discussed opinion in the mass media that the number of people with anxiety, depression and other affective states is increasing year to year implies a relative increase in these disorders over the past decades. Nevertheless, the study of literary sources has provided multifaceted estimates of the prevalence of psychosocial factors (PSF). Due to the different recording methods in epidemiological studies, the heterogeneity of the data is too high to make a proper comparison. According to the available epidemiological findings, one-third of the population of the United States and European countries is susceptible to anxiety disorders [1]. At the same time, the prevalence of psychosocial factors depending on sex is also different. Negative psychological characteristics (e.g., anxiety and depression) are twice as common in women and often have a more severe form and an earlier onset [2].

The impact of PSF on health is unequal in terms of gender. For example, depressive disorders are on the list of the leading widespread diseases in the world among women, but not men, according to Global Burden Diseases (2002) [3]. And this may be an echo of other common negative psychosocial factors, such as high anxiety, vital exhaustion, and stress in the family and workplace. A number of these states are inextricably linked to the XX or XY genotype or are due to sex differences in functioning (i.e., susceptibility to diseases). For other psychological factors, there is a clear link to work and social environment, which differs for both sexes [4, 5].

Cardiovascular effects of stress and other psychological factors may also differ in women and men [6]. Large-scale studies show that particular psychosocial characteristics, such as stress or depression, are associated with cardiovascular health to the same degree in men and women, while others, i.e., vital exhaustion, anxiety signs and low life satisfaction, are associated with heart disease rates in women but not in men.

Analysis of recent studies and meta-analyses [7] indicates that social gradient, as a mediator, as well as the sex differences, boost the effect of psychosocial characteristics on cardiovascular health.

Different levels of PSF are not always adverse, but can also serve as protective factors concerning physical and mental health. Thus, a favourable profile of social contacts with relatives or friends is associated with favourable indicators of mental health and serves as a barrier to depression and perceived stress. In addition, the social support received from friends is positively correlated with the lifestyle, in particular, with intensive physical activities [8]. The accumulation of data on the influence of psychosocial factors on the risk of cardiovascular events is a prerequisite for the creation of authoritative working groups and the development of international regulations and recommendations [9]. Yet the question of the impact of gender differences remains unresolved.

In Russia, such studies are rare, but the differences in the studied population and the tools used do not allow us to give comparative estimates in the dynamics of the prevalence of PSF. Moreover, there are no available cohort studies at all.

Our study identified gender differences in the prevalence and dynamics of affective states over a long period, i.e., 23 years, and determined their impact on the risk of developing CVD (such as arterial hypertension, myocardial infarction, stroke) among the population aged 25–64.

2. Methods

This study is based on the survey of the male and female population living in one of the districts of Novosibirsk (Russia). The research was carried out within the framework of screenings conducted in 1994–1995, 2003–2005, 2013–2016, and 2016–2017.

In 1994–1995, the third screening under the WHO program Multinational Monitoring of Trends and Determinants of Cardiovascular Disease – Optional Psychosocial Sybstudy (MONICA-MOPSY) examined individuals aged 25–64 (n = 1527, 43% men, mean age – 44.85 ± 0.4 years, response rate – 77.3%) [10].

Another international project HAPIEE (Health, Alcohol and Psychosocial Factors in Eastern Europe) in 2003–2005 examined 45–64-year-old individuals (n = 1650, 34.9% of men, mean age – 54.25 ± 0.2 year, response rate – 66.5%) [11].

In 2013–2016, a survey of a random representative sample aged 25–44 was conducted as part of screening studies under the budgeting scheme of The Institute of Internal and Preventive Medicine, state reg. no. 01201282292 (n = 975, 43.8% men, mean age 34.5 ± 0.4 years, response rate – 71.5%).

In 2016–2017, the International PCDR project (The International Project on Cardiovascular Disease in Russia) examined 35–64-year-old individuals (n = 663, 41.3% men, mean age – 51.95 ± 0.32 years, response rate – 73.6%). The study surveyed the residents of the same district of Novosibirsk as in the previous years.

All samples were formed based on electoral rolls using a random number table. We used a random mechanical selection method. The general examination was conducted according to the standard methods accepted in epidemiology and included in the program. The methods were strictly standardised and conformed to the requirements of the MONICA project protocol. The material was validated and processed under the WHO program MONICA-psychosocial in the Information Collection Center of the MEDIS Institute in Munich, Germany (Institut für Medizinische Informatik und Systemforschung). Quality control was carried out in MONICA quality control centres: Dundee (Scotland), Prague (Czech Republic), Budapest (Hungary). The results presented were considered satisfactory.

2.1 Psychosocial testing

Anxiety traits levels were assessed using the Spielberger test (Anxiety subscale, as a personality trait). Interpretation of the data was based on the following criteria: the assessment of a trait of anxiety less than 30 corresponded to low anxiety (LAL); the score from 31 to 44 was a sign of moderate anxiety (MAL); and a score of more than 45 indicated high anxiety level (HAL).

A depression scale blank, i.e., the MOPSY test (Depression Scale, MMPI Adopted by MONICA protocol), consisting of 15 questions, was used to assess depression. For each question, there are two answers: "I agree" and "I disagree". The severity of depression was evaluated as no depression (ND), moderate (MD), or major (major D).

The vital exhaustion level was studied using the MOPSY questionnaire (Maastricht Vital Exhaustion Questionnaire). The test consisted of 14 statements. To respond to each statement, there are 3 answers: "yes", "no", "I don't know". The level of vital exhaustion was estimated as no vital exhaustion (NVE), moderate vital exhaustion (MVE), or high vital exhaustion (HVE).

Hostility (Hostility Scale, Cook-Medley test). The test consisted of 20 statements. 2 answers, "agree" and "disagree", were provided to respond to each statement. Hostility expression was assessed as low, moderate, or high.

Social support (Berkman-Syme test) [12]. A 17-point index of close contacts (ICC) was determined. It was evaluated as low, moderate, or high. Social Network Index (SNI), consisting of 9 points, was assessed as low, moderate-1, moderate-2, or high.

The subjects were asked to answer the scale questions on their own according to the given instructions. Individuals who did not fill out the questionnaire were not included in the sample.

2.2 Endpoints

The study identified the following "endpoints": the first cases of arterial hypertension (AH), myocardial infarction (MI), and stroke. All MI cases were recorded under the WHO epidemiological program Register of acute myocardial infarction, conducted in Novosibirsk from 1978 to the present day [13]; newly occuring cases of hypertension and stroke were recorded during the observation of the cohort. Sources used to identify cases of AH and stroke included population-based cohort study (annually), medical history, hospital discharge, medical records in polyclinics or general practices documents, death certificates, interviews with relatives, pathological and forensic reports. AH was defined as a condition in which SBP was 140 mmHg and above and/or DBP – 90 mmHg and/or antihypertensive medication was taken.

2.3 Participants

The object for the study of CVD risk was the cohort formed from the number of 25–64-year-old individuals examined at the III MONICA-psychosocial screening. The prospective follow-up period for the participants was 16 years (1994–2010). A total of 384 women and 190 men, with a baseline age of 25–64 years without CVD or DM at the time of screening, were included in the analysis. Over 16 years, the cohort had 15 cases of first-onset MI in women and 30 in men, and 35 cases of the first-onset stroke in women and 22 in men. During the same period, 229 cases of first-time AH were detected in women and 46 cases in men.

3. Results and discussion

3.1 Sex differences in the dynamics of psychosocial factors from 1994 to 2017

The results of the study showed that high levels of anxiety traits were present in two-third of the female population aged 25–64 in 1994 (**Table 1**). Whereas among men, high anxiety was found in less than half of those surveyed. Among the male population in 1994, the frequency of high anxiety increased linearly from younger to older age groups. In contrast, among women, high levels of AT were more common in the younger age groups of 25–34 and 35–44. Between 2003 and 2005, the maximum HAL values among both sexes, except for men in the 45–54 year group, were observed. In 2013–2016, there was a significant decrease in the prevalence of HAL in young groups in both sexes (**Table 1**). By 2016–2017, only the female population of 35–64-year- olds had consolidated such a favourable trend, but in men, the prevalence of high anxiety was back to 1994 levels. Thus, for the first time, the frequency of HAL among men 35–44 years was higher than in women of the same age group, although the differences did not reach statistical significance. The increase in anxiety levels among men is likely due to peak values of social tensions amid the economic crisis that began to gain momentum after 2014. Subsequently, we should expect similar changes among the female population.

The study of sex differences in epidemiological studies in the United States showed that the prevalence of anxiety changed slightly from 1990 to 2003 and averaged about 30% among women and 20% among men [14, 15]. This is lower

DOI: http://dx.doi.org/10.5772/intechopen.99767

Levels		25–34 years				35–44 years				45–54 years				55–64 years				25–64 years			
		M		F		M		F		M		F		M		F		M		F	
		N	%	N	%	N	%	N	%	N	%	N	%	N	%	N	%	N	%	N	%
Low	1994	12	6.8	0	0	4	2.2	1	0.6	0	0	1	0.5	0	0	2	1.2	16	4.5	1	0.3
Moderate		96	54.9	56	35.4	86	48.6	48	30.2	57	42	85	46.2	67	39.6	76	45	182	51.7	104	32.8
High		67	38.3	102	64.6	87	49.2	110	69.2	79	58	98	53.3	102	60.4	91	53.8	154	43.8	212	66.9
Total		175	100	158	100	177	100	159	100	136	100	184	100	169	100	169	100	352	100	317	100
		χ^2 = 28.982 df = 2 p < 0.001				χ^2 = 14.338 df = 2 p = 0.001				χ^2 = 1.39 df = 2 p = 0.499				χ^2 = 3.193 df = 2 p = 0.203				χ^2 = 15.937 df = 2 p < 0.001			
Low	2005									7	2.3	2	0.4	8	2.9	0	0	15	2.6	2	0.2
Moderate										135	44.4	113	20.4	79	29	70	13.5	214	37.2	183	17
High										162	53.3	439	79.2	185	68	450	86.5	347	60.2	889	82.8
Total										304	100	554	100	272	100	520	100	576	100	1074	100
										χ^2 = 65 df = 2 p = 0.0001				χ^2 = 45.98 df = 2 p < 0.001				χ^2 = 14.51 df = 2 p < 0.001			
Low	2013	31	18.8	15	7	29	11.1	15	4.5									60	14.1	30	5.5
Moderate		97	58.8	113	53.1	145	55.3	141	42.1									242	56.7	254	46.4
High		37	22.4	85	39.9	88	33.6	179	53.4									125	29.3	264	48.2
Total		165	100	213	100	262	100	335	100									427	100	548	100
		χ^2 = 19.89 df = 2 p = 0.0001				χ^2 = 27 df = 2 p = 0.0001												χ^2 = 45.6 df = 2 p = 0.0001			
Low	2017					2	2.9	10	11.2	3	4	15	10.3	7	3	8	5.4	12	4.5	33	8.6
Moderate						33	47.8	38	42.7	45	56	53	36.3	57	48.7	72	48.3	135	50.8	163	42.4
High						34	49.3	41	46.1	32	40	78	53.4	53	45.3	69	46.3	119	44.7	188	49
Total						69	100	89	100	80	100	146	100	117	100	149	100	266	100	384	100
						χ^2 = 3.869 df = 2 p > 0.05				χ^2 = 9.418 df = 2 p < 0.01				χ^2 = 0.060 df = 2 p > 0.05				χ^2 = 6.740 df = 2 p = 0.035			

Abbreviations: M- males; F – females; N – numbers (absolute).

Table 1.
Gender differences in the dynamic of anxiety traits levels in age groups of a population aged 25–64 years in 1994–2017.

than presented in our study. Similarly, a comparison of data from the European Union showed no significant change in the rates of anxiety disorders between 2005 and 2011. Anxiety was more often recorded among the female population, but its prevalence, on the contrary, was higher among middle-aged Europeans [1, 16]. Significant differences in prevalence are related to the use of different instruments to assess anxiety in our study [17].

Depression (D) occurred in more than half of the female population aged 25–64 in 1994 (**Table 2**). The prevalence of D among men was less than 30%. At the same time, the frequency of major depression among women is 4 times higher on average than among men ($p < 0.001$). The prevalence of major D in 1994 in men increased with age and was unexpectedly higher among 45–54-year-olds. Among women of 45–54 years old, major D in 2003 increased by 2% over 1994, but the 4-fold drop in major D in the 55–64-year-olds group was reflected in a decline in the overall average major depression rates of that period. In 2013, in the young-age population, there was an increase in the high prevalence of major D among men, and we observed a tendency of the narrowing gap in the prevalence of depression with the female population. In 2017, high levels of major D persisted among men and women in the younger age group of 35–44 years old, and even an explosive increase in major D was found in the category of 55–64-year-old women. At the same time, the proportion of individuals with no D in the population aged 45–64 years of both sexes was higher than in 1994.

Sex distribution was studied in 2006–2009 and 2013–2015 as part of the first and second waves of the European health interview survey (EHIS). The proportion of people suffering from depressive disorders among women was higher than among men in each of the EU member states [18]. Portugal recorded the largest gender gap: the proportion of Portuguese women with chronic depression was 11.3% higher than men. The third wave of the European health interview survey (EHIS) was scheduled to start in 2019, but the COVID-19 pandemic is delaying new findings to help understand the current trend in the prevalence of depression depending on sex and age in the Eurozone.

The prevalence of high VE in 1994 was 2 times higher among women than men in the open population aged 25–64 (14.6% and 31%, for men and women of 25–64 years old, respectively; $p < 0.001$). In 1994, both men and women showed a non-linear increase in the frequency of high VE from younger to older age groups (**Table 3**). Between 2003 and 2005, the increase in average levels of VE compared to 1994 reduced the proportion of those who did not experience vital exhaustion. The gender gap in high VE levels was heterogeneous across age groups. The 2013–2016 trend for a significant decrease in high and average VE levels in men and women in 2017 remained only in the 35–44-year-olds group. However, in older age categories, the decrease in VE occurred only among the female population of 45–64 years old, whereas in men of this age, the levels of vital exhaustion did not decrease, but, on the contrary, slightly increased compared to 2003. Then, for the first time in the entire 23-year follow-up period, men were more likely to report VE than women (16.9% and 15.6% for men and women of 35–64 years old, respectively, n.s.).

According to The Copenhagen City Heart Study, the prevalence of medium and high VE levels measured between 1991 and 1994 was 25% in the population, of which 58.5% were women. It should be noted that in this study, the examined population was quite old: the average age was 60 [19]. In a large-scale epidemiological study in the United States, high levels of VE were observed in 24% of the participants, and average levels of VE were found in 44% of the surveyed. Women were more likely than men to report high VE levels [20].

More than half of the male and female population have high or average levels of hostility (**Table 4**). At the same time, the prevalence of hostility in 1994 was

Levels		25–34 years				35–44 years				45–54 years				55–64 years				25–64 years			
		M		F		M		F		M		F		M		F		M		F	
		N	%	N	%	N	%	N	%	N	%	N	%	N	%	N	%	N	%	N	%
Major	1994	1	0.6	10	9.7	3	1.8	18	13.6	9	6.9	1	2.9	6	4	8	18.6	19	3.1	37	11.8
Moderate		39	23.4	44	42.7	39	23.9	53	40.2	35	26.9	17	48.6	44	29.5	20	46.5	157	25.8	134	42.8
No D		127	76	49	47.6	121	74.2	61	46.2	86	66.2	17	48.6	99	66.4	15	34.9	433	71.1	142	45.4
Total		167	100	103	100	163	100	132	100	130	100	35	100	149	100	43	100	609	100	313	100
		$\chi^2 = 28.674$ df = 2 $p < 0.001$				$\chi^2 = 29.695$ df = 2 $p < 0.001$				$\chi^2 = 6.219$ df = 2 $p = 0.045$				$\chi^2 = 18.210$ df = 2 $P < 0.001$				$\chi^2 = 66.724$ df = 2 $p < 0.001$			
Major	2005									4	1.3	28	5.1	11	4	22	4.2	15	2.6	50	4.7
Moderate										75	24.7	179	32.3	62	22.8	161	31	137	23.8	340	31.7
No D										225	74	347	62.6	199	73.2	337	64.8	424	73.6	684	63.7
Total										304	100	554	100	272	100	520	100	576	100	1074	100
										$\chi^2 = 15.036$ df = 2 $p = 0.001$				$\chi^2 = 6.088$ df = 2 $P = 0.048$				$\chi^2 = 17.541$ df = 2 $p < 0.001$			
Major	2013	11	6.7	36	16.9	29	11.1	54	16.1									>40	9.4	90	16.4
Moderate		36	21.8	50	23.5	54	20.6	97	29									90	21.1	147	26.8
No D		118	71.5	127	59.6	179	68.3	184	54.9									297	69.5	311	56.8
Total		165	100	213	100	262	100	335	100									427	100	548	100
		$\chi^2 = 9.97$ df = 2 $p = 0.007$				$\chi^2 = 11.08$ df = 2 $p = 0.004$												$\chi^2 = 18.531$ df = 2 $p < 0.001$			
Major	2017					8	11.6	11	12.4	3	4	14	9.5	4	3.4	30	20.1	15	5.6	55	14.3
Moderate						11	15.9	22	24.7	17	21	36	24.7	29	24.8	31	20.8	57	21.4	89	23.2
No D						50	72.5	56	62.9	60	75	96	65.8	84	71.8	88	59.1	194	73	240	62.5
Total						69	100	89	100	80	100	146	100	117	100	149	100	266	100	384	100
						$\chi^2 = 1.980$ df = 2 $p = 0.372$				$\chi^2 = 3.239$ df = 2 $p = 0.199$				$\chi^2 = 16.430$ df = 2 $p < 0.001$				$\chi^2 = 13.779$ df = 2 $p < 0.002$			

Abbreviations: M- males; F – females; N – numbers (absolute); D – depression.

Table 2.
Gender differences in the dynamic of depression levels in age groups of a population aged 25–64 years in 1994–2017.

Levels		25–34 years				35–44 years				45–54 years				55–64 years				25–64 years			
		M		F		M		F		M		F		M		F		M		F	
		N	%	N	%	N	%	N	%	N	%	N	%	N	%	N	%	N	%	N	%
High	1994	8	4.8	23	22.3	23	13.9	45	33.3	29	22.5	10	25	29	19.3	26	44.8	89	14.6	104	31
Moderate		80	48.5	49	47.6	78	47.3	63	46.7	65	50.4	17	42.5	95	63.3	19	32.8	318	52.2	148	44
No VE		77	46.7	31	30.1	64	38.8	27	20	35	27.1	13	32.5	26	17.3	13	22.4	202	33	84	25
Total		165	100	103	100	165	100	135	100	129	100	40	100	150	100	58	100	609	100	336	100
		χ^2 = 21.085 df = 2 p = 0.001				χ^2 = 20.967 df = 2 p = 0.001				χ^2 = 0.785 df = 2 p = 0.675				χ^2 = 17.991 df = 2 p < 0.001				χ^2 = 36 df = 2 p < 0.001			
High	2005									50	16.4	172	31	59	21.7	148	28.5	109	18.9	320	29.8
Moderate										174	57.2	303	54.7	157	57.7	314	60.4	331	57.5	617	57.4
No VE										80	26.3	79	14.3	56	20.6	58	11.2	136	23.6	137	12.8
Total										304	100	554	100	272	100	520	100	576	100	1074	100
										χ^2 = 31.794 df = 2 p < 0.001				χ^2 = 14.38 df = 2 p = 0.001				χ^2 = 4.086 df = 2 p = 0.13			
High	2013	7	4.2	24	11.3	19	7.3	65	19.4									26	6.1	89	16.2
Moderate		52	31.5	82	38.5	91	34.7	135	40.3									143	33.5	217	39.6
No VE		106	64.2	107	50.2	152	58	135	40.3									258	60.4	242	44.2
Total		165	100	213	100	262	100	335	100									427	100	548	100
		χ^2 = 10.112 df = 2 p = 0.006				χ^2 = 26.23 df = 2 p = 0.001												χ^2 = 35.77 df = 2 p = 0.001			
High	2017					4	5.8	10	11.2	14	17.5	17	11.6	27	23.1	33	22.1	45	16.9	60	15.6
Moderate						22	31.9	38	42.7	19	23.7	68	46.6	56	47.9	67	45	97	36.5	173	45.1
No VE						43	62.3	41	46.1	47	58.8	61	41.8	34	29	49	32.9	124	46.6	151	39.3
Total						69	100	89	100	80	100	146	100	117	100	149	100	266	100	384	100
						χ^2 = 4.425 df = 2 p > 0.05				χ^2 = 11.401 df = 2 p < 0.01				χ^2 = 0.451 df = 2 p > 0.05				χ^2 = 4.927 df = 2 p = 0.086			

Abbreviations: M- males; F – females; N – numbers (absolute); VE – vital exhaustion.

Table 3.
Gender differences in the dynamic of vital exhaustion levels in age groups of a population aged 25–64 years in 1994–2017.

Levels		25–34 years				35–44 years				45–54 years				55–64 years				25–64 years			
		M		F		M		F		M		F		M		F		M		F	
		N	%	N	%	N	%	N	%	N	%	N	%	N	%	N	%	N	%	N	%
High	1994	52	31.7	48	46.6	53	33.8	54	40	37	30.3	15	37.5	50	33.6	24	41.4	192	32.4	141	42
Moderate		25	15.2	26	25.2	37	23.6	38	28.1	24	19.7	7	17.5	27	18.1	15	25.9	113	19.1	86	25.6
Low		87	53.4	29	28.2	67	42.6	43	31.9	61	50	18	45	72	48.4	19	32.8	287	48.4	109	32.4
Total		164	100	103	100	157	100	135	100	122	100	40	100	149	100	58	100	592	100	336	100
		χ^2 = 16.08 df = 2 p < 0.001				χ^2 = 3.622 df = 2 p = 0.001				n.s.				n.s.				χ^2 = 22.58 df = 2 p < 0.001			
High	2005									138	45.4	189	34.1	111	40.8	183	35.2	249	43.2	372	34.6
Moderate										58	19.1	132	23.8	51	18.8	120	23.1	109	18.9	252	23.5
Low										108	35.5	233	42.1	110	40.4	217	41.7	218	37.8	450	41.9
Total										304	100	554	100	272	100	520	100	576	100	1074	100
										χ^2 = 10.657 df = 2 p = 0.005				n.s.				n.s.			
High	2013	61	37	62	29.1	90	34.4	100	29.9									151	35.4	162	29.6
Moderate		46	27.9	45	21.1	70	26.7	85	25.4									116	27.2	130	23.7
Low		58	35.2	106	49.8	102	38.9	150	44.8									160	37.5	256	46.7
Total		165	100	213	100	262	100	335	100									427	100	548	100
		χ^2 = 8.103 df = 2 p = 0.017				n.s.												χ^2 = 8.451 df = 2 p = 0.015			
High	2017					22	31.9	27	30.3	20	25	50	34.2	46	39.3	42	28.2	88	33.1	119	31
Moderate						32	46.4	26	29.2	22	27.5	26	17.8	24	20.5	38	25.5	78	29.3	90	23.4
Low						15	21.7	36	40.4	38	47.5	70	47.9	47	40.2	69	46.3	100	37.6	175	45.6
Total						69	100	89	100	80	100	146	100	117	100	149	100	266	100	384	100
						χ^2 = 7.365 df = 2 p < 0.05				n.s.				n.s.				χ^2 = 4.687 df = 2 p = 0.096			

Abbreviations: M- males; F – females; N – numbers (absolute).

Table 4.
Gender differences in the dynamic of hostility levels in age groups of a population aged 25–64 years in 1994–2017.

unexpectedly higher among the female population in all age groups. However, in further follow-up periods, from 2003 to 2017, men showed higher levels of hostility compared to women. This reinforces our theory that trajectories in the prevalence of psychosocial characteristics change during periods of changing socio-economic patterns in society. Between 2013 and 2016, the trend in the prevalence of men over women with high hostility was consolidated by reducing its prevalence among the female population to historically low values of less than 30% in the 25–34- and 35–44-year-olds groups. In 2017, this trend was also recorded in the older age groups, where the lowest levels of high hostility were observed among men of 45–54 years old and women of 55–64 years old for the entire observation period between 1994 and 2017.

What makes our results unique is that reports on the prevalence of affective states are limited and more commonly cited in clinical groups. Concerning the frequency of hostility in other populations, the most informative is the CARDIA study, which included more than 5,000 men and women aged 18–30. At the time of the initial survey (1985–1986), the high level of hostility was 23.4% in the study population, the average was 52.3%, and was more common among men, compared to women [21].

Sex differences in the dynamics of social support levels are presented in **Tables 5** and **6**. The higher prevalence of low close contact (ICC) among men, compared to women, was reported in both the youngest 25–34-year-olds group (63.8% vs. 57.7%) and older age groups of 45–54 and 55–64 (64% vs. 54%, respectively) in 1994. In 2003 and 2013, there was a downward trend in the frequency of the low close contact index to 46–50%, although ICC levels did not differ depending on sex. In 2017, on the contrary, women were 14.4% more likely to show a lack of social support, in comparison with men, and completely levelled the emerging favourable trend of 2013.

The prevalence of a low social network index (combined indicator: low and moderate-1) in the open population among men and women aged 25–64 was equally high in 1994 and between 2003 and 2005. Between 2013 and 2016, there was an unstable trend toward an increase in the level of social ties among young age groups of both sexes. Later, over a short period, this trend reversed, marking an unfavourable increase, predominantly among the female population of 35–64 years old, reaching, on average, 75% of the values in the frequency of the low index of social ties. Such differences are explained by the fact that women have better social connections and receive support from multiple sources, but satisfaction with close contacts is reflected in the perception of social support and the effect on health [22, 23].

3.2 Gender effect in the risk of AH in individuals with unfavourable levels of PSF

In our study of the risk of AH development depending on PSF levels, we obtained the following results. Among men and women with HAL, the risk of AH was higher in the "stronger sex", with an increased risk demonstrated in the first five years of follow-up (**Figure 1**). The magnitude of risk in men was maximum after 10 years of follow-up (HR = 5.75), and in women in the first five years – HR = 2.38 (95% CI: 1.13–4.99). And this is despite the fact that the prevalence of HAL is higher in women. Indeed, BigData analysis showed that age and male sex are associated risk factors for AH in individuals with anxiety disorders [24]. In a multivariate model adjusted for social characteristics and age, the risk of AH was also higher among men (HR = 4.57; 95% CI:2.07–10.08). While age was a determinant of AH risk in women (HR = 7.93; $p < 0.01$ for the oldest age category), marital

Levels		25–34 years				35–44 years				45–54 years				55–64 years				25–64 years			
		M		F		M		F		M		F		M		F		M		F	
		N	%	N	%	N	%	N	%	N	%	N	%	N	%	N	%	N	%	N	%
Low	1994	102	63.8	82	57.7	85	55.9	86	60.6	79	64.2	72	54.1	102	64.6	71	54.2	368	62	311	56.8
Moderate		39	24.4	50	35.2	44	28.9	45	31.7	33	26.8	52	39.1	37	23.4	55	42	153	25.9	202	36.9
High		19	11.9	10	7	23	15.1	11	7.7	11	8.9	9	6.8	19	12	5	3.8	72	12.1	35	6.4
Total		160	100	142	100	152	100	142	100	123	100	133	100	158	100	131	100	593	100	548	100
		$\chi^2 = 5.27$ df = 2 p = 0.072				n.s.				n.s.				$\chi^2 = 14.85$ df = 2 p < 0.001				$\chi^2 = 22.603$ df = 2 p < 0.001			
Low	2005									140	46.1	298	53.8	129	47.4	251	48.3	269	46.7	549	51.1
Moderate										141	46.4	231	41.7	118	43.4	240	46.2	259	45	471	43.9
High										23	7.6	25	4.5	25	9.2	29	5.6	48	8.3	54	5
Total										304	100	554	100	272	100	520	100	576	100	1074	100
										$\chi^2 = 6.567$ df = 2 p = 0.038				n.s.				n.s.			
Low	2013	79	47.9	95	44.6	130	49.6	167	49.9									209	48.9	262	47.8
Moderate		66	40	96	45.1	105	40.1	141	42.1									171	40	237	43.2
High		20	12.1	22	10.3	27	10.3	27	8.1									47	11	49	8.9
Total		165	100	213	100	262	100	335	100									427	100	548	100
		n.s.				n.s.												n.s.			
Low	2017					34	49.3	49	55.1	38	47.5	98	67.1	49	41.9	83	55.7	121	45.5	230	59.9
Moderate						30	43.5	32	36	35	43.75	46	31.5	53	45.3	55	36.9	118	44.4	133	34.6
High						5	7.2	8	8.9	7	8.75	2	1.4	15	12.8	11	7.4	27	10.1	21	5.5
Total						69	100	89	100	80	100	146	100	117	100	149	100	266	100	384	100
						n.s.				$\chi^2 = 12.537$ df = 2 p < 0.01				n.s.				$\chi^2 = 14.554$ df = 2 p < 0.001			

Abbreviations: M- males; F – females; N – numbers (absolute).

Table 5.
Gender differences in the dynamic of close contact index in age groups of a population aged 25–64 years in 1994–2017.

Levels		25–34 years				35–44 years				45–54 years				55–64 years				25–64 years			
		M		F		M		F		M		F		M		F		M		F	
		N	%	N	%	N	%	N	%	N	%	N	%	N	%	N	%	N	%	N	%
Low	1994	122	76.3	111	78.2	113	74.4	110	77.4	94	72.9	104	78.2	128	81.6	98	74.8	457	76.4	423	77.2
Moderate		28	17.5	28	19.7	33	21.7	29	20.4	26	20.2	23	17.3	21	13.4	31	23.7	108	18.1	111	20.3
High		10	6.3	3	2.1	6	3.9	3	2.1	9	7	6	4.5	8	5.1	2	1.5	33	5.5	14	2.5
Total		160	100	142	100	152	100	142	100	129	100	133	100	157	100	131	100	598	100	548	100
		$\chi^2 = 15.894$ df = 3 p = 0.001				n.s.				n.s.				$\chi^2 = 7.217$ df = 2 p = 0.028				$\chi^2 = 6.867$ df = 2 p = 0.033			
Low	2005									233	76.7	444	80.2	202	74.3	416	80	435	75.5	860	80.1
Moderate										59	19.4	97	17.5	61	22.4	90	17.3	120	20.8	187	17.4
High										12	3.9	13	2.3	9	3.3	14	2.7	21	3.7	27	2.5
Total										304	100	554	100	272	100	520	100	576	100	1074	100
										n.s.				n.s.				$\chi^2 = 5.001$ df = 2 p = 0.083			
Low	2013	98	59.4	123	57.8	158	60.3	212	63.3									256	60	335	61.1
Moderate		53	32.1	71	33.3	88	33.6	99	29.6									141	33	170	31
High		14	8.5	19	8.9	16	6.1	24	7.2									30	7	43	7.9
Total		165	100	213	100	262	100	335	100									427	100	548	100
		n.s.				n.s.												n.s.			
Low	2017					53	73.6	66	68	46	56.8	119	85	67	65.1	97	70.3	166	64.8	282	75.2
Moderate						16	22.2	23	23.7	29	35.8	19	13.6	31	30.1	34	24.6	76	29.7	76	20.3
High						3	4.2	8	8.2	6	7.4	2	1.4	5	4.9	7	5.1	14	5.5	17	4.5
Total						72	100	97	100	81	100	140	100	103	100	138	100	256	100	375	100
						n.s.				$\chi^2 = 22.212$ df = 2 p < 0.001				n.s.				$\chi^2 = 8.175$ df = 2 p = 0.017			

Abbreviations: M- males; F – females; N – numbers (absolute).

Table 6.
Gender differences in the dynamic of social networks index in age groups of a population aged 25–64 years in 1994–2017.

status was also important in men: divorced and widowed appeared to be more vulnerable (HR = 4.30 and HR = 4.84, respectively; p for all <0.001).

The risk of AH in men with D was high already in the first 5 years of follow-up observations, 6.7 times higher, gradually decreasing 10 and 16 years after screening, but it remained significant. In women, a significant cohort outcome was determined only 10 years after screening and was 1.7 times higher for those with depression. Multivariate analysis also identified a higher risk of AH among men rather than women: HR = 5.3 and HR = 1.4 (95%CI:1.04–1.98), respectively. As with high anxiety, women's risk was higher in the older age groups of 45–54 and of 55–64, significantly outpacing men in these categories, reaching HR = 6.9. At the same time, the mean level of education was a protective factor for women (HR = 0.56; $p < 0.05$). In men, everything is different. Divorced (HR = 3.0), those with primary education (HR = 5.6), and manual labour workers (HR = 2.8) with D had higher risks of AH compared with married men with higher education and higher occupational status (the white-collars, e.g., engineers and technicians, managers) (p for all <0.05).

Similarly revealing, in terms of gender differences, is a recent report by Kao W. T. et al. (2019). In this 10-year study, men with depression had a higher risk of AH than those without D [25]. In women, the results were contradictory: some risk models showed a decrease in the development of AH among women with depression; but using a model adjusted for other covariates, they showed an increased risk of AH in women, compared with individuals without D. The authors considered social factors to be among the many reasons for the higher risk of AH among men rather than women.

The maximum risk of hypertension in men with VE was recorded in the first five years from the start of the study HR = 3.2 (95% CI:1–7.3). Further, this risk decreased but remained significant by the end of the follow-up period. Women with VE had a 2-fold higher risk of AH after 5 years of observation, but after 10 years it was no longer statistically significant. In the multivariate model, the risk of AH was also higher in the male cohort HR = 2.9 (95%CI:1–7.9). In women, the social parameters (i.e. marital status, education, occupational status) and age included in the model reduced the risk to a greater extent than in men, although it remained significant, HR = 1.34 (95% CI:0.99–1.82). Age over 34 years (HR = 2.3) and primary education (HR = 1.8) were additional predictors of AH risk among women with VE. In the ARIC Study, the highest quartile of VE was also associated with lower educational attainment and higher systolic BP [20]. In men, the age limit was significantly higher (over 54 years old), but the increase in risk at this age was more than 5 times higher for people with VE as well. In addition, divorce played a significant role in the occurrence of AH in men with VE (HR = 3.3). This is probably the case when VE is a potential response to intractable problems in life and the inability to adapt to prolonged exposure to psychological stressors [26].

The risk of developing AH, during the first 5 years of follow-up, was already 2 times higher in both men and women with a low index of close contacts (ICC) as compared to those with higher indices. Among those with low social network indices (SNI), the risk of developing AH was 5.9 times higher among men and 1.8 times higher among women in the first 5 years of follow-up. The multivariate model retained a statistically significant risk of developing AH only in men with low ICC (HR = 1.2). At the same time, the marital status "unmarried" (i.e. single/divorced/widowed) significantly increased the risk level to the limit of 7.1 times (for widowers). It should be noted that in widowed women, the risk of AH was also significant (HR = 2.7 95% CI: 1.03–7.35), although not as high as in men.

In women, there was also a tendency of an increased 2-fold risk of AH among those who had primary education (p = 0.06).

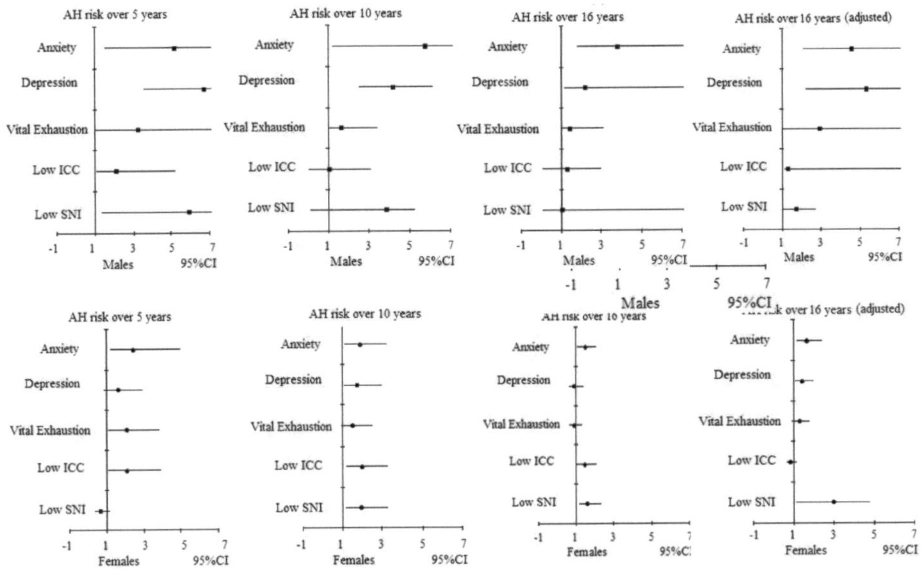

Figure 1.
Gender differences in risk of an arterial hypertension incidence in a cohort aged 25–64 with anxiety traits, depression, vital exhaustion and low social support. Abbreviations: AH- arterial hypertension; CI- confidence interval; ICC – Index of close contacts; SNI – Social network index.

The effect of low social ties on the risk of AH in the multivariate model was 1.7 times higher in men and 2.9 times higher in women. The effect of marital status "single" was statistically significant only in men, as well as heavy physical labour, which increased the risk by almost 3 times. However, the initial level of educational attainment was statistically significant for both sexes: the risk of AH was 1.4 times higher in men and 2 times higher in women with low SNI. In both sexes, age was a more significant risk factor because it had a linear effect on the risk of AH, being the maximum in the age group of 55–64, reaching HR = 8 in women.

In our study, marital status "unmarried" (divorced, single, or widowed) determined the extreme degree of social isolation in men with low ICC / SNI, which was reflected in a higher risk of AH in them, compared to the "tender gender", where marital status was not always a significant risk factor [27]. In the ELSA study (n = 8310), loneliness remained a significant predictor of cardiovascular events regardless of sociodemographic factors and social isolation; even after the inclusion of traditional RFS to the model, the association between loneliness and CVD was maintained [28].

3.3 Gender effect in the risk of MI in individuals with unfavourable levels of PSF

The risk of myocardial infarction for 16 years of follow-up was slightly higher among women with high anxiety compared to men (HR = 4.19 and HR = 3.7, respectively), but the inclusion of social characteristics and age in the model increased the risk value among women to HR = 5.16 (p for all <0.05). In men, the risk in the multivariate model decreased but remained significant HR = 1.79 (**Figure 2**). A great risk share in this model was explained by age over 54; however, these associations were not statistically significant in women.

The risk of a heart attack in men with depression was 2 and in women 2.5 times higher. In the multivariate model, the risk of MI in men was reduced but remained significant, and in women with D, statistics were no longer valid. In the age group

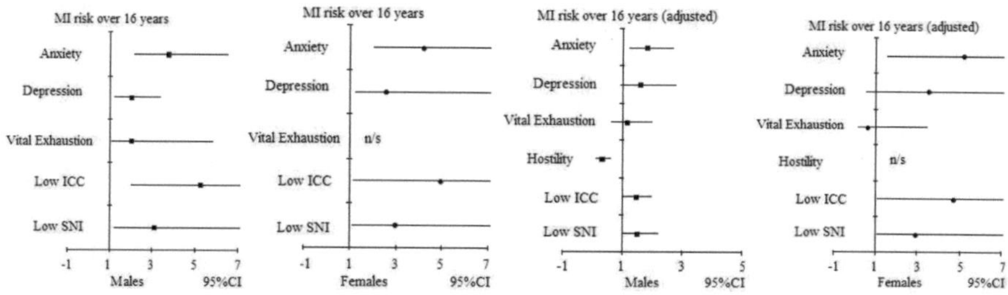

Figure 2.
Gender differences in risk of myocardial infarction incidence in a cohort aged 25–64 years with anxiety traits, depression, vital exhaustion, hostility and low social support. Abbreviations: CI- confidence interval; ICC – Index of close contacts; MI- myocardial infarction; SNI – Social network index.

of 55–64, the risk of MI was highest in men (HR = 6.8) and women (HR = 6.3). Marital status "single" (HR = 6), primary education (HR = 3.2), and manual labour (HR = 6.7) were predictors of high risk of MI in men with D (p for all <0.05). No such associations were found in women.

A recent publication of the ESC 2018 working group cites several studies concerning sex differences in the risk of coronary heart disease (CHD) and CVD mortality [9]. Studies of young population samples (under 40) found that the effect of depression on the risk of CHD was higher among women than in men. In the NHANES III study, a history of major depression was associated with an almost 15-fold increased risk of CHD in women and 3.5-fold in men [29]. This confirms our earlier findings [30], but in our present study, the sex differences were not as significant in risk.

In the simple risk model, VE did not affect the development of MI in women, whereas in men it was 2 times higher compared to those in whom vital exhaustion was not found. The multivariate model reduced the magnitude of risk after adjusting for socio-demographic characteristics, but the statistical significance for men remained the same. Living out of wedlock, age over 44, and blue-collar occupations were associated with a 3–7-fold increase in risk for men. Divorced status in women also increased the risk of myocardial infarction (5 times higher).

In our study, the moderate to high levels of hostility reduced the risk of MI by 70%. However, some social characteristics changed this ratio unfavourably. Living out of wedlock has been associated with the risk of MI in men who demonstrate hostility. The increase in risk was particularly significant among the widowed (12 times higher). Primary education and age over 44 also increased the risk of MI. Executive positions combined with hostility is associated with a 9-fold increased risk of MI compared to engineering professions. No significant associations and effects on the risk of MI in women with hostility during the 16-year follow-up period were found.

A recent meta-analysis assessing the impact of hostility showed that anxiety, depression, and psychological stress, but not anger or hostility, were associated with CHD risk in women. In men, on the contrary, anger is one of the leading psychosocial risk factors for cardiovascular events [31]. Our study complements these conclusions by showing that the risk of IM is manifested only in a certain social environment.

The risk of MI in individuals with low indices of close contacts and social ties was significantly higher but did not differ significantly depending on sex, slightly predominating in men. At the same time, the lack of close contacts increased the risk more significantly (5 times), rather than a poor social network (3 times). Interestingly, the multivariate model practically did not weaken the risk of MI in women, which increased significantly among women with low ICC and primary education (HR = 15.4). In men, primary education had a comparatively smaller effect on risk, giving preference to age, living out of wedlock (single, divorced, widowed status), and having an engineering or technician occupation, or physical labour. Similar associations were found for the social network index (SNI) in the multivariate model, where the risk of MI was higher in women compared to men. In contrast to close contacts, the lack of social connections combined with age, primary education and physical labour increased the risk of MI – 3-3.7 times in women. For men, such factors as marital status “single”, age, primary education, and physical labour remained significant. Importantly, low SNI combined with a mid-level executive position also increased the risk of MI (2.5 times). A similar effect was not observed in women.

3.4 Gender effect in the risk of stroke in individuals with unfavourable levels of PSF

The risk of stroke was higher among men with HAL, HR = 4.43 (95% CI:2.8–6.9), rather than among women, HR = 3.5. In the multivariate model, the risk of stroke was lower for men than for women. Adverse changes in marital status (divorce or death of a spouse), as well as age over 54 years, were associated with an increase in the risk of stroke (3.8–5.8 times higher) in men, but not women.

Stroke is the fourth leading cause of death in the female population [32]. Recent studies indicate an independent influence of anxiety in stroke risk [33, 34]. This confirms the results obtained earlier [35]. The overall risk of stroke according to the meta-analysis, which included 950 thousand participants, was 1.24. It is reported that individuals with more severe anxiety may have a higher risk [36]. In multivariate models, a higher risk of stroke was observed among men, people with low education attainment, and those living out of wedlock [32], as well as in our study. Our study confirms the need to consider the social gradient in terms of the effect of PSF on the risk of CVD in the general population.

Depression increased the risk of stroke more strongly in men (by 5.8 times) than in women (HR = 4.6). However, including social and demographic variables in the model increased the risk of stroke in women 8.5 times. At the same time, the combination of age over 54 years with depression increased the risk of stroke (6.9 times in women, and 3.1 times in men). Depression in widowed men with primary education increased the risk more than 8 times. A tendency toward increased risk was observed in men with D in low-skilled jobs.

A meta-analysis of more than 17 cohort studies found a 1.34-fold increase in the risk of stroke among people with depression [37], which again confirms our results [30]. In this analysis, the differences in risk among men and women were not so significant (HR = 1.49 and 1.35), which may be explained by a shift in the evaluation due to differences between studies, since some studies were performed among the male population [38]. Yet individual studies show a significantly higher risk of stroke in women than in men [39]. In addition, the influence of age is also significant, increasing the effect of depression in the group of people under 65 years (**Figure 3**) [39].

Vital exhaustion increased the risk of stroke equally in men and women in both the simple and multivariate models, although the inclusion of social and demographic characteristics reduced the risk value; it remained high: 2.6 times higher in men and 2.53 times higher in women in the multivariate model. The age of 55–64 years was significant in the development of stroke, increasing the risk in men 2.4 times, in women 2.9 times. Marital status and educational attainment were associated with stroke risk only in men, but not in women. Being divorced and having an

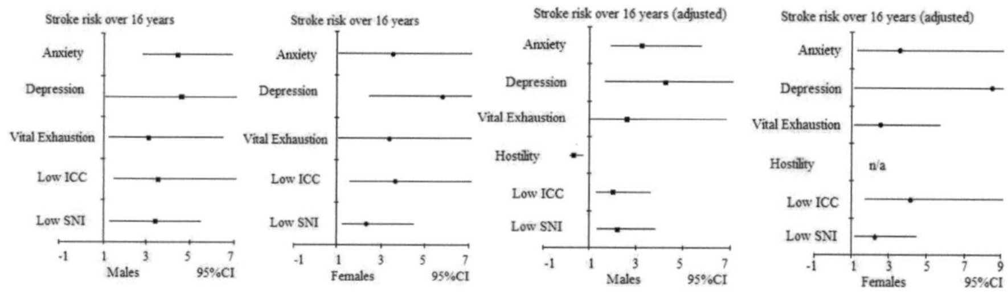

Figure 3.
Gender differences in risk of stroke incidence in a cohort aged 25–64 years with anxiety traits, depression, vital exhaustion, hostility and low social support. Abbreviations: CI- confidence interval; ICC – Index of close contacts; SNI – Social network index.

elementary level of education increased the risk of stroke in the cohort of men by 3.8–4.8 times. The tendency toward risk is also observed among widows.

Gender differences in stroke risk were also studied in the Copenhagen City Heart Study. The researchers found that women with high levels of VE had a 2.27-fold risk of stroke, which was slightly reduced in a multivariate analysis. Yet no association was found with stroke in men with VE. A longer cohort study might have levelled the gender difference in this longitudinal study: it estimated 6–9 years in this study [40].

Hostility in men has a negative association with stroke risk (HR = 0.29, 95% CI:0.1–0.7). Divorce, primary education, and the age of 55–64 are associated with a 3.2–4.6-fold increase in the risk of stroke. The maximum risk values were observed among pensioners (HR = 14.5) in comparison with executives. There was no association with stroke in women with hostility during the 16-year follow-up period.

The low level of close contacts increased the risk of stroke to the same degree in men and women – 3.5 times. But a poor social network (low SNI) was more important for men, increasing the risk of stroke 3.4 times, and for women 2.3 times. Adding social parameters and age to the analysis reduced the risk value in men with low ICC to HR = 2 (95% CI:1.27–3.61), while the risk of stroke increased 4.13-fold in women. Only women with higher education and a favourable level of close contact were resistant to the risk of stroke. In men, only primary education was associated with a twofold risk of stroke. Moreover, being a divorced or widowed blue-collar was associated with an increased risk of stroke in men but not women. However, age over 54 was critically important in the risk of stroke in both sexes, but with a greater magnitude among women (HR = 5.19; $p < 0.05$).

In contrast to the simple model, in the multivariate Cox model, SNI increased the risk of stroke in the same way in men and women (2.2 times). As in the case of low ICC, any level of education attainment, apart from higher education, increased the risk of stroke in women; while in men, only primary education was significant, in case of poor social ties. Women aged 55–64 were 2 times more likely than men of the same age group to have a stroke. Yet occupational status, as well as marital status, were statistically significant only in men. Being a blue-collar worker and having the status of a divorced or a widower, combined with a low SNI, increased the risk of stroke 4.8–6.9 times. Literary sources show that the socially isolated, i.e., deprived of social contacts and not participating in social activities, lonely or not satisfied with the quality of their social contacts, have a 30% higher risk of CHD, stroke and early mortality [41]. Such studies only add to the significance of the influence of the social gradient described in our previous works [42].

4. Conclusions

In the period from 1994 to 2003/05, our study registered high levels of negative psychological characteristics, which prevailed among women. The favourable trend of 2013 in the reduction of affective states reversed shortly. By 2017, younger men for the first time began reporting higher levels of anxiety and vital exhaustion than women. For 23 years, against the background of an increase in the proportion of people of both sexes without negative psychological conditions, the gender gap in the frequency of major depression decreased. Such multifaceted trends are due to a decrease in the average levels of PSF in our study.

It is worth mentioning that an increased level of hostility in the Russian/Siberian population is associated with a negative risk of stroke. It can be assumed that a low level of hostility is probably not the most advantageous, from an evolutionary point of view, tool of adaptability in the conditions of the permanent crisis in Russia in the post-Soviet period. At the same time, high anxiety, as a personality trait, develops in character over many years, activates biological mechanisms and leads to the development of cardiovascular events. This also applies to other psychosocial factors. It should be pointed out that the increase in the risk of CVD is observed already in the first 5 years after the initial study and remains significant for a long period – 16 years in both sexes. The magnitude of the risk depends on gender. Its higher values were determined in men with unfavourable levels of PSF in the development of AH and stroke. Yet the inclusion of social characteristics to the model often changed this ratio, weakening the risk magnitude in men, but maintaining the same or increasing in women. This is explained by the high sensitivity of men to living outside wedlock, increasing the risk of CVD among divorced and, especially, widowed (6–8 times). In women, such associations were not typical. Obviously, more men benefit from being married rather than women who have to bear the domestic burden. These explanations can be found in our earlier works. The influence of occupational status was also decisive for men. Working professions are associated with a higher risk of CVD in men compared to engineers, technicians and managers. In women, the prognostically unfavourable factor was the initial level of education attained and age over 44 years in combination with affective states. Among men, the impact of these factors was less significant.

Author details

Valery V. Gafarov[1,2], Dmitriy O. Panov[1,2]*, Elena A. Gromova[1,2], Igor V. Gagulin[1,2], Almira V. Gafarova[1,2] and Eldar A. Krymov[1,2]

1 Institute of Internal and Preventive Medicine – Branch of Institute of Cytology and Genetics RAS, Novosibirsk, Russian Federation

2 Collaborative Laboratory of Cardiovascular Diseases Epidemiology, Novosibirsk, Russian Federation

*Address all correspondence to: dimitriy2004@inbox.ru

IntechOpen

© 2021 The Author(s). Licensee IntechOpen. This chapter is distributed under the terms of the Creative Commons Attribution License (http://creativecommons.org/licenses/by/3.0), which permits unrestricted use, distribution, and reproduction in any medium, provided the original work is properly cited.

References

[1] Bandelow B., Michaelis S. Epidemiology of anxiety disorders in the 21st century. Dialogues Clin Neurosci. 2015;17(3):327-335. doi:10.31887/DCNS.2015.17.3/bbandelow

[2] Albert P. R. Why is depression more prevalent in women? J Psychiatry Neurosci. 2015;40(4):219-221. doi: 10.1503/jpn.150205

[3] Mathers C. D., Bernard C., Moesgaard Iburg K., M. Inoue, Ma Fat D., Shibuya K., Stein C., Tomijima N., Xu H. Global Burden of Disease in 2002: data sources, methods and results. Global Program on Evidence for Health Policy, Discussion Paper No.54. Geneva: World Health Organization; 2003. https://www.who.int/healthinfo/paper54.pdf

[4] Gafarov V. V., Gromova E. A., Panov D. O., Gagulin I. V., Gafarova A. V. Gender Differences in Dynamic of Family Stress Indicators in Population Aged 25-64 Years from 1988 To 2017. Medical & Clinical Research. 2021; 6(4): 520-526. DOI: 10.33140/MCR.06.04.09

[5] Gafarov V. V., Panov D. O., Gromova E. A., Krymov E. A., Gagulin I. V., Gafarova A. V. Gender differences in dynamic of job stress as cardiovascular risk factor in population aged 25-64 years from 1988 to 2017. Journal of Cardiology Research Review & Reports. 2021;2(2):1-12. DOI: 10.47363/JCRRR/2021(2)142

[6] Mathews L., Ogunmoroti O., Nasir K., Blumenthal R. S., et al. Psychological Factors and Their Association with Ideal Cardiovascular Health Among Women and Men. Journal of Women's Health. 2018;27(5): 709-715. https://doi.org/10.1089/jwh.2017.6563.

[7] Tillmann, T. Psychosocial and socioeconomic factors in the development of cardiovascular disease: a study of causality, mediation, international variation, and prediction in predominantly Eastern European settings. Doctoral thesis (Ph.D); UCL (University College London); 2018: 366 p.

[8] Ocsovszky Z., Rafael B., Martos T., Csabai M., Bagyura Z., Sallay V., Merkely B. A társas támogatás és az egészséges életmód összefüggései [Correlation of social support and healthy lifestyle (In Hungarian)]. Orv Hetil. 2020;161(4):129-138. doi: 10.1556/650.2020.31625.

[9] Vaccarino V., Badimon L., Bremner J.D., Cenko E., Cubedo J., Dorobantu M., Duncker D.J., Koller A., Manfrini O., Milicic D., Padro T., Pries A.R., Quyyumi A.A., Tousoulis D., Trifunovic D., Vasiljevic Z., de Wit C., Bugiardini R.; ESC Scientific Document Group Reviewers. Depression and coronary heart disease: 2018 position paper of the ESC working group on coronary pathophysiology and microcirculation. Eur Heart J. 2020;41 (17):1687-1696. doi: 10.1093/eurheartj/ehy913.

[10] Tunstall-Pedoe H., Kuulasmaa K., Tolonen H., Davidson M., Mendis S. with 64 other contributors for The WHO MONICA Project. MONICA Monograph and Multimedia Sourcebook. World's largest study of heart disease, stroke, risk factors, and population trends 1979–2002. Edited by H. Tunstall-Pedoe. WHO: Geneve; on-line publication. Available for: http://apps.who.int/iris/bitstream/10665/42597/1/9241562234.pdf.

[11] UCL department of epidemiology and public health Central and Eastern Europe research group HAPIEE study. Available at: http://www.ucl.ac.uk/easteurope/hapiee-cohort.htm.

[12] Gafarov V., Panov D., Gromova E., Krymov E., Gagulin I., Gafarova A. Male and Female Trajectories of Social Isolation in Russia from 1994 To 2017. Journal of Clinical Epidemiology and Toxicology. 2021;2(1):1-6. doi: 10.47363/JCET/2021(2)107.

[13] Gafarov V.V., Pak V.A., Gagulin I. V., Gafarova A.V. Epidemiology and prevention of chronic non-communicable diseases for 2 decades and during the socio-economic crisis in Russia. Novosibirsk: SB RAMS, 2000. 284 p.

[14] National Institute of Mental Health. Statistics. Prevalence of Any Anxiety Disorder Among Adults. Available at: https://www.nimh.nih.gov/health/statistics/any-anxiety-disorder.shtml

[15] McLean C.P., Asnaani A., Litz B.T., Hofmann S.G. Gender differences in anxiety disorders: prevalence, course of illness, comorbidity and burden of illness. J Psychiatr Res. 2011; 45(8): 1027-1035. doi:10.1016/j.jpsychires.2011.03.006

[16] Wittchen H.U., Jacobi F., Rehm J., Gustavsson A., Svensson M., Jönsson B., Olesen J., Allgulander C., Alonso J., Faravelli C., Fratiglioni L., Jennum P., Lieb R., Maercker A., van Os J., Preisig M., Salvador-Carulla L., Simon R., Steinhausen H.C. The size and burden of mental disorders and other disorders of the brain in Europe 2010. Eur Neuropsychopharmacol. 2011; 21 (9):655-79. doi: 10.1016/j.euroneuro.2011.07.018.

[17] Gafarov V. V., Panov D. O., Gromova E. A., Krymov E. A., Gagulin I. V., Gafarova A. V. Sex Differences and Trends in Prevalence of Anxiety, Depression and Vital Exhaustion in Russia / Siberia from1994 To 2017. International Journal of Medical Science and Clinical Invention. 2021;8(3): 5288-5298. doi: 10.18535/ijmsci/v8i03.06.

[18] European health interview survey (EHIS). Eurostat Statistics Explained. Online Publication. Available at: https://ec.europa.eu/eurostat/statistics-explained/index.php?title=Glossary:European_health_interview_survey_(EHIS).

[19] Islamoska S., Ishtiak-Ahmed K., Hansen Å.M., Grynderup M.B., Mortensen E.L., Garde A.H., Gyntelberg F., Prescott E.I.B., Török E., Waldemar G., Nabe-Nielsen K. Vital Exhaustion and Incidence of Dementia: Results from the Copenhagen City Heart Study. J Alzheimers Dis. 2019;67(1): 369-379. doi: 10.3233/JAD-180478.

[20] Williams J.E., Mosley T.H. Jr., Kop W.J., Couper D.J., Welch V.L., Rosamond W.D. Vital exhaustion as a risk factor for adverse cardiac events (from the Atherosclerosis Risk In Communities [ARIC] study). Am J Cardiol. 2010;105(12):1661-1665. doi: 10.1016/j.amjcard.2010.01.340.

[21] Yan L.L., Liu K., Matthews K.A., Daviglus M.L., Ferguson T.F., Kiefe C.I. Psychosocial factors and risk of hypertension: the Coronary Artery Risk Development in Young Adults (CARDIA) study. JAMA. 2003;290(16): 2138-48. doi: 10.1001/jama.290.16.2138.

[22] Antonucci T.C., Akiyama H. An examination of sex differences in social support among older men and women. Sex Roles. 1987;17: 737-749. DOI: 10.1007/BF00287685.

[23] Robles T.F., Slatcher R.B., Trombello J.M., McGinn M.M. Marital quality and health: A meta-analytic review. Psychological bulletin. 2014; 140(1):140-187. DOI: 10.1037/a0031859.

[24] Wu E.L., Chien I.C., Lin C.H. Increased risk of hypertension in patients with anxiety disorders: A population-based study. Journal of Psychosomatic Research. 2014;77(6): 522-527. doi: 10.1016/j.jpsychores.2014.10.006.

[25] Kao W.T., Chang C.L., Lin C.H., Wu S.L., Lin S.L., Lung F.W. Gender Disparity in the Risk of Hypertension in Subjects with Major Depressive Disorder. Front Psychiatry. 2019; 10: 541. doi: 10.3389/fpsyt.2019.00541.

[26] Frestad D., Prescott E. Vital exhaustion and coronary heart disease risk: A systematic review and meta-analysis. Psychosom Med. 2017; 79:260–272.

[27] Gafarov V., Panov D., Gromova E., Gagulin I., Gafarova A. The Risk of Hypertension Over 16 Years and Family and Job Stress in Female Population 25 – 64 Years in Russia/Siberia. EC Cardiology. 2017; 3(1):05-13.

[28] Bu F., Zaninotto P., Fancourt D. Longitudinal associations between loneliness, social isolation and cardiovascular events. Heart. 2020; 0:1–6. doi:10.1136/heartjnl-2020-316614.

[29] Vaccarino V. Psychosocial risk factors in women: Special reference to depression and posttraumatic stress disorder. In: Orth-Gomer K., Vaccarino V., Schneiderman N., Deter H.C., eds. Psychosocial Stress and Cardiovascular Disease in Women: Concepts, Findings and Future Perspectives. Switzerland: Springer International Publishing; 2015, pp. 63 – 86.

[30] Gafarov V.V., Panov D.O., Gromova E.A., Gagulin I.V., Gafarova A.V. The influence of depression on risk development of acute cardiovascular diseases in the female population aged 25-64 in Russia. Int J Circumpolar Health. 2013; 72(1): 21223. DOI: 10.3402/ijch.v72i0.21223

[31] Smaardijk V.R., Maas A.H.E.M., Lodder P., Kop W.J., Mommersteeg P. M.C. Sex and gender-stratified risks of psychological factors for adverse clinical outcomes in patients with ischemic heart disease: A systematic review and meta-analysis. Int J Cardiol. 2020; 302: 21-29. doi: 10.1016/j.ijcard.2019.12.014.

[32] Bushnell C.D., Chaturvedi S., Gage K.R., Herson P.S., Hurn P.D., Jiménez M.C., Kittner S.J., Madsen T.E., McCullough L.D., McDermott M., Reeves M.J., Rundek T. Sex differences in stroke: Challenges and opportunities. J Cereb Blood Flow Metab. 2018 Dec;38 (12):2179-2191. doi: 10.1177/0271678X18793324.

[33] Lambiase M.J., Kubzansky L.D., Thurston R.C. Prospective study of anxiety and incident stroke. Stroke. 2014; 45(2): 438-43. doi: 10.1161/STROKEAHA.113.003741.

[34] Portegies M.L., Bos M.J., Koudstaal P.J., Hofman A., Tiemeier H. W., Ikram M.A. Anxiety and the Risk of Stroke: The Rotterdam Study. Stroke. 2016;47(4):1120-3. doi: 10.1161/STROKEAHA.115.012361.

[35] Gafarov V.V., Gromova H.A., Gagulin I.V., Ekimova Y.C., Santrapinskiy D.K. Arterial hypertension, myocardial infarction and stroke: risk of development and psychosocial factors. Alaska Med. 2007; 49(2 Suppl): 117-9.

[36] Pérez-Piñar M., Ayerbe L., González E., Mathur R., Foguet-Boreu Q., Ayis S. Anxiety disorders and risk of stroke: A systematic review and meta-analysis. Eur Psychiatry. 2017 Mar; 41: 102-108. doi: 10.1016/j.eurpsy.2016.11.004.

[37] Dong J.Y., Zhang Y.H., Tong J., Qin L.Q. Depression and risk of stroke: a meta-analysis of prospective studies. Stroke. 2012; 43(1): 32-7. doi: 10.1161/STROKEAHA.111.630871.

[38] Majed B., Arveiler D., Bingham A., Ferrieres J., Ruidavets J.B., Montaye M., Appleton K., Haas B., Kee F., Amouyel P., Ducimetiere P., Empana J. P.; PRIME Study Group. Depressive

symptoms, a time-dependent risk factor for coronary heart disease and stroke in middle-aged men: the PRIME Study. Stroke. 2012; 43(7):1761-7. doi: 10.1161/STROKEAHA.111.645366.

[39] Seifert C.L., Poppert H., Sander D., Feurer R., Etgen T., Ander K.H., Pürner K., Brönner M., Sepp D., Kehl V., Förstl H., Bickel H. Depressive symptoms and the risk of ischemic stroke in the elderly–influence of age and sex. PLoS One. 2012; 7(11):e50803. doi: 10.1371/journal.pone.0050803.

[40] Kornerup H., Marott J.L., Schnohr P., Boysen G., Barefoot J., Prescott E. Vital exhaustion increases the risk of ischemic stroke in women but not in men: results from the Copenhagen City Heart Study. J Psychosom Res. 2010; 68:131–137. doi: 10.1016/j.jpsychores.2009.08.009.

[41] Valtorta N.K., Kanaan M., Gilbody S., et al. Loneliness and social isolation as risk factors for coronary heart disease and stroke: systematic review and meta-analysis of longitudinal observational studies. Heart. 2016; 102: 1009-1016. DOI: 10.1136/heartjnl-2015-308790.

[42] Gafarov V.V., Panov D.O., Gromova E.A., Gagulin I.V., Gafarova A.V. The influence of social support on risk of acute cardiovascular diseases in female population aged 25-64 in Russia. Int J Circumpolar Health. 2013; 72:21210. doi: 10.3402/ijch.v72i0.21210.

Chapter 2

Vascular Calcification and Cardiovascular Risk in Chronic Kidney Disease: A Problem That Is Here to Stay

Eduarda Castanheiro Esteves Carias,
Roberto Calças Marques and Ana Paula Andrade da Silva

Abstract

Cardiovascular disease is the primary cause of morbidity and mortality in chronic kidney disease (CKD) population, particularly in end stage renal disease (ESRD). This could be explained in part due to the presence of traditional cardiovascular risk factors, such as older age, hypertension, dyslipidemia and diabetes, but is also associated with nontraditional cardiovascular risk factors related to CKD, like inflammation, anemia, abnormal calcium and phosphate metabolism and extracellular fluid volume overload, which may contribute to intimal or medial wall arterial calcification. Vascular calcification (VC) is a dynamic process, resulting from the dysregulation of the balance of molecules that promote and those that inhibit this course. It is important for clinicians to both acknowledge and recognize the pathways and risk factors of VC in order to improve cardiovascular health in CKD patients. This chapter will focus on the biology of VC, the association with CKD, risk factor modification, screening and prevention of VC and cardiovascular disease in CKD patients.

Keywords: vascular calcification, cardiovascular disease, chronic kidney disease, mineral metabolism

1. Introduction

Vascular Calcification (VC) refers to the ectopic deposition of calcium phosphate crystals in arterial walls [1, 2]. This is a process that can be seen in all arteries with a distinction made based on the offended layer of the wall – medial or intimal – with different explaining mechanisms [3]. Besides vessel walls, other tissues like cardiac valves can also show calcifications [1, 4, 5].

In 1855, Virchow described the VC as "artery ossification", precisely in patients with renal disease [3, 6]. More recent, studies showed the same findings in Egyptian mummies [7].

In fact, with current molecular knowledge, we understand that mineralization of the tunica media, the type of VC associated with CKD and its mineral disturbances [8], occurs with trans-differentiation of muscle cells to bone cells, in a process one could call ossification [9, 10]. On the origin of those cellular changes, several factors interact to put in motion a series of events that will result in an active promotion of mineral deposition [1, 11, 12].

VC increases with age [13] and it is associated with many diseases such as diabetes [14], cardiovascular diseases (CVD) [8, 15], some genetic diseases [2, 16] and particularly CKD [8, 17–19]. In the latter, VC is observed in early stages, progresses with the renal impairment and affects almost every dialysis patient [20], even in the absence of traditional risk factors of hypertension, obesity, dyslipidaemia and smoking [21, 22]. For calcification to happen, an unregulated state of bone ossification induction and the loss of many molecules that are believed to be osteogenesis inhibitors, must occur [11, 12]. In CKD, the culprit appointed by many recent studies is another of its complications – the mineral disturbance [11].

Cardiovascular (CV) events are tightly related to the CKD population, with high incidence of sudden cardiac death, arrhythmia, congestive heart failure and stroke, corresponding to the most common cause of death, especially in dialysis patients [2, 20, 23]. VC progression and severity [24] is directly associated with these CV events and its related mortality [21] due to arterial calcification and its consequences, like ventricular hypertrophy or micro-embolic disease [10, 23, 25]. This explains the high prevalence of cardiac events and mortality even in patients without the traditional cardio-vascular risk factors [8, 10].

Until now, no study came to the conclusion that VC directly causes CV events [26]. Moreover, VC has some features in common with arterial aggression leading to CVD [26, 27]. For that reason, there are still some who argue that VC is a consequence and not the cause for CVD [28–30].

This chapter will focus on the biology of vascular calcification and the association with chronic kidney disease.

2. The biology of vascular calcification

The calcification of the vasculature refers to the pathological deposition of phospho-calcium minerals in the arteries, leading to its stiffness [19] and thickening, as a result of a complex interaction of factors [4, 23]. Regardless of that, phospho-calcium can spontaneously precipitate [31]. Oversaturation increases of those ions concentrations and acidic environment favors their precipitation with a formation of various intermediates minerals, gradually bigger, until the least soluble, **hydroxyapatite** (HA) which will then crystalize [32]. The deposition of this crystal, or **nucleation process**, occurs chiefly in the apoptotic cells [9, 17, 33] or in mineral containing vesicles [34], which will then release more calcium to extracellular matrix (ECM), promoting more apoptosis when entering the neighboring cells, in a vicious cycle [32].

2.1 Calcification types

The histological location of that deposition and the pathobiology has made a distinction between types of calcifications [4, 35]. This phenomenon can arise in: i) the inner layer of endothelial and connective subendothelial tissue of arteries, ii) the medial muscular layer, iii) in the cardiac valves (resulting in valve sclerosis and stenosis) and iv) calcific uremic arteriolopathy, previously known as calciphylaxis [3]. These are the calcifications referring to the vascular system, of which we will focus on the first two. Besides VC, other extra-skeletal calcifications may happen [3, 36].

Atherosclerosis, an accumulation of calcium in the intimal layer of large and medium sized arteries, is observed following a long inflammatory process and as a last stage of that series of events [23, 37, 38]. It involves the infiltration of macrophages in the epithelial and subepithelial connective tissue and the formation of a lipid plaque [3, 23]. Hence, it is related to dyslipidaemia, arterial hypertension and tabagism, but also with age [8].

In **medial calcific sclerosis** (MCS) or **Mönckeberg's medial arteriosclerosis**, the target of calcification is the muscular medial layer of elastic or muscular arteries, and posteriorly, fibrosis, stiffness and thickening ensues [36, 37, 39]. This form is widely related to mineral imbalance, and it is seen in diabetes, some rare genetic diseases [40] and strongly related to CKD [17, 37]. This is the form to which we will be referring to.

It is important to point out that atherosclerosis is due to inflammation and lipid deposition and for that depends on the so-called traditional CV factors (dyslipidaemia, arterial hypertension and tabagism) while medial VC does not [23, 41, 42]. In atherosclerosis, plaque calcification creates areas of different compliance [23, 39, 43, 44]. It ultimately leads to plaque rupture and acute vessel obstruction and is more closely associated with an increase in mortality [23, 43, 45, 46].

The association of MCS and mortality was brought up by many studies but not yet proven to be a cause-effect [28, 29] and some opinions still diverge, as we will discuss ahead. Research efforts have improved our knowledge on the molecular mechanisms involved, showing a passive process of physicochemical reaction resulting in vesicles [17, 47]. As stated earlier, apoptotic debris are good mineral nucleation sites but extracellular vesicles (EV) are regarded as having much higher mineralization potential [48].

Cells capable of osteo-transdifferentiation include not only vascular smooth muscle cells (VSMC) in the media, but also miofibroblasts in the adventitia, pericytes under endothelial cells (related to atherosclerosis), multipotent vascular mesenchymal cells and cardiac valve interstitial cells [42, 49, 50]. EVs, originally termed matrix vesicles, are nanoparticles of cellular origin, heterogeneous in size, shape and content, with two origins: membrane budding or in an endosomal pathway where multivesicular bodies fuse with the plasma membrane and then releases to the ECM by the regulation of sphingomyelin 3 [1, 17, 47, 51]. These EVs are designated exosomes [1, 52]. These vesicles are known for many decades to be related to bone mineralization but only recently were identified in VC. Indeed, EV's membrane have affinity to matrix proteins and, contrary to non-calcifying vesicles, contain phosphatidilserin (acidic phospholipid) and calcium-channel annexin family molecules in the membrane, responsible for the vesicle's release. Annexin-6 has been described as a regulator of VC in vivo [1, 37, 47, 53].

EV's release is promoted by high levels of calcium and their calcifying potential depends on its altered content compared to normal vesicles, with lower calcification modulating proteins – which we will analyze in detail later –, higher calcium and phosphate content, lipids, microRNAs, matrix metalloproteinases (MMP) for matrix digestion and alkaline phosphatase (ALP), which normally is not present in vascular tissue. ALP releases free inorganic phosphate (Pi) – enhancing more crystal formation [47].

The nucleation of HA begins inside the vesicles, with molding crystals' size and shape, and continues with the of in the ECM. Even tough origin and release of EVs are still poorly understood, vesicles are regarded as nucleating foci for VC [52, 54].

2.2 Transdifferentiation of VSMC

The unregulated osteogenesis is owed to the influence of external and internal factors (age, inflammation, toxins, CKD or diabetes) that induce transformation of VSMC to osteogenic cells responsible for a pathological mineralization [23, 37, 54, 55].

Gene silencing lead to the loss of contractile properties by the underexpression of α-smooth muscle actin (SMA) and smooth muscle protein 22 (SM2) – the de-differentiation of VSMCs – whereas the upregulation of several genes coding for bone-like cells, give VSMCs the **osteogenic characteristics** [48, 49, 56]:

- **ALP** – enzyme responsible for the increasing Pi availability needed for crystal formation. ALP in soft tissues is a marker of ectopic calcium deposits [49, 57].

- **Collagen I** – implicated in the ECM remodeling and HA deposition as described [58].

- **Osteopontin (OPN)** – it is a binding-calcium particle (preventing HA formation) and a pro-inflammatory agent. It is thought that the cleavage of OPN under osteogenic circumstances by MMPs, may disrupter its equilibrium rendering an inflammatory and angiogenic role and involved in proliferation and migration of calcifying VSMCs [59].

- **Osteocalcin and Osteonectin** – increased in calcifying cells but with role on VC yet to be demonstrated [3, 25].

- **RANK-L** – Receptor activator of nuclear factor KB ligand. RANK is a member of tumor necrosis factor (TNF) receptor family, expressed by osteoclasts and increased in medial VC where it promotes VSMC calcification (demonstrated in vitro). The mechanism is the upregulation of a pathway of transdifferentiation. It also promotes osteoclast activity, responsible for osteoporosis [13].

2.3 Loss of calcification inhibitors

Along with the aforementioned change in phenotype, the loss of calcification inhibitors must take place concomitantly for the end-result of VC [58]. These are referred as the calcifying protein inhibitors preventing HA harm to ECM and cells [37].

They are herein described:

- **Matrix Gla Protein (MGP)** – Vitamin K dependent protein (VKDP), expressed in several tissues and in VSMCs. The activated molecule has a glutamic γ-carboxylation [55]. In normal states, the carboxylate MGP binds and inhibits crystal formation and prevents osteoblastic transformation. The unbalance toward the uncarboxylated inactive form is present in VC and is assumed to be a procalcifying agent [47]. Because of its vitamin K dependence for the γ-carboxylation of glutamic residues, anti-cumarinic medications (anti-vitamin K) may disrupt its normal quantities [58, 60].

- **Gla-Rich Protein (GRP)** – GRP is the newest member of the vitamin K-dependent protein (VKDP) family, first identified in sturgeon calcified cartilage and characterized by the presence of an unprecedented 15 putative calcium-binding Gla residues in human [61]. It is considered a negative regulator of osteogenic differentiation [62], a modulator of calcium availability in the ECM [61, 63], and an inhibitor of calcification in the CV [64] and articular systems [65]. GRP calcium binding properties [61, 66] and association to calcification processes [61, 63–67] indicates that its function might be associated with prevention of calcium-induced signaling pathways and direct mineral-binding to inhibit crystal formation/maturation. GRP is also involved in the mineralization-competence of VSMCs derived EVs and possibly associated with the fetuin-A/MGP calcification inhibitory system [64].

- **Fetuin-A (Fet-A)** – also known as α2-Heremans-Schimd glycoprotein, is a potent anti-calcification glycoprotein in circulation [34]. Binds crystals therefore preventing its growth and the formation of insoluble nanoparticles [68, 69]. The complexes formed with crystals – primary calciprotein particles (CPP-1) – are more easily eliminated by the reticuloendothelial system than normal calciparticles and with less toxicity to those cells [70]. The re-arrangement of the CPP-1 in terms of form and crystal features will make a particle believed to be more cytotoxic and VC-inducing, called secondary CPP (CPP-2) [37]. Fet-A is linked with reduction of inflammatory response and oxidative stress produced by calcification. As seen, it is diminished in EVs responsible for VC [49]. Studies shown Fet-A to be decrease in serum of CKD patients, with age, restrictive diet, low weight and aerobic exercise [58]. Despite being phospho-calcium containers impeding its growth and deposition, CPPs are cytotoxic particles and in case of impaired elimination it is believed to be responsible for the inflammation state and premature aging seen on CKD.

- **Osteoprogerin (OPG)** – binds RANK-L preventing its binding to RANK and its effects: osteoclastic differentiation and medial calcification [58, 71].

- **Pyrophosphate (PPi)** – prevents the formation of phospho-calcium crystals in the extracellular environment [58, 71].

2.4 Regulation: Signaling pathways

Different, complex and not fully understood molecular pathways activate the changes described in the pathobiology of VC [4]. Many of those factors have more than one implication in VC and a lot of them interact with each other. There is a "perfect storm" [25, 49] behind VC. Hereby we analyze the mechanism and the signals involved with the onset of VC.

- **Runx2/Cbaf** – The transcriptional promoter activity of Runt-related **transcriptor factor-2,** also known as Core-binding factor subunit α1, is responsible for the underexpression of muscle fibers causing the de-differentiation process of VSMCs [72]. Together with the downstream **Osterix gene** it is responsible for the upregulation of the aforementioned Osteocalcin, Osteopontin (OPN), Osteonectin, ALP, Collagen I, RANK-L and also sclerostin, since all of them have a binding site for cbaf in their genes/promoters [49, 58]. These promoters regulate genes involved with the cell cycle for lineage determination, interacting in order to enhance osteoblastic/osteochondrogenic protein characteristics and osteogenic lineage commitment of the VSMCs [73]. This mechanism is related with age, CKD, diabetes type 2, inflammation and with toxins like uremic products [37, 72].

- **Wnt pathway** – in this signal transduction pathway, several glycoproteins (Wnts) are capable of activating specific membrane receptor complexes, responsible for the dephosphorylated stabilization of ß-catenin that leads to the intracellular signaling of transcription factors activation [13, 74]. Different receptors are involved but low-density related protein receptors (LRP) 5 and

6 were described as involved in the pathway resulting in activation of Runx2 and Osterix by ß-catenin, in a way not yet clarified [13, 58]. There are many proteins to regulate Wnt cascade like sclerostin, which binds to the membrane receptor thus inhibiting it, and **MSX-2** homeobox that promotes paracrine Wnt signals [13, 49]. It is also implied in the cell-cycle, proliferation, lineage commitment and regulation of apoptosis and its activation is related to TNF-α, oxidative stress and hyperphosphatemia [13, 58].

- **The Bone Morphogenetic Protein-2 (BMP-2)** – a cytokine of TGF-ß family and a mediator of VC. By activating its membrane receptor can activate (by phosphorylation) co-regulatory proteins of the Smad family and will put, together with Runx2, the cascade of events in motion [42, 58]. Both BMP-2 and BMP-4 receptors can phosphorylate and activate that cascade toward osteoblastic/chondrocyte's formation and prevent mesenchymal cells transformation in (normal) VSMCs or adipocytes. It is crucial for VC to happen, since neither BMPs nor Runx2 are able to put the osteogenesis machinery in motion alone [13, 58].

- **TGF-ß** – upregulated when elastosis develops, like BMPs, can promote the transducing of osteogenic genes with Runx2 activation [58].

- **RANK/RANK-L/OPG pathway** – the already mentioned TNF-α family receptor, RANK activation results in the activation of NF-κB transcription factor. Involved in cellular responses to aggressions like free radicals, oxidized LDL cholesterol or some cytokines and it was linked to VC in some studies. It also increases BMP-4 expression and so, activates Runx2 [58]. As discussed, RANK-L is the activator of receptor RANK and OPG competes with RANK-L, preventing the pathway activation. So, RANK signaling depends on RANK-L:OPG ratio but also indirectly of the regulatory factor Runx2, capable of promoting RANK-L expression [25, 71].

- **ENPP1/PPi/ALP axis** – as discussed, PPi opposes crystal formation whereas ALP is a crystal-promotor by hydrolysing PPi and making it a source of phosphor (Pi) [47]. In a complex interaction of several enzymes, PPi is formed by Ectonucleotide Pyrophosphatase/Phosphodiesterase-1 enzyme (ENPP1) from adenosine triphosphate (ATP). Another membrane enzyme – Progressive Ankylosis Protein (ANK) – makes PPi available to the extracellular environment where it can prevent Pi to mineralize. An overexpression of ENPP1, ANK and ALP gives the continuous exaggerated production and release of PPi to the ECM, for posterior destruction by ALP [36, 47, 57, 58].

Vitamin D can induce such activity. ATP Binding Cassette Subfamily C member 6 (ABCC6) and ecto-5′-nucleotidase (NT5E) genes encode for the intermediary enzymes in the formation and degradation of ATP to AMP and ultimately, adenosine; These several enzymes are related to genetic calcifying diseases [58].

- **Phosphate and calcium status** – increased concentrations of these ions result in the formation of either crystals or nanoparticles with proteins, as referred. Transient or continuous elevated extracellular phosphate, in any form, has cytotoxicity consequences: it can lead to apoptosis because of ROS burden, an important calcifying event; and it can activate the digesting MMPs responsible for elastolysis [4, 13, 75]. Elevated calcium concentrations facilitate phosphate entry and is linked to calcification even in normal phosphoric quantities. Both calcium and Pi are related with Runx2 activation [13, 17, 47]. HA crystals, nanoparticles or free phosphate can render the same results. In fact, it has been proposed that cell-internalized CPPs with low fetuin-A are the most common event and that they can be detected circulating in CKD patients' blood, as they do not in healthy individuals [32].

- **MicroRNAs (miRNAs)** – regulate gene expression by targeting translated mRNAs and altering its traducing to proteins. EVs are known to have miRNAs and there have been new studies on this matter [47].

On the other hand, it is of notice that for the installation of VC, there is a role to be played by the concomitant loss of several osteogenesis antagonizing molecules, such as [58]:

- **MGP, GRP and Fet-A** – the carboxylated forms not only bind calcium but also inhibit BMPs impeding BMPs-BMP receptor activation.

- **BMP-7** – apart from the other BMPs, it does not promote Runx2 but the expression of smooth muscle fibers, antagonizing the VSMC differentiation. Because of that, the loss of its action will possibly increase VC risk [58, 72].

- **Sclerostin** – a glycoprotein with expression promoted by Runx2 and OSX is not consistently associated with VC and its role is to be fully explained, but it was however identified as an inhibitor of the Wnt cascade in its signal activation by ß-catenin and therefore inhibiting osteogenesis [58].

- **Adiponectin** – an adipocyte's hormone, restricts osteoblastic differentiation by 1/p38 receptors signaling pathway [40].

A complex myriad of factors may offend the vessel wall's cells such as: elastolysis, cytokines, ROS, oxidized lipids, glucose, uremic molecules, BMPs and circulating calciprotein particles (CCPs). These will ignite signaling pathways like the Wnt pathway, resulting in the trans-differentiation of VSCM by the action

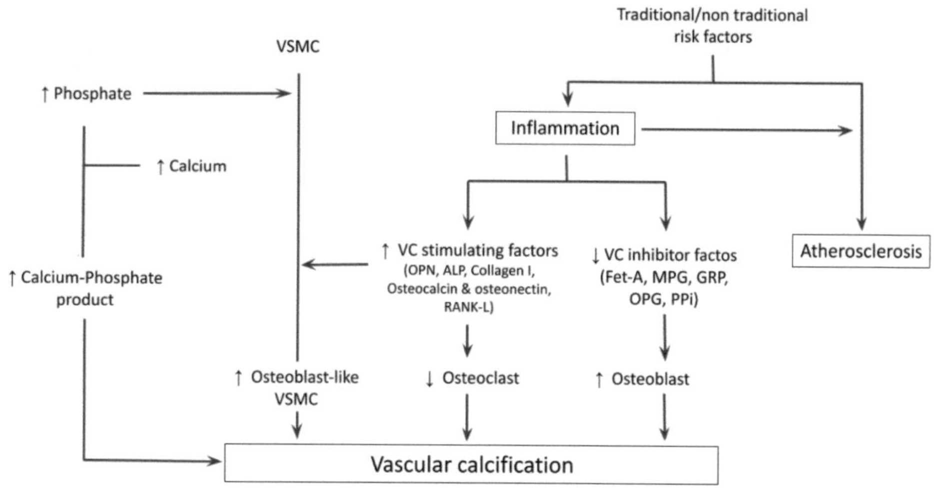

Figure 1.
Mechanisms of vascular calcification. ALP: Alkaline phosphatase; Fet-A: Fetuin-A; GRP: Gla-rich protein; MGP: Matrix Gla protein; OPN: Osteopontin; OPG: Osteoprotegerin; PPi: Pyrophosphate; RANK-L: Receptor activator of nuclear factor KB*- ligand; VC: Vascular calcification; VSMC: Vascular smooth muscle cells. (Adapted from Dellegrottaglie et al. [28].)*

of transcription factor Runx2. Deposition of minerals is promoted in the matrix, either in vesicles or apoptotic bodies. As this occurs, a loss of calcification inhibitors will pose no obstruction to the process.

Ultimately, the stiffness caused by this remodeling of the medial layer will result in ventricular hypertrophy [19, 49].

Figure 1 resumes the before mentioned pathways and mechanisms implied in the vascular calcification process.

3. Vascular calcification in chronic kidney disease

Cardiovascular disease is the leading cause of death in patients with CKD, especially among those with end stage renal disease (ESRD) [76, 77]. This high cardiovascular risk may be in part due to excess VC [78, 79].

The prevalence of vascular calcification in CKD patients increases with progressively decreasing kidney function and is greater than the general population [21, 80]. In patients with estimated glomerular filtration rate (eGFR) less than 60 mL/min/1.73 m2 and not on dialysis, VC is known to be present in 47 to 83%. In dialysis adult patients, coronary artery calcification (CAC) has been detected in 51–93% and valvular calcification in 20–47% [2, 5, 81].

Increased CV risk may be due to CAC, with remarkably high prevalence in patients undergoing dialysis [8, 76, 82, 83]. It can be said that 20-year-old patients in dialysis have the same CV mortality risk as 80–90 year-old non-diabetic and non-uraemic subjects [82]. This may be associated with dialysis vintage, the intake of supplemental calcium, particularly with calcium-containing phosphate binders, and the mean calcium-phosphorus ion product.

3.1 Clinical significance

The diagnosis of CKD–Mineral Bone Disease (MBD) includes the detection of extra-osseous calcification, such as arterial, valvular, and myocardial calcification [5].

The clinical significance of vascular calcification depends on the site (ie, medial or intimal) and type of the affected arteries. Intimal calcification is associated with the formation and progression of atherosclerotic lesions and is associated with the development of plaques and occlusive lesions as in coronary artery disease, cerebrovascular disease, and peripheral vascular disease [9].

Tunica media calcification was initially considered to be clinically non-significant [9]. However, it was later demonstrated in CKD and ESRD patients that was associated with decreased vascular distensibility and increased vessel stiffness and pulse pressure with consequent progression of intimal lesions [9, 11, 84–86]. London et al. conducted a study including 202 HD patients which showed that medial calcification had major impact on clinical outcome, being an independent prognostic marker for all cause and CV mortality in chronic HD patients independently of classical atherogenic factors, with close association to time on HD [8].

3.1.1 Coronary artery calcification

Coronary artery calcification (CAC) is common and progressive in young adults with ESRD who are undergoing dialysis [21]. Some studies reveal an association between CAC and CVD in this population [80, 83].

Coronary artery calcification score, measured noninvasively by electron-beam computed tomography (EBCT), was found to be an independent predictor of overall mortality in dialysis patients [87]. In one study with 39 patients undergoing HD, those with CAC had higher serum phosphorus concentrations, higher calcium–phosphorus ion product in serum, and their daily intake of calcium-containing phosphate-binding agents was nearly two times greater than those without calcification [21].

3.1.2 Large-vessel calcification

Calcification of aorta and other large arteries is associated with increased arterial stiffness. This will cause lack of distensibility, leading to hypertension and increased pulse pressure, both risk factors for left ventricular dysfunction and heart failure among CKD patients [85, 88].

3.2 Risk factors

The higher prevalence of traditional CV risk factors, such as older age, hypertension, dyslipidemia and diabetes, and the presence of nontraditional CV risk factors related to CKD (anemia, abnormal calcium and phosphate metabolism, extracellular fluid volume overload, electrolyte imbalance) may explain the high occurrence of CVD and contribute to intimal or medial wall calcification in patients with kidney failure [28].

3.2.1 Demographic features and time on dialysis

Vascular calcification is associated with the increasing age and time on dialysis [21, 89, 90]. A study with 134 patients on HD, peritoneal dialysis and with stage 4 CKD demonstrated that age and male gender were important determinants of VC [77, 91].

3.2.2 Mineral metabolism

Disorders of mineral metabolism may promote CV calcification, contributing to higher CVD and mortality in patients with kidney failure or ESRD. Several observational studies have noted an association between mineral and bone disorders with adverse outcomes, most notably with increased phosphate levels (increased risk of VC, cardiomyopathy, and mortality) [11, 22, 92, 93].

Hyperphosphatemia, uremia, hyperglycemia and other metabolites may initiate the process of VC by transforming vascular smooth muscle cells to a chondrocyte or osteoblast-like cell. In dialysis patients, this process is accelerated in the setting of the common presence of high calcium, high phosphorus, and abnormal bone remodeling [91].

3.2.2.1 Hyperphosphatemia and hypercalcemia

Epidemiological studies have shown that hyperphosphatemia is associated with unexpectedly high rates of CV events and death in ESRD patients [94].

Hyperphosphatemia is a strong inducer of VC by inducing smooth muscle cells to undergo an osteochondrogenic phenotype change through a mechanism requiring sodium-dependent phosphate cotransporters [11]. In a group of 43 patients receiving peritoneal dialysis studied by MDCT at baseline and after 1 year of follow-up, Stompor and colleagues reported a significant correlation between changes in coronary calcium score and mean values of phosphate and calcium–phosphate product [95]. A study with uremic rats fed with high phosphate diet showed that aortic medial calcification could be blocked by treatment with the phosphate binder, sevelamer [96].

Lowering serum phosphate levels with a non-calcium containing phosphate binder slows progression of VC in pre-dialysis and ESRD patients [97–99]. In pre-dialysis patients, treatment with calcium carbonate did not enhance the progression of CAC, as it has been observed in patients on dialysis [97].

3.2.2.2 Oral calcium intake

In dialysis patients, the use of calcium-based phosphate binders is strongly associated with development and progression of CAC, due to the ingestion of large amounts of calcium and the consequent hypercalcemia [97]. Therefore, a positive calcium balance may increase the risk of calcium overload and CV calcification and it should be taken into account when calcium salts are prescribed. Discontinuation or dose reduction of calcium-based phosphate binders is suggested in the presence of hypercalcemia, CV calcification, adynamic bone disease, and/or low serum PTH levels [90].

Phosphate binding and lowering of serum phosphate can be achieved with calcium-based or non-calcium-based binders. A meta-analysis including 11 randomized trials (4622 patients) showed that patients assigned to non-calcium-based binders had a 22% reduction in all-cause mortality compared with those assigned to calcium-based phosphate binders in patients with CKD [100].

3.2.2.3 Dialysate calcium

The exposure to high calcium concentrations may influence the development of low–turnover bone disease and CAC in HD patients. A randomized controlled study showed that lowering Ca exposure through dialysate (dialysate Ca concentration of 1.25 mmol/L vs. 1.75 mmol/L) attenuates progression of CAC and improves low bone turn-over in HD patients with baseline PTH levels ≤300 pg./ml [101].

3.2.2.4 Secondary hyperparathyroidism and adynamic bone disease

Both secondary hyperparathyroidism (SHPT) high-turnover renal osteodystrophy and adynamic bone disease have been associated with VC. In a group of 58 ESRD patients on HD, bone-histomorphometry characteristics were compared with the arterial calcification (AC) scores. High AC scores were associated with bone histomorphometry values, suggestive of low bone activity and adynamic bone disease. This indicates that therapeutic interventions associated with excessive decrease of parathyroid activity favors lower bone turnover and adynamic bone disease that, in combination with interventions that increase the Ca balance, could influence the development and progression of AC [102].

3.2.2.5 Vitamin D and calcimimetic agents

A major complication of SHPT is renal osteodystrophy, in association with alterations in calcium and phosphorus metabolism leading to CV calcification. Active vitamin D compounds and calcimimetic agents are used to treat SHPT in dialysis patients. Untreated vitamin D deficiency has been associated with increased VC, in part due to accelerated development of atherosclerosis [103, 104]. In these patients, vitamin D supplement may have a protective benefit against VC by decreasing endothelial injury, inactivating renin-angiotensin-aldosterone system, decreasing insulin resistance, lowering cholesterol, inhibiting foam cell and cholesterol efflux in macrophages, and modulating vascular regeneration [105]. Excessive administration of vitamin D has been also associated with increased VC, possibly related to hypercalcemia and an elevated calcium-phosphate product. Cinacalcet has the ability to simultaneously lower PTH, calcium, phosphorus, and CaxP in patients with SHPT [106]. In a study, Cinacalcet plus low-dose active vitamin D derivatives attenuated vascular and cardiac valve calcification [107].

3.2.2.6 Hypomagnesemia and FGF-23

Hypomagnesemia has been associated with increased VC [23, 108, 109]. In a population with diabetes mellitus type 2 and mild to moderate CKD, hypomagnesemia was found to be an independent predictor of mitral valve calcification and intima media thickness [110].

3.2.2.7 Oral vitamin K antagonists

The vitamin K-dependent MGP, despite not being related to blood coagulation cascade, is affected by Vitamin K antagonists (VKA) and is considered a strong inhibitor of calcification of arterial vessel wall and cartilage [111]. Warfarin (a VKA) is a risk factor for calcific uremic arteriolopathy, necrotizing skin condition observed in dialysis patients, associated with extremely high mortality rates [11, 112, 113].

3.2.3 Diabetes

Many studies have shown that diabetes is a risk factor for VC in patients without CKD. In patients with eGFR <60 mL/min/1.73 m2 who were not on dialysis, diabetes also increased the risk of VC from 3.5 to 55.7% [114].

3.2.4 Dyslipidemia

Dyslipidemia increases the risk of VC in patients without CKD, via induction of inflammation and endothelial/vascular smooth muscle cell damage by oxidized lipids [115, 116]. Beneficial effects of sevelamer on VC may be related to its lipid-lowering effects [99].

3.2.5 Other molecules

Serum Gla-Rich Protein (GRP) levels were found to progressively decrease from stage 2 to stage 4 CKD. A multivariate analysis study identified that decreased eGFR, low levels of GRP, and high levels of fibroblast growth factor-23 (FGF-23) were associated with higher VC score and pulse pressure. These results indicate an association between GRP, renal dysfunction and CKD-mineral and bone disorder. The relationship between low levels of GRP and VC suggests a future potential utility for GRP as an early marker of vascular damage in CKD [117]. Once uremic CPPs and EVs are important players in the mechanisms of widespread calcification in CKD, GRP could have a role as an inhibitory factor, preventing calcification at systemic and tissue levels. Possible future approaches targeting the increase of γ-carboxylated GRP bioavailability could represent promising therapeutics [118].

3.3 Detection

The recognition of vascular or valvular calcification in patients with CKD stages G3a–G5D places them with highest cardiovascular risk [119]. The early diagnosis of VC and the identification of its cause raises hope for therapeutic intervention that might reduce CVD in patients with CKD.

Various noninvasive methods, such as ultrasound, fluoroscopy, and digital subtraction angiography, have been used to detect and measure VC [28]. Currently, EBCT and multidetector computed tomography (MDCT) are excellent methods to detect and quantify VC [28], with their results being stronger predictors of a cardiovascular event in normal population [28, 119]. Bursztyn and colleagues reported a twofold greater progression in coronary calcium score (measured by MDCT) in hypertensive patients with CKD, than in hypertensive patients with normal renal function [120].

A number of noninvasive methods, which are more easily and available techniques, can also be used to detect the presence or absence of valvular calcification, like lateral abdominal radiograph and echocardiogram [119]. The simplest technique is plain radiography, which demonstrates pipe-stem calcification of the tunica media and more irregular, patchy calcifications of the internal elastic lamina. However, this is an insensitive method and does not quantify the severity of VC [8].

Several scores, based on plain radiographic imaging or CT scans, are used in clinical studies to calcium quantification and scoring:

- **Agatston score** - quantifies CAC detected by an unenhanced low-dose cardiac CT scan. The Agatston score allows for early risk stratification for a major adverse cardiac event.

- **Adragão score** – the Adragão score quantifies calcification of the iliac, femoral, radial and digital arteries observed on plain radiographs of the hands and pelvis. The final value ranges between 0 and 8 points (0 to 4 in the pelvis and 0 to 4 in the hands). VC score ≥ 3 had an almost fourfold higher risk of cardiovascular mortality, representing a simple and inexpensive tool for assessing the cardiovascular risk related to VC in HD patients [121].

In the Study of Mineral and Bone Disorders that included 742 patients with nondialysis CKD stages 3–5 from 39 centers in Spain, VC assessment using Adragão Score was independently associated with all-cause and cardiovascular mortality as well as a shorter hospitalization event–free period [122].

- **Kauppila score** – This score quantifies the severity of lumbar aortic calcifications observed on a lateral abdominal radiograph ranging from the T-10 vertebra to the first two sacral vertebrae. A score of 1 to 3 is assigned based on extent of calcification (ie, one-third, two-thirds, or more than two-thirds of the vertebra).

3.4 Treatment

The approach to decrease the progression of VC can be influenced by treatment. Given that VC is associated with increased cardiovascular risk and the pathogenesis seems to be related to CKD-MBD abnormalities and atherosclerosis, the treatment should focus on the prevention of arterial lesions, correcting the several traditional and non-traditional pro-atherogenic risk factors responsible for arterial injury, mainly calcium and phosphate balance [5, 29].

Some experimental studies have suggested that the administration of magnesium prevents VC, not only reducing the deposition of calcium, but also inhibiting osteogenic transdifferentiation, and may be considered an important and realistic approach to potentially reduce the risk for VC and subsequent cardiovascular complications in CKD patients. Clinical trials are warranted to further assess the clinical relevance of magnesium in this regard [123, 124].

In patients with CKD G3a–G5D, decisions about phosphate-lowering treatment should be based on progressively or persistently elevated serum phosphate, as mentioned earlier [119].

In the management of moderate to severe secondary hyperparathyroidism, current treatment options consist of the oral administration of intestinal phosphate binders, oral or intravenous calcitriol or active vitamin D analogs, and the oral or intravenous calcimimetic agents (cinacalcet and etacalcetide) [125].

4. Conclusions

The high incidence of multiple traditional and non-traditional risk factors predisposes advanced CKD and dialysis patients to a considerable burden of CVD. This chapter has summarized the biology of VC, highlighting the processes of mineralization, the effects of local inflammation, and the available evidence about risk factors modification, prevention and screening in CKD. Clinicians must understand the limitations of the current evidence and adapt specific therapeutic strategies to the individual patient. Future research into modifiable, non-traditional risk factors with emphasis on mineral bone metabolism is warranted and we look forward to their clinical application and improvement of CVD outcomes in CKD patients.

Conflict of interest

The authors declare no conflict of interest.

Author details

Eduarda Castanheiro Esteves Carias†, Roberto Calças Marques†
and Ana Paula Andrade da Silva*
Department of Nephrology, Centro Hospitalar Universitário do Algarve, Faro, Portugal

*Address all correspondence to: anapassionara@gmail.com

† Joint first authorship.

IntechOpen

© 2021 The Author(s). Licensee IntechOpen. This chapter is distributed under the terms of the Creative Commons Attribution License (http://creativecommons.org/licenses/by/3.0), which permits unrestricted use, distribution, and reproduction in any medium, provided the original work is properly cited.

References

[1] Kapustin AN, Chatrou MLL, Drozdov I, Zheng Y, Davidson SM, Soong D, et al. Vascular smooth muscle cell calcification is mediated by regulated exosome secretion. Circ Res. 2015;116(8):1312-1323.

[2] Lanzer P, Boehm M, Sorribas V, Thiriet M, Janzen J, Zeller T, et al. Medial vascular calcification revisited: Review and perspectives. European Heart Journal. 2014. p. 1515-25.

[3] Bover J, Górriz JL, Ur Na-Torres P, Lloret MJ, Ruiz-García C, Dasilva I, et al. Revista de la Sociedad Española de Nefrología Detection of cardiovascular calcifications: Is it a useful tool for nephrologists? Nefrología. 2016;336(66).

[4] Wu M, Rementer C, Giachelli CM. Vascular calcification: An update on mechanisms and challenges in treatment. Calcif Tissue Int. 2013;93(4):365-373.

[5] KDIGO. KDIGO clinical practice guideline for the diagnosis, evaluation, prevention, and treatment of Chronic Kidney Disease-Mineral and Bone Disorder (CKD-MBD). Kidney Int Suppl. 2009;76(113): S1-130.

[6] Virchow R. Cellular pathology. As based upon physiological and pathological histology. Philadelphia J B Lippincott. 1863;566.

[7] Allam AH, Thompson RC, Wann LS, Miyamoto MI, Nur El-Din AEH, El-Maksoud GA, et al. Atherosclerosis in ancient egyptian mummies: The horus study. JACC Cardiovasc Imaging. 2011;4(4):315-327.

[8] London GM, Guerin AP, Marchais SJ, Metivier F, Pannier B, Adda H. Arterial media calcification in end-stage renal disease: impact on all-cause and cardiovascular mortality. NephrolDialTransplant [Internet]. 2003;18(931-509):1731-1740. Available from: http://ndt.oxfordjournals.org/cgi/doi/10.1093/ndt/gfg414

[9] Shanahan CM, Cary NRB, Salisbury JR, Proudfoot D, Weissberg PL, Edmonds ME. Medial localization of mineralization-regulating proteins in association with Monckeberg's sclerosis: Evidence for smooth muscle cell-mediated vascular calcification. Circulation. 1999;100(21):2168-2176.

[10] Jono S, McKee MD, Murry CE, Shioi a, Nishizawa Y, Mori K, et al. Phosphate regulation of vascular smooth muscle cell calcification. Circ Res. 2000;87(7): E10–E17.

[11] Giachelli CM. The emerging role of phosphate in vascular calcification. Kidney Int. 2009;75(9):890-897.

[12] Shroff RC, McNair R, Skepper JN, Figg N, Schurgers LJ, Deanfield J, et al. Chronic Mineral Dysregulation Promotes Vascular Smooth Muscle Cell Adaptation and Extracellular Matrix Calcification. J Am Soc Nephrol [Internet]. 2010;21(1):103-112. Available from: http://www.jasn.org/cgi/doi/10.1681/ASN.2009060640

[13] Leopold JA. Vascular calcification an age-old problem of old age. Circulation. 2013;127(24):2380-2382.

[14] Shurraw S, Majumdar SR, Thadhani R, Wiebe N, Tonelli M. Glycemic control and the risk of death in 1,484 patients receiving maintenance hemodialysis. Am J Kidney Dis [Internet]. 2010;55(5):875-84. Available from: http://www.ncbi.nlm.nih.gov/pubmed/20346561

[15] Niskanen L, Siitonen O, Suhonen M, Uusitupa MI. Medial artery calcification predicts cardiovascular mortality in patients with NIDDM. Diabetes Care [Internet]. 1994;17(11):1252-6. Available from: http://www.ncbi.nlm.nih.gov/pubmed/7821163

[16] Pérez-Hernández N, Aptilon-Duque G, Blachman-Braun R, Vargas-Alarcón G, Rodríguez-Cortés AA, Azrad-Daniel S, et al. Vascular Calcification: Current Genetics Underlying This Complex Phenomenon. Chinese medical journal. 2017. p. 1113-21.

[17] Shanahan CM, Crouthamel MH, Kapustin A, Giachelli CM. Arterial calcification in chronic kidney disease: Key roles for calcium and phosphate. Circulation Research. 2011. p. 697-711.

[18] Chen W, Melamed ML. Vascular calcification in predialysis CKD: Common and deadly. Clinical Journal of the American Society of Nephrology. 2015;10(4):551-553.

[19] Vlachopoulos C, Aznaouridis K, Stefanadis C. Prediction of Cardiovascular Events and All-Cause Mortality With Arterial Stiffness. A Systematic Review and Meta-Analysis. J Am Coll Cardiol. 2010;55(13):1318-1327.

[20] Stevens LA, Djurdjev O, Cardew S, Cameron EC, Levin A. Calcium, Phosphate, and Parathyroid Hormone Levels in Combination and as a Function of Dialysis Duration Predict Mortality: Evidence for the Complexity of the Association between Mineral Metabolism and Outcomes. J Am Soc Nephrol. 2004;15(3):770-779.

[21] Goodman WG, Goldin J, Kuizon BD, Yoon C, Gales B, Sider D, et al. Coronary-artery calcification in young adults with end-stage renal disease who are undergoing dialysis. N Engl J Med [Internet]. 2000;342(20):1478-1483. Available from: http://www.ncbi.nlm.nih.gov/entrez/query.fcgi?cmd=Retrieve&db=PubMed&dopt=Citation&list_uids=10816185

[22] Block GA, Klassen PS, Lazarus JM, Ofsthun N, Lowrie EG, Chertow GM. Mineral metabolism, mortality, and morbidity in maintenance hemodialysis. J Am Soc Nephrol [Internet]. 2004;15(8):2208-18. Available from: http://www.ncbi.nlm.nih.gov/pubmed/15284307

[23] Vervloet M, Cozzolino M. Vascular calcification in chronic kidney disease: different bricks in the wall? Kidney International. 2017. p. 808-17.

[24] Sigrist M, Bungay P, Taal MW, McIntyre CW. Vascular calcification and cardiovascular function in chronic kidney disease. Nephrol Dial Transplant [Internet]. 2006;21(3):707-14. Available from: http://www.ncbi.nlm.nih.gov/pubmed/16263735

[25] Mizobuchi M, Towler D, Slatopolsky E. Vascular calcification: the killer of patients with chronic kidney disease. J Am Soc Nephrol [Internet]. 2009;20(7):1453-64. Available from: http://www.ncbi.nlm.nih.gov/pubmed/19478096

[26] Fang Y, Ginsberg C, Sugatani T, Monier-Faugere MC, Malluche H, Hruska KA. Early chronic kidney disease-mineral bone disorder stimulates vascular calcification. Kidney Int. 2014;85(1):142-150.

[27] Brandenburg VM, Ketteler M, Rodriguez M. Ten years of progress in our understanding of uremic vascular calcification and disease: A decade summarized in 20 steps. Kidney International Supplements. 2011. p. 116-21.

[28] Dellegrottaglie S, Saran R, Rajagopalan S. Vascular calcification in patients with renal failure: Culprit or innocent bystander? Cardiology Clinics. 2005. p. 373-84.

[29] Zoccali C, London G. Con: Vascular calcification is a surrogate marker, but not the cause of ongoing vascular disease, and it is not a treatment target in chronic kidney disease. Nephrol Dial Transplant [Internet]. 2015;30(3):352-357. Available from: http://www.ncbi.nlm.nih.gov/pubmed/25712936%5Cnhttp://ndt.oxfordjournals.org/cgi/doi/10.1093/ndt/gfv021

[30] Shanahan CM. Inflammation ushers in calcification: A cycle of damage and protection? Circulation. 2007;116(24):2782-2785.

[31] Schlieper G, Aretz A, Verberckmoes SC, Kruger T, Behets GJ, Ghadimi R, et al. Ultrastructural Analysis of Vascular Calcifications in Uremia. J Am Soc Nephrol [Internet]. 2010;21(4):689-696. Available from: http://www.jasn.org/cgi/doi/10.1681/ASN.2009080829

[32] Kuro-o M. Klotho and the aging process. Korean Journal of Internal Medicine. 2011. p. 113-22.

[33] Proudfoot D, Skepper JN, Hegyi L, Bennett MR, Shanahan CM, Weissberg PL. Apoptosis regulates human vascular calcification in vitro: Evidence for initiation of vascular calcification by apoptotic bodies. Circ Res. 2000;87(11):1055-1062.

[34] Reynolds JL, Joannides AJ, Skepper JN, Mcnair R, Schurgers LJ, Proudfoot D, et al. Human vascular smooth muscle cells undergo vesicle-mediated calcification in response to changes in extracellular calcium and phosphate concentrations: A potential mechanism for accelerated vascular calcification in ESRD. J Am Soc Nephrol. 2004;15(11):2857-2867.

[35] Demer LL, Tintut Y. Vascular calcification: Pathobiology of a multifaceted disease. Circulation. 2008. p. 2938-48.

[36] Nicoll R, Henein M. Arterial calcification: A new perspective? International Journal of Cardiology. 2017. p. 11-22.

[37] Din UAAS El, Salem MM, Abdulazim DO. Vascular calcification: When should we interfere in chronic kidney disease patients and how? World J Nephrol [Internet]. 2016;5(5):398. Available from: http://www.wjgnet.com/2220-6124/full/v5/i5/398.htm

[38] Aikawa E, Nahrendorf M, Figueiredo JL, Swirski FK, Shtatland T, Kohler RH, et al. Osteogenesis associates with inflammation in early-stage atherosclerosis evaluated by molecular imaging in vivo. Circulation. 2007;116(24):2841-2850.

[39] London GM. Cardiovascular Disease in Chronic Renal Failure: Pathophysiologic Aspects. Seminars in Dialysis. 2003. p. 85-94.

[40] Rutsch F, Nitschke Y, Terkeltaub R. Genetics in arterial calcification: Pieces of a puzzle and cogs in a wheel. Circulation Research. 2011. p. 578-92.

[41] Wang M, Jiang L, Monticone RE, Lakatta EG. Proinflammation: The key to arterial aging. Trends in Endocrinology and Metabolism. 2014. p. 72-9.

[42] Boström K, Watson KE, Horn S, Wortham C, Herman IM, Demer LL. Bone morphogenetic protein expression in human atherosclerotic lesions. J Clin Invest. 1993;91(4):1800-1809.

[43] Maldonado N, Kelly-Arnold A, Vengrenyuk Y, Laudier D, Fallon JT, Virmani R, et al. A mechanistic analysis of the role of microcalcifications in atherosclerotic plaque stability: potential implications for plaque rupture. Am J Physiol Heart Circ Physiol [Internet]. 2012;303(5):H619-H628. Available from: http://www.ncbi.nlm.nih.gov/pubmed/22777419%5Cnhttp://www.pubmedcentral.nih.gov/articlerender.fcgi?artid=PMC3468470

[44] Huang H, Virmani R, Younis H, Burke AP, Kamm RD, Lee RT. The impact of calcification on the biomechanical stability of atherosclerotic plaques. Circulation. 2001;103(8):1051-1056.

[45] Abdelbaky A, Corsini E, Figueroa AL, Fontanez S, Subramanian S, Ferencik M, et al. Focal arterial inflammation precedes subsequent calcification in the same location: A longitudinal FDG-PET/CT study. Circ Cardiovasc Imaging. 2013;6(5):747-754.

[46] Sallam T, Cheng H, Demer LL, Tintut Y. Regulatory circuits controlling vascular cell calcification. Cellular and Molecular Life Sciences. 2013. p. 3187-97.

[47] Cui L, Houston DA, Farquharson C, MacRae VE. Characterisation of matrix vesicles in skeletal and soft tissue mineralisation. Bone. 2016. p. 147-58.

[48] Shanahan CM. Autophagy and matrix vesicles: New partners in vascular calcification. Kidney International. 2013. p. 984-6.

[49] Shroff R, Long DA, Shanahan C. Mechanistic Insights into Vascular Calcification in CKD. J Am Soc Nephrol [Internet]. 2013;24(2):179-189. Available from: http://www.jasn.org/cgi/doi/10.1681/ASN.2011121191

[50] Lin C-S, Lue TF. Defining Vascular Stem Cells. Stem Cells Dev [Internet]. 2013;22(7):1018-1026. Available from: http://online.liebertpub.com/doi/abs/10.1089/scd.2012.0504

[51] Viegas CSB, Rafael MS, Enriquez JL, Teixeira A, Vitorino R, Luís IM, et al. Gla-rich protein acts as a calcification inhibitor in the human cardiovascular system. Arterioscler Thromb Vasc Biol. 2015;35(2):399-408.

[52] Krohn JB, Hutcheson JD, Martínez-Martínez E, Aikawa E. Extracellular vesicles in cardiovascular calcification: Expanding current paradigms. Journal of Physiology. 2016. p. 2895-903.

[53] Thouverey C, Malinowska A, Balcerzak M, Strzelecka-Kiliszek A, Buchet R, Dadlez M, et al. Proteomic characterization of biogenesis and functions of matrix vesicles released from mineralizing human osteoblast-like cells. J Proteomics. 2011;74(7):1123-1134.

[54] Lu KC, Wu CC, Yen JF, Liu WC. Vascular calcification and renal bone disorders. Scientific World Journal. 2014.

[55] Lee D. Vascular calcification: Inducers and inhibitors. Materials Science and Engineering B: Solid-State Materials for Advanced Technology. 2011. p. 1133-41.

[56] Paloian NJ, Giachelli CM. A current understanding of vascular calcification in CKD. AJP Ren Physiol [Internet]. 2014;307(8):F891–F900. Available from: http://ajprenal.physiology.org/cgi/doi/10.1152/ajprenal.00163.2014

[57] Golub EE, Boesze-Battaglia K. The role of alkaline phosphatase in mineralization. Current Opinion in Orthopaedics. 2007. p. 444-8.

[58] Evrard S, Delanaye P, Kamel S, Cristol JP, Cavalier E, Arnaud J, et al. Vascular calcification: From pathophysiology to biomarkers. Clinica Chimica Acta. 2014. p. 401-14.

[59] Scatena M, Liaw L, Giachelli CM. Osteopontin: A multifunctional molecule regulating chronic inflammation and vascular disease. Arteriosclerosis, Thrombosis, and Vascular Biology. 2007. p. 2302-9.

[60] Luo G, Ducy P, McKee MD, Pinero GJ, Loyer E, Behringer RR, et al. Spontaneous calcification of arteries and cartilage in mice lacking matrix GLA protien. Nature. 1997;386(6620): 78-81.

[61] Viegas CSB, Simes DC, Laizè V, Williamson MK, Price PA, Cancela ML. Gla-rich Protein (GRP), a new vitamin K-dependent protein identified from sturgeon cartilage and highly conserved in vertebrates. J Biol Chem.2008. 283:36655-36664.

[62] Surmann-Schmitt C, Dietz U, Kireva T, Adam N, Park J, Tagariello A, Onnerfjord P, Heinegård D, Schlötzer-Schrehardt U, Deutzmann R, von der Mark K, Stock M. Ucma, a novel secreted cartilage-specific protein with implications in osteogenesis. J Biol Chem. 2008. 283:7082-7093.

[63] Viegas CSB, Cavaco S, Neves PL, Ferreira A, João A, Williamson MK, Price PA, Cancela ML, Simes DC. Gla-rich protein (GRP) is a novel vitamin K dependent protein present in serum and accumulated at sites of pathological calcifications. Am J Pathol. 2009. 175:2288-2298.

[64] Viegas CS, Rafael MS, Enriquez JL, Teixeira A, Vitorino R, Luís IM, Costa RM, Santos S, Cavaco S, Neves J, Macedo AL, Willems BA, Vermeer C, Simes DC. Gla-rich protein acts as a calcification inhibitor in the human cardiovascular system". Arterioscler Thromb Vasc Biol. 2015. 35(2):399-408.

[65] Cavaco S, Viegas CS, Rafael MS, Ramos A, Magalhães J, Blanco FJ, Vermeer C, Simes DC. Gla-rich protein is involved in the cross-talk between calcification and inflammation in osteoarthritis. Cell Mol Life Sci. 2016. 73:1051-1065.

[66] Viegas CSB, Herfs M, Rafael MS, Enriquez JL, Teixeira A, Luís I, van 't Hoofd C, João A, Maria VL, Cavaco S, Ferreira A, Serra M, Theuwissen E, Vermeer C, Simes, DC. Gla-rich protein is a potential new vitamin K target in cancer: Evidences for a direct GRP-mineral interaction, Biomed Res Int. 2014; doi:10.1155/ 2014/340216.

[67] Rafael MS, Cavaco S, Viegas CSB, Santos S, Ramos A, Willems B, Herfs M, Theuwissen E, Vermeer C, Simes DC. (2014) Insights into the association of Gla-rich protein and osteoarthritis, novel splice variants and γ-carboxylation status. Mol Nutr Food Res. 58:1636-1646.

[68] Schafer C, Heiss A, Schwarz A, Westenfeld R, Ketteler M, Floege J, et al. The serum protein alpha 2-Heremans-Schmid glycoprotein/ fetuin-A is a systemically acting inhibitor of ectopic calcification. J Clin Invest [Internet]. 2003;112(3):357-366. Available from: http://www.ncbi.nlm.nih.gov/ pubmed/12897203%5Cnhttp://www. ncbi.nlm.nih.gov/pmc/articles/ PMC166290/pdf/JCI0317202.pdf

[69] Ketteler M, Bongartz P, Westenfeld R, Wildberger JE, Mahnken AH, Böhm R, et al. Association of low fetuin-A (AHSG) concentrations in serum with cardiovascular mortality in patients on dialysis: a cross-sectional study. Lancet (London, England) [Internet]. 2003;361(9360):827-33. Available from:

http://www.ncbi.nlm.nih.gov/pubmed/12642050

[70] Dautova Y, Kozlova D, Skepper JN, Epple M, Bootman MD, Proudfoot D. Fetuin-A and albumin alter cytotoxic effects of calcium phosphate nanoparticles on human vascular smooth muscle cells. PLoS One [Internet]. 2014;9(5):e97565. Available from: http://www.ncbi.nlm.nih.gov/pubmed/24849210%5Cnhttp://journals.plos.org/plosone/article/asset?id=10.1371/journal.pone.0097565.PDF

[71] Vassalle C, Mazzone A. Bone loss and vascular calcification: A bi-directional interplay? Vascular Pharmacology. 2016. p. 77-86.

[72] Moe SM, Duan D, Doehle BP, O'Neill KD, Chen NX. Uremia induces the osteoblast differentiation factor Cbfa1 in human blood vessels. Kidney Int. 2003;63(3):1003-1011.

[73] Lin ME, Chen T, Leaf EM, Speer MY, Giachelli CM. Runx2 Expression in Smooth Muscle Cells Is Required for Arterial Medial Calcification in Mice. Am J Pathol. 2015;185(7):1958-1969.

[74] Cai T, Sun D, Duan Y, Wen P, Dai C, Yang J, et al. WNT/β-catenin signaling promotes VSMCs to osteogenic transdifferentiation and calcification through directly modulating Runx2 gene expression. Exp Cell Res. 2016;345(2):206-217.

[75] Sage AP, Tintut Y, Demer LL. Regulatory mechanisms in vascular calcification. Nature Reviews Cardiology. 2010. p. 528-36.

[76] Greenland et al. ACCF/AHA Expert Consensus Document on Coronary Artery Calcium Scoring; J Am Coll Cardiol; 2007 Jan 23;49(3):378-402. doi: 10.1016/j.jacc.2006.10.001

[77] Sigrist, MK; Taal, MW; et al; Progressive Vascular Calcification over 2 Years Is Associated with Arterial Stiffening and Increased Mortality in Patients with Stages 4 and 5 Chronic Kidney Disease. Clin J Am Soc Nephrol 2: 1241-1248, 2007. doi: 10.2215/CJN.02190507

[78] Alani, H.; Tamimi, A.; Tamimi, N. Cardiovascular co-morbidity in chronic kidney disease: Current knowledge and future research needs. World J. Nephrol. 2014, 3, 156-168; doi: 10.5527/wjn.v3.i4.156

[79] Cozzolino, M.; Mangano, M.; Stucchi, A.; Ciceri, P.; Conte, F.; Galassi, A.; Cardiovascular disease in dialysis patients. Nephrol. Dial. Transpl. 2018, 33, iii28–iii34; DOI:10.1093/ndt/gfy174

[80] Liu, M.; Li, X.C.; Lu, L.; Cao, Y.; Sun, R.R.; Chen, S.; Zhang, P.Y. Cardiovascular disease and its relationship with chronic kidney disease. Eur. Rev. Med. Pharmacol. Sci. 2014, 18, 2918-2926.

[81] Meema HE, Oreopoulos DG, deVeber GA, Arterial calcifications in severe chronic renal disease and their relationship to dialysis treatment, renal transplant, and parathyroidectomy, Radiology. 1976;121(2):315; DOI: 10.1148/121.2.315

[82] Goldsmith, D; et al; How important and how treatable is vascular stiffness as a cardiovascular risk factor in renal failure?, Nephrol Dial Transplant (2002) 17: 965-969; https://doi.org/10.1093/ndt/17.6.965

[83] Raggi P, et al; Cardiac Calcification in Adult Hemodialysis Patients A Link Between End-Stage Renal Disease and Cardiovascular Disease?; Journal of the American College of Cardiology; Vol. 39, No. 4, 2002; doi: 10.1016/s0735-1097(01)01781-8

[84] Lehto S, Niskanen L, Suhonen M et al. Medial artery calcification. A neglected harbinger of cardiovascular complications in non-insulin-dependent diabetes mellitus; Arterioscler Thromb Vasc Biol 1996; 16: 978-983; DOI: 10.1161/01.atv.16.8.978

[85] Nitta K, Akiba T, Suzuki K, et al. Assessment of coronary artery calcification in hemodialysis patients using multi-detector spiral CT scan; Hypertens Res 2004;27(8):527-533; DOI: 10.1291/hypres.27.527

[86] Moody, WE; Edwards, NC; et al; Arterial disease in chronic kidney disease; Heart. 2013; Mar;99(6):365-72; doi:10.1136/heartjnl-2012-302818

[87] Matsuoka M, et al; Impact of high coronary artery calcification score (CACS) on survival in patients on chronic hemodialysis; Clin Exp Nephrol (2004) 8:54-58, Japanese Society of Nephrology 2004, DOI 10.1007/s10157-003-0260-0

[88] Ohishi M, Tatara Y, et al.; The combination of chronic kidney disease and increased arterial stiffness is a predictor for stroke and cardiovascular disease in hypertensive patients; Hypertens Res. 2011;34(11):1209. Epub 2011 Aug 4, doi: 10.1038/hr.2011.117

[89] Goldsmith DJ, Covic A, Sambrook PA, Ackrill P; Vascular calcification in long-term haemodialysis patients in a single unit: a retrospective analysis; Nephron. 1997;77(1):37; doi: 10.1159/00019024

[90] McCullough PA, Sandberg KR, Dumler F, Yanez JE, Determinants of coronary vascular calcification in patients with chronic kidney disease and end-stage renal disease: a systematic review, J Nephrol. 2004;17(2):205

[91] Moe, S.M; Chen N.X.; Mechanisms of Vascular Calcification in Chronic Kidney Disease, J Am Soc Nephrol 19: 213-216, 2008. doi: 10.1681/ASN.2007080854

[92] Karohl C, Raggi P; Approach to Cardiovascular Disease Prevention in Patients With Chronic Kidney Disease; Current Treatment Options in Cardiovascular Medicine (2012) 14:391-413 DOI 10.1007/s11936-012-0189-2

[93] Covic A, Kothawala P, et al.; Systematic review of the evidence underlying the association between mineral metabolism disturbances and risk of all-cause mortality, cardiovascular mortality and cardiovascular events in chronic kidney disease; Nephrol Dial Transplant, 2009 May;24(5):1506-1523. doi: 10.1093/ndt/gfn613

[94] Locatelli, F., Pozzoni, P., et al. (2003). Epidemiology of cardiovascular risk in patients with chronic kidney disease. Nephrology, Dialysis, Transplantation, 18(Suppl 7), vii2–vii9; DOI: 10.1093/ndt/gfg1072

[95] Stompor TP, Pasowicz M, Sulowicz W, et al. Trends and dynamics of changes in calcification score over the 1-year observation period in patients on peritoneal dialysis. Am J Kidney Dis 2004;44(3):517-528; https://doi.org/10.1053/j.ajkd.2004.05.029

[96] Cozzolino M, Dusso AS, Liapis H et al. The effects of sevelamer hydrochloride and calcium carbonate on kidney calcification in uremic rats. J Am Soc Nephrol 2002; 13: 2299-2308; DOI: 10.1097/01.asn.0000025782.24383.0d

[97] Russo D, Miranda I, Ruocco C et al. The progression of coronary artery calcification in predialysis patients on calcium carbonate or sevelamer; Kidney Int 2007; 72: 1255-1261; doi: 10.1038/sj.ki.5002518

[98] Block GA, Spiegel DM, Ehrlich J et al. Effects of sevelamer and calcium on coronary artery calcification in patients new to hemodialysis. Kidney Int 2005; 68: 1815-1824; doi: 10.1111/j.1523-1755.2005.00600.x

[99] Chertow GM, Burke SK, Raggi P. Sevelamer attenuates the progression of coronary and aortic calcification in hemodialysis patients. Kidney Int 2002; 62: 245-252; DOI: 10.1046/j.1523-1755.2002.00434.x

[100] Jamal SA, Vandermeer B, et al.; Effect of calcium-based versus non-calcium-based phosphate binders on mortality in patients with chronic kidney disease: an updated systematic review and meta-analysis; Lancet volume 382, issue 9900, P1268-1277, october 12, 2013; http://dx.doi.org/10.1016/S0140-6736(13)60897-1

[101] Ercan Ok, Gulay Asci, et al.; Reduction of Dialysate Calcium Level Reduces Progression of Coronary Artery Calcification and Improves Low Bone Turnover in Patients on Hemodialysis; J Am Soc Nephrol 27: 2475-2486, 2016. doi: 10.1681/ASN.2015030268

[102] London G.M.; et al; Arterial Calcifications and Bone Histomorphometry in End-Stage Renal Disease, J Am Soc Nephrol 15: 1943-1951, 2004; DOI: 10.1097/01.ASN.0000129337.50739.48

[103] de Boer I, Kestenbaum B, et al.; 25-hydroxyvitamin D levels inversely associate with risk for developing coronary artery calcification, J Am Soc Nephrol. 2009;20(8):1805. Epub 2009 May 14; doi: 10.1681/ASN.2008111157

[104] London GM, Guérin AP, et al.; Mineral metabolism and arterial functions in end-stage renal disease: potential role of 25-hydroxyvitamin D deficiency; J Am Soc Nephrol. 2007;18(2):613. Epub 2007 Jan 3, DOI: https://doi.org/10.1681/ASN.2006060573

[105] Hou YC, Liu WC, et al.; Role of Vitamin D in Uremic Vascular Calcification; Biomed Res Int. 2017;2017:2803579. Epub 2017 Feb 12; doi: 10.1155/2017/2803579.

[106] Messa P, Macario F, et al., The OPTIMA Study: Assessing a New Cinacalcet (Sensipar/Mimpara) Treatment Algorithm for Secondary Hyperparathyroidism; Clin J Am Soc Nephrol 3: 36-45, 2008 doi: 10.2215/CJN.03591006

[107] Raggi P, Chertow GM, et al.; The ADVANCE study: a randomized study to evaluate the effects of cinacalcet plus low-dose vitamin D on vascular calcification in patients on hemodialysis, Nephrol Dial Transplant (2011) 26: 1327-1339 doi: 10.1093/ndt/gfq725

[108] Ishimura E, Okuno S, et al.; Significant association between the presence of peripheral vascular calcification and lower serum magnesium in hemodialysis patients Clin Nephrol, 2007 Oct;68(4):222-227. doi: 10.5414/cnp68222.

[109] Molnar AO, Biyani M, et al.; Lower serum magnesium is associated with vascular calcification in peritoneal dialysis patients: a cross sectional study; BMC Nephrol. 2017;18(1):129. Epub 2017 Apr 6; doi: 10.1186/s12882-017-0549-y

[110] Silva AL, Gundlach K, et al.; Low Magnesium Levels and FGF-23 Dysregulation Predict Mitral Valve Calcification as well as Intima Media Thickness in Predialysis Diabetic Patients; International Journal of Endocrinology Volume 2015, Article ID 308190, 10 pages; http://dx.doi.org/10.1155/2015/308190

[111] Schurgers LJ, Barreto DV, et al.; The circulating inactive form of matrix gla protein is a surrogate marker for vascular calcification in chronic kidney disease: a preliminary report; lin J Am Soc Nephrol. 2010;5(4):568. Epub 2010 Feb 4; doi: 10.2215/CJN.07081009

[112] McCarthy JT; El-Azhary RA; et al; Survival, Risk Factors, and Effect of Treatment in 101 Patients With Calciphylaxis; Mayo Clin Proc. 2016;91(10):1384; DOI: 10.1016/j.mayocp.2016.06.025

[113] Fine A, Zacharias J; Calciphylaxis is usually non-ulcerating: risk factors, outcome and therapy; Kidney Int. 2002;61(6):2210; DOI: 10.1046/j.1523-1755.2002.00375.x

[114] Kramer H, Toto R, Peshock R, Cooper R, Victor R; Association between chronic kidney disease and coronary artery calcification: the Dallas Heart Study; J Am Soc Nephrol. 2005;16(2):507. Epub 2004 Dec 15; doi: 10.1681/ASN.2004070610. Epub 2004 Dec 15

[115] Parhami F, Basseri B, Hwang J, Tintut Y, Demer LL; High-density lipoprotein regulates calcification of vascular cells; Circ Res. 2002;91(7):570; doi: 10.1161/01.res.0000036607.05037.da

[116] Tamashiro M, Iseki K, et al.; Significant association between the progression of coronary artery calcification and dyslipidemia in patients on chronic hemodialysis; Am J Kidney Dis. 2001;38(1):64; doi: 10.1053/ajkd.2001.25195

[117] Silva AP, Viegas C, et al.; Gla-Rich Protein (GRP) as an Early and Novel Marker of Vascular Calcification and Kidney Dysfunction in Diabetic Patients with CKD: A Pilot Cross-Sectional Study; J. Clin. Med. 2020, 9, 635; doi:10.3390/jcm9030635

[118] Viegas, CB, Santos L; et al.; Chronic Kidney Disease Circulating Calciprotein Particles and Extracellular Vesicles Promote Vascular Calcification - A Role for GRP (Gla-Rich Protein); Arterioscler Thromb Vasc Biol DOI: 10.1161/ATVBAHA.117.310578

[119] KDIGO. KDIGO clinical practice guideline for the diagnosis, evaluation, prevention, and treatment of Chronic Kidney Disease-Mineral and Bone Disorder (CKD-MBD). Kidney International Supplements (2017) 7, 1-59

[120] Bursztyn M, Motro M, Grossman E, et al. Accelerated coronary artery calcification in mildly reduced renal function of high-risk hypertensives: a 3-year prospective observation. J Hypertens 2003;21(10):1953-1959.

[121] Adragao, T; Pires A, et al; A simple vascular calcification score predicts cardiovascular risk in haemodialysis patients, Nephrol Dial Transplant (2004) 19: 1480-1488 DOI: 10.1093/ndt/gfh217

[122] Gorriz, JL; Molina, P; et al; Vascular Calcification in Patients with Nondialysis CKD over 3 Years; Clinical Journal of the American Society of Nephrology. 2015;10(4): 654-666; DOI: https://doi.org/10.2215/CJN.07450714

[123] Ter Braake, AD; Tinnemans, PT; et al; Magnesium prevents vascular calcification in vitro by inhibition of hydroxyapatite crystal formation; Scientific Reports (2018), 8(1); DOI:10.1038/s41598-018-20241-3

[124] Bai, Y; Zhang, J; et al; Magnesium prevents β-glycerophosphate-induced calcification in rat aortic vascular smooth muscle cells. Biomedical Reports (2015) 3(4), 593-597; DOI: 10.3892/br.2015.473

[125] Block, GA; Bushinsky, DA; et al. Effect of Etelcalcetide vs Cinacalcet on Serum Parathyroid Hormone in Patients Receiving Hemodialysis With Secondary Hyperparathyroidism. JAMA 2017; 317(2), 156; DOI: 10.1001/jama.2016.19468

Chapter 3

Genetic Polymorphisms and Their Interactions with the Risk Factors of Cardiovascular Diseases: Review Chapter

Joseph Musonda Chalwe, Christa Grobler and Wilna Oldewage-Theron

Abstract

Cardiovascular diseases (CVDs) have been reported to have a complex pathogenesis by a number of studies. Atherosclerosis and inflammation have been established as the main contributors to CVDs. Furthermore, genetic polymorphisms have been identified and found to have a correlation with an individual's susceptibility to developing CVD. Some of these polymorphisms and corresponding cardiovascular risk (CVR) factors include: C174G (Interleukin (IL)-6 association), methylenetetrahydrofolate reductase (MTHFR) C667T/A1298C (hyperhomocysteinaemia), VII R353Q (coagulation factor VII association) and rs247616/rs1968905/rs1270922 (cholesteryl ester transfer protein (CEPT) - cholesterol metabolism) amongst others. At a time when disease prediction, diagnosis and prognosis are still being investigated, these polymorphisms have the potential for use in these areas as well as opening more opportunities in the understanding of CVD. The objective of this chapter was to review the current knowledge about the relationship between genetic polymorphisms and cardiovascular disease.

Keywords: cardiovascular disease, cardiovascular risk, genetic, polymorphisms

1. Introduction

Cardiovascular diseases (CVDs) are a group of disorders affecting the heart and blood vessels and include coronary heart disease (CHD), cerebrovascular disease, peripheral arterial disease, rheumatic heart disease, congenital heart disease, deep vein thrombosis and pulmonary embolism [1]. The pathogenesis of CVD is mainly attributed to atherosclerosis which starts with a progressive alteration and deposit of plaque in the inner walls of the arteries [2]. It also involves the interaction of blood cells, vascular wall, lipoprotein and immune system, leading to the development of CVD [2, 3]. Atherosclerosis is characterised by arterial wall thickening and a loss of elasticity [3]. Atherosclerotic plaque consists of a soft yellow lesion (mostly consisting of lipids) and covered with a white fibrous cap [4], resulting in clinically important complications such as mechanical obstruction of the blood vessel, thrombosis and weakening of the underlying endothelial layer leading to aneurysm formation [5]. Atherosclerosis has a complicated pathogenesis. It has been reported that both lipoprotein retention and inflammatory cellular components are involved in the development of a plaque. It has long been accepted that low-density lipoprotein cholesterol (LDL-C) is a causal agent for atherosclerosis. Furthermore, monocytes and foam cells have been associated with the advancement of atherosclerotic disease [3, 6, 7]. Alkhalil and Choudhury [6] reported that structures outside vascular intima and media are also linked to atherosclerosis. Pathologically the progression of the lesion is as follows: from endothelial injury and dysfunction to fatty streak to fibrotic plaque to an eventual complicated lesion [8]. Atherosclerosis is thus a multifactorial progressive disorder that clinically manifests mostly during middle age or even later in life [8, 9]. Elderly people usually have poor endothelial healing with prolonged exposure to various risk factors as well as alterations in blood vessels, which increase the probability of a cardiovascular event [8–10].

2. Cardiovascular risk biomarkers

Several genetic and environmental factors have been shown to play a significant role in the progression of CVDs [11, 12]. Moreover, there is a close interlink between CVD and obesity, dyslipidaemia, oxidative stress, inflammation and hypertension to mention a few. Each of these biomarkers have mechanisms and pathways that have been reported to directly or indirectly lead to CVD [13]. Every population has distinct genetic and ethnic dynamics that contributes to the CVR of the population [14, 15]. CVDs are the foremost causes of death worldwide [1], with low and middle income countries currently experiencing the highest prevalence and mortality rates [16]. For this reason, recent data suggests that population-based CVR profiling is necessary for successful risk determination, disease prevention and treatment [1, 14, 15]. The Multinational Monitoring of Trends and Determinants in Cardiovascular Disease (MONICA) by WHO [17] and the MORGAM (Monica Risk, Genetics, Archiving and Monograph) [18] Project defined a wide range of biomarkers for CVR. These different classifications [19] are summarised in **Table 1**.

Biomarker	Description
Inflammation	
high-sensitivity C-reactive protein (hs-CRP)	An acute phase protein, a biomarker of the inflammatory reaction and an important risk marker for CVD [20]
Interleukin (IL)-6	A pro-inflammatory cytokine, anti-inflammatory myokine and inducer of CRP synthesis, associated with increased CVR [21]
Tumour necrosis factor (TNF)-α	A pro-inflammatory cytokine that accelerates the progression of CVDs [22]
Interleukin (IL)-1	A cytokine extremely expressed in several CVDs and contributes to their pathogenesis [23]
Interleukin (IL)-11-receptor antagonist	A stromal cell-derived cytokine capable of both pro- and anti-inflammatory ability linked to CVR [24]
Interleukin (IL)-10	An anti-inflammatory cytokine, stimulating inflammatory resolution and deflects endothelial dysfunction [25]
Interleukin (IL)-18	A pro-inflammatory cytokine that stimulates interferon (IFN)-γ production and a link to CVR [26]
Neopterin	A pteridine that indicates pro-inflammatory immune status, disease severity and prognosis in CVD [27]
Dyslipidaemia	
Total cholesterol (TC)	A sterol organic molecule who's variability in circulation has been associated with a higher risk of CVD [28]

Biomarker	Description
Low-density lipoprotein cholesterol (LDL-C)	A type of cholesterol that plays a vital role in plaque formation and increased LDL-C levels are correlated with CVR [29]
High-density lipoprotein cholesterol (HDL-C)	A lipoprotein that has shown a protective effect on inflammation, oxidation, angiogenesis and glucose homeostasis. For this reason, low HDL-C levels have been reported to increase CVR [30]
Lipoprotein (a) (Lp-(a))	A protein that carries cholesterol in blood and has demonstrated to be an independent and CVR factor for the advancement of CVD [31]
Apolipoprotein B (Apo B)	A structural protein that transports very low-density lipoprotein (VLDL-C) and shown as a marker of atherogenic potential and CVR [32]
Apolipoprotein A-I (Apo A-I)	A primary component of HDL-C which has been shown to have an association with premature CVD [33]
Paraoxonase-1 (PON1)	A high-density lipoprotein-associated esterase that has been reported to have a direct and an indirect relationship with CVDs [34]
Metabolic biomarkers	
Glucose	A monosaccharide who's elevated levels signify diabetes which is associated with CVR due to increased atherosclerosis [35]
Insulin	A key anabolic hormone of the body. Insulin resistance is exemplified by deficiencies in the uptake and oxidation of glucose. The increase in levels of insulin have repeatedly been associated with CVD [36]
Haemoglobin A1c (HbA1c)	This is a form of haemoglobin that is chemically attached to a sugar (glycated haemoglobin). It's used to diagnose diabetes. Hyperglycaemia is associated with CVR [37]
Adiponectin	An adipokine with anti-inflammatory and cardiovascular-protective properties which can prevent atherosclerosis. Decreased levels of adiponectin have been linked to increased CVR [38]
Ferritin	A blood protein that stores iron and has been reported as a risk factor for CVD [39]
Leptin	An adipocyte-derived adipokine that has been demonstrated to stimulate oxidative stress, inflammation, thrombosis, arterial stiffness and angiogenesis amongst others. These effects lead to the development of CVDs [40]
Oxidative stress	
Myeloperoxidase (MPO)	A cationic protein in neutrophils that stimulates the production of oxidants that trigger tissue damage. These oxidation processes contribute to atherosclerosis associating increased MPO with CVR [41]
Homocysteine	A non-proteinogenic α-amino acid that plays a key role in the synthesis of amino acids methionine and cysteine. It has been reported as an independent risk factor CVD [42]
Vitamin B12	A coenzyme in the remethylation process of homocysteine. Low levels of vitamin B12 may therefore lead to hyperhomocysteinaemia and increased CVR [43]
Holotranscobalamin (holoTC)	A cobalamin that transports vitamin B12 into the cells by binding to a specific receptor and has been shown to have an association with CVD [44]
Haemostasis	
Fibrinogen	A protein that is vital for proper blood clot formation. Elevated levels of fibrinogen are associated with CVR [45]
Factor VII	A protein that produces blood clots in the coagulation cascade. Several studies have associated increased factor VII activity with CVR, as it results in a pro-thrombotic state. Whilst other studies have reported contradicting results [46]

Biomarker	Description
Factor VIII: von Willebrand factor complex	A blood-clotting protein that is also called anti-hemophilic factor. A link between increased circulating levels of Factor VIII: von Willebrand complex and an increased risk of developing CVD has been reported [47]
Anti-thrombin III & D-Dimer	A fibrin breakdown product and marker of activated coagulation that has been associated with the advancement of atherothrombosis and eventually CVD [48]. Antithrombin III inhibits abnormal blood clot formation. Low levels are linked to CVR [49].
Renal function	
Creatinine	A breakdown product of creatine phosphate from muscle and protein metabolism that is measured to assess renal function and is elevated in renal damage or failure. Chronic kidney disease and renal failure are associated with an increased CVR due to the excess release of renin [50]
Microalbuminuria (MA)	A constant elevation of albumin in urine. It signifies endothelial dysfunction and is therefore associated with CVR [51]
Cystatin-C	A low molecular-weight protein who's increased circulating concentrations appear to have an increased CVR [52]
Necrosis	
Troponin 1	A protein found in skeletal and heart (cardiac) muscle fibres that regulate muscular contraction. Increased levels Troponin 1 are strongly associated with the incidence of CVD [53]
Creatine kinase-MB (CK-MB)	An isoenzyme that is found mainly in heart muscle cells. It has been linked to hypertension [54]
Other	
Vitamin D	A secosteroid that increases intestinal absorption of calcium, magnesium and phosphate. It controls inflammatory and immune responses (anti-inflammatory effect). Decreased levels of vitamin D have been associated with increased CVR [55]
Folate	It's also known as vitamin B_9 and is involved in the metabolism of homocysteine as a coenzyme. A decrease in the levels of folate is hence associated with CVR [56]
Intercellular adhesion molecule-1 (ICAM-1)	A cell adhesion molecule expressed by several cell types. Increased levels of circulating endothelial ICAM-1 are associated with endothelial activation and atherosclerosis, therefore increased CVR [57]
Vascular cell adhesion molecule (VCAM-1)	A cell adhesion molecule expressed by vascular endothelial cells that has been directly associated with the development of CVD [57]

Table 1.
Classification of CVD risk biomarkers.

3. Genetic polymorphisms

Despite being complex disorders CVDs are preventable. Coronary heart disease, hypertonia, and thrombophilia are some examples of these disorders, that have been shown to develop from a combination of genetic mutations and environmental factors [58, 59]. Fiatal *et al.*, [59] reported that the current advances in the genomics of CVDs have created opportunities for the use of predisposition genetic polymorphisms for prevention, diagnosis and treatment in the future. Multiple polymorphisms (**Table 2**) have been identified as contributing factors to CVR, namely: C174G (IL-6 association) [62], methylenetetrahydrofolate reductase (MTHFR) C667T/A1298C (hyperhomocysteinaemia) [131], VII R353Q (coagulation factor VII association) [113], rs247616/rs1968905/rs1270922 (cholesteryl ester transfer protein

Gene (*Homo sapiens*)	Location	Exons	Succinct
Inflammatory markers			
hs-CRP gene	Chromosome 1: q23.2	3	This gene encodes a pentraxin protein which regulates the complement. It's been shown to play a role in a number of host defence related functions. The concentration of this protein increases in reaction to tissue injury, infection, or in a cytokine storm inflammatory response. Inflammation is involved in atherosclerosis and the thinning of blood vessels due to the accumulation of lipids. This is subsequently associated with CVD [60, 61].
IL-6 gene	Chromosome 7: 7p15.3	6	The promotor region of the IL-6 gene has been the focal point for IL-6 polymorphism investigations (Hu et al., 2018, Ou *et al.*, 2018). This gene encodes cytokines that play a role in inflammation and the maturation of B cells. Furthermore, the resulting protein (endogenous pyrogen) has been demonstrated to cause a fever in people with autoimmune diseases or infections (Hu *et al.*, 2018, Ou *et al.*, 2018, [62, 63].
TNF-α gene	Chromosome 6: 6p21.33	4	Macrophages produce the proinflammatory cytokine encoded by this gene. It regulates processes such as cell proliferation, apoptosis, lipid metabolism, and coagulation by binding to receptors TNFRSF1A/TNFR1 and TNFRSF1B/TNFBR. It's been reported in conditions such as autoimmune diseases, insulin resistance, psoriasis, rheumatoid arthritis ankylosing spondylitis, tuberculosis, autosomal dominant polycystic kidney disease, cancer and CVD [64–66].
IL-1 beta gene	Chromosome 2: 2q14.1	7	This gene encodes an interleukin 1 cytokine protein that is proteolytically converted to its active form by caspase 1 (CASP1/ICE). Activated macrophages secrete this protein. The functions and link to the development of CVD are similar to the TNF-α gene [67, 68].
IL-11-receptor antagonist gene	Chromosome 19: 19q13.42	5	This gene encodes cytokines that belong to the gp130 family. These cytokines lead to the production of multi-subunit receptors which stimulate the T-cell-dependent maturation of immunoglobulin-producing B cells. It's also involved in the proliferation of cells [69, 70].

Gene (*Homo sapiens*)	Location	Exons	Succinct
IL-10 gene	Chromosome 1: 1q32.1	7	This gene encodes a cytokine that is secreted by monocytes and lymphocytes. It's involved in maintaining tissue homeostasis and inflammation. Additionally, it improves B cell survival, proliferation, and antibody production [71, 72].
IL-18 gene	Chromosome 11: 11q23.1	6	This gene encodes a proinflammatory cytokine that belongs to the IL-1 family. It is present as a precursor of macrophages and keratinocytes. It functions to regulate both innate and acquired immunity. It's been demonstrated in autoimmune, inflammatory and infectious diseases [73–75].
Neopterin gene			The gene expression for NO is stimulated by immune cells. For this reason, its known as a marker for the activation of the immune system. Tetrahydrobiopterin is essential for elevated concentrations of NOS. It's been reported to have a protective role in in cases of brain damage and inflammation [76].
Dyslipidaemia			
LDLR gene	Chromosome 19: 19p13.2	18	The low-density lipoprotein receptor (LDLR) gene family is made up of proteins that are found on the surface of cells that play a crucial role in endocytosis. After binding to the cell membrane, the molecules are taken into the cell where metabolism and cholesterol synthesis take place (TC, LDL-C, HDL-C). Changes in this gene have been linked to the development of conditions like familial hypercholesterolemia [77–79].
Lp-(a) gene	Chromosome 6: 6q25.3-q26	39	This gene is expressed in the liver. It encodes serine proteinase, an enzyme that suppresses the tissue-type plasminogen activator I activity. The encoded protein is involved atherogenesis which produces fragments that leads to atherosclerotic lesions and promote thrombogenesis. An increase in plasma levels of this protein has been correlated to atherosclerosis and CVD [80–82].
Apo B gene	Chromosome 2: 2p24.1	29	The product of this gene plays a role in the metabolism of lipids (chylomicrons, LDL, VLDL and triglycerides). It exists in two forms, apoB-48 and apoB-100, even though they have a common N-terminal sequence. This gene and changes in its sequence have been reported to trigger hypobetalipoproteinaemia, normotriglyceridaemic hypobetalipoproteinaemia, and hypercholesterolaemia to mention a few [83, 63].

Gene (*Homo sapiens*)	Location	Exons	Succinct
Apo A-I gene	Chromosome 11: 11q23.3	4	The protein encoded by this gene is Apo A-I which forms most of HDL-C in the circulation. It functions to enhance the transportation of TC from the tissues to the liver for excretion. This gene and associated mutations have been shown to cause conditions such HDL-C deficiencies, Tangier disease, and non-neuropathic amyloidosis amongst others [84, 85].
PON1 gene	Chromosome 7: 7q21.3	9	The protein encoded by this gene belongs to the paraoxonase family and has been known to show evidence of lactonase and ester hydrolase activity. It is produced in the kidney and binds to HDL-C when released. CVDs and diabetic retinopathy have been linked to this gene and its mutations [86, 87].
Cholesterol ester transfer protein (CETP) gene	Chromosome 16: 16q13	17	This protein coding gene is located on chromosome 16 position 16q13 *(H. sapiens).* It translates a hydrophobic glycoprotein that plays a vital role in the reversal of cholesterol transport [88], [89]. The CETP gene has 17 exons and its variants have been studied to assess their associations to risks such as CVDs and potential benefits as a pharmacological agent [90, 91].
Metabolic Biomarkers			
GLUT4 gene (SLC2A4)	Chromosome 17: 17p13.1	11	The protein encoded by this gene is a glucose transporter. It belongs to the solute carrier family 2 (facilitated glucose transporter). It regulates how the adipocytes and muscles take insulin-stimulated glucose. A link between this gene and diabetes mellitus has been demonstrated [92, 93].
INS gene	Chromosome 11: 11p15.5	3	Insulin is encoded by this gene. It regulates how carbohydrates and lipids are metabolised. It enhances how glucose is absorbed into the liver and muscle cells after being bound to the insulin receptor (INSR). Variants in the sequence of this gene have been reported and linked to the development of various forms of diabetes mellitus [94, 95].
Resistin (RETN) gene	Chromosome 19: 19p13.2	4	The protein encoded by this gene is resistin. It belongs to the family of resistin-like genes with distinct 10 cys identical spacing. This hormone is secreted by adipocytes and has been known to inhibit the ability of insulin to stimulate glucose uptake. It has also been linked to obesity and type II diabetes [96, 97].

Gene (*Homo sapiens*)	Location	Exons	Succinct
Adiponectin, C1Q And Collagen Domain Containing (ADIPOQ) gene	Chromosome 3: 3q27.3	4	This gene encodes a protein that has a similar composition to collagens X and VIII and complement factor C1q. It's primarily found in adipose tissue. The biological processes this gene is involved in are metabolic and hormonal processes. Adiponectin deficiency has been correlated with this gene and its variants [98, 99].
Ferritin Heavy Chain 1 (FTH1) gene	Chromosome 11: 11q12.3	4	The ferroxidase enzyme is encoded by this gene. It stores iron and is made up of 24 subunits of the heavy and light ferritin chains. Mutations have been reported to affect iron transport and secretion in tissues. Consequently, this results in conditions such as neurodegenerative diseases [100, 101].
Leptin (LEP) gene	Chromosome 7: 7q32.1	3	Leptin is encoded by the LEP gene. The adipocytes secrete this protein, and it is responsible for maintaining energy homeostasis after binding to leptin receptors. Polymorphisms in this gene cause obesity and type 2 diabetes mellitus. It's also been demonstrated in haematopoiesis, immune regulation and inflammation [102, 103].
Oxidative stress			
Myeloperoxidase (MPO) gene	Chromosome 17: 17q22	12	This gene encodes the haem protein MPO. It's present in polymorphonuclear leukocytes where it functions in host defences. It secrets hypohalous acids that are pivotal to the microbicidal activity of neutrophils. Elevated levels of MPO have been associated with CVDs [104, 105].
Methylenetetrahydrofolate reductase (MTHFR) gene	Chromosome 1: 36.22	12	This protein facilitates the conversion of 5,10-methylenetetrahydrofolate to a co-substrate for homocysteine remethylation to methionine known as 5-methyltetrahydrofolate. The physiological functions of MTHFR include folate metabolism, DNA methylation and the stability of DNA to mention a few [106–108].
Transcobalamin (TCN2) gene	Chromosome 22: 22q12.2	9	This gene encodes transcobalamin. This protein transports cobalamin belonging to the vitamin B12-binding protein family. Variations in the TCN2 gene have been associated with transcobalamin deficiency [109, 110].

Gene (*Homo sapiens*)	Location	Exons	Succinct
Haemostasis			
Fibrinogen gene			
Factor VII gene	Chromosome 13: 13q34	10	It is a coagulation factor VII protein coding gene with 10 exons. Despite the variability in the findings due to small sample populations, various studies have been conducted on the R353Q polymorphism, factor VII conditions and its association to CVD [111–113]. This gene is crucial for haemostasis and is transported in circulation as a zymogen. It is activated by proteolysis which further stimulates the coagulation cascade by transforming factor IX to factor IXa and/or factor X to factor Xa [114].
Factor VIII gene	Chromosome X: Xq28	27	This gene encodes a protein that participates in blood-clotting (intrinsic pathway). It produces two isoforms. Isoform 1 (large glycoprotein) links with von Willebrand factor in a noncovalent complex while variant 2 (small protein) is crucial for coagulant activity. Mutations in this gene lead to haemophilia A, a prevalent recessive X-linked coagulation disorder [115, 116].
Serpin Family C Member 1 (SERPINC1) gene	Chromosome 1: 1q25.1	9	This gene encodes antithrombin III. This is a protease inhibitor belonging to the serpin superfamily. It participates in the blood coagulation cascade by inhibiting the activity of certain proteins (heparin). Studies have identified variations in this gene which result in antithrombin-III deficiency which presents a potent risk for thrombosis [117, 118].
Renal function			
Cystatin 3 (CST3) gene	Chromosome 20: 20p11.21	4	This gene encodes Cystatin-C belonging to the cysteine protease inhibitors family. There are three classifications of this family, namely: type 1 cystatins (stefins), type 2 cystatins and the kininogens. They regulate various chemical reactions by being enzyme blockers. Defects in this gene have been linked to amyloid angiopathy. The amount of protein that is produced in both atherosclerotic and aneurysmal aortic lesions is reduced confirming its role in CVD [119, 120].
Necrosis			
Troponin I3 (TNNI3) gene	Chromosome 19: 19q13.42	8	The protein encoded by this gene is Troponin I (TnI) which is exclusively found in the cardiac muscle. It's one of the three proteins (TnI, troponin T (TnT) and troponin C (TnC)) making up the troponin complex of the thin filaments of striated muscle. The troponin complex, in the presence of calcium, regulate the contraction of cardiac muscles. Familial hypertrophic cardiomyopathy type 7 (CMH7) and familial restrictive cardiomyopathy (RCM) are a result of variations in this gene. Elevated TnI levels is used as a marker for myocardial injury [121, 122].

Gene (*Homo sapiens*)	Location	Exons	Succinct
Creatine Kinase, M-Type (CKM) gene	Chromosome 19: 19q13.32	8	This gene encodes Creatine Kinase (CK), a cytoplasmic enzyme, that plays a role in energy homeostasis. CK reversibly catalyses the transfer of phosphate between Adenosine triphosphate (ATP) and various phosphagens like creatine phosphate. It's been reported as a significant marker for myocardial infarction [123, 124].
Other			
Vitamin D receptor (VDR) gene	Chromosome 12: 12q13.11	12	The vitamin D3 receptor is encoded by this gene. This receptor enables normal reaction to vitamin D by the body. Vitamin D functions to regulate how calcium and phosphate are absorbed from the intestines into circulation. This is significant for normal formation of bones and teeth. Changes in this gene are related with type II vitamin D-resistant rickets [125, 126].
Intercellular adhesion molecule-1 (ICAM-1) gene	Chromosome 19: 19p13.2	7	ICAM-1 is a cell surface glycoprotein that is encoded by the ICAM-1 gene. It's a member of the immunoglobulin superfamily. Usually found on endothelial cells and immune. The concentrations of this glycoprotein become elevated once cytokines have been stimulated (CD18) [127, 128].
Vascular cell adhesion molecule (VCAM-1) gene	Chromosome 1: 1p21.2	9	This gene belongs to the Ig superfamily and encodes, VCAM-1, a transmembrane glycoprotein. It is produced on cytokine-activated endothelium where it facilitates leukocyte-endothelial cell adhesion and signal transduction. VCAM-1 is involved in atherosclerosis progression [129, 130].

Table 2.
Genes controlling the CVR factors.

(CEPT) - cholesterol metabolism) [132, 133], Angiotensinogen (AGT) M235T (hypertension) [134], G308A (pro-inflammatory) [135], A522T (dyslipidaemia) [136] and rs9939609 (obesity predisposition) [137]. Most of the studies investigating genetic polymorphisms associated with CVD in the past 10 years have been conducted in populations of different ancestry and ethnicity [58, 59]. Identifying populations that are at risk of developing CVDs may assist in developing prevention programs which may reduce disease progression. However, there is a paucity of information about CVR and genetic polymorphisms [59]. The aim of this chapter was thus to review the literature investigating the prevalence of the various CVR factors in relation to their genetic polymorphisms.

4. Relationship between some common polymorphisms and corresponding CVR factors

4.1 Inflammatory markers

4.1.1 C174G polymorphism (IL-6)

The C174G polymorphism is a mutation that triggers a change in the nucleotide bases from guanine to cytosine at position 174 in the promoter region of the IL-6 gene [138, 139]. This is known as a single-nucleotide substitution (SNP) of one base for another and has been demonstrated to affect the transcription of IL-6. The findings on the frequency of the highest genotype are conflicting partly due to differences in the ethnicity of the study populations. Nevertheless, the reported genotypes CC, G allele and GG have all been associated with an increase in serum IL-6 levels where they induce a transcriptional inflammatory response [62, 139, 140]. This SNP influences the physiology of the IL-6 gene resulting in variations of circulating IL-6 concentrations. Elevated IL-6 levels have been reported in a wide range of inflammation-associated disease states such as CVR, diabetes mellitus risk, rheumatoid arthritis, COVID-19, celiac disease and psoriasis to mention a few [62, 138–140].

4.2 Dyslipidaemia

4.2.1 rs247616, rs1968905 and rs1270922 polymorphisms (CETP)

The CETP polymorphisms (rs247616, rs1968905 and rs1270922) are SNPs that occur as a result of substitutions in their nucleotide bases [89, 133]. These polymorphisms have previously been used to determine the CETP levels in a CVD population [133]. Mutations in the CETP gene have been found to cause hyperalphalipoproteinaemia 1 (HALP1). Furthermore, it's also been shown that different variants code for distinct isoforms within this gene. This eventually influences the metabolism of HDL-C [89]. Reports on the link between the CETP polymorphisms, CVR and the concentrations of CETP through LDL-C are inconsistent [89, 132, 133].

4.3 Metabolic biomarkers

4.3.1 Gly972Arg polymorphism

The Gly972Arg polymorphism occurs as a result of a substitution between glycine and arginine (GGG ↔ AGG substitutions) in codon 972 (G972R). It has been demonstrated that this mutation is involved in the development of type 2 diabetes mellitus (type 2 DM) [141]. This is due to the fact that it's been described to influence tyrosine phosphorylation at a specific site of IRS-1 which may lead to the development of insulin resistance (IR) and impair insulin secretion [142]. The Gly972Arg polymorphism has been investigated in a number of studies and found to have a high prevalence in type 2 diabetic subjects and other conditions like obesity [143, 144].

4.4 Oxidative stress

4.4.1 C677T and A1298C polymorphisms (MTHFR)

The *MTHFR* C677T polymorphism is a SNP where cytosine (C) is replaced with thymine (T) at position 677 resulting in the gene to code for valine as opposed to alanine at exon 4. The change between alanine and valine nucleotide bases happens on codon 222 resulting in this polymorphism sometimes being described as Ala222Val polymorphism. It has been reported to have the alleles heterozygous *C677T and* homozygous *T667T* which are mutant, whereas the homozygous *C677C* is a wild type allele [145–149].

The A1298C polymorphism causes a change where glutamate is substituted with an alanine at position 429. Each of these genotypes have been shown to reduce the MTHFR enzymatic activity resulting in the methyl group to be unavailable for attachment to homocysteine in order to generate methionine. Hyperhomocysteinaemia has been reported in the development of a number of conditions, for example, CVR, chronic myeloid leukaemia (CML), multiple abortions, autism, osteoporosis, multiple sclerosis, psoriasis, and Alzheimer's disease [106, 108, 135, 145, 146].

4.5 Haemostasis

4.5.1 R353Q polymorphism (factor VII)

In the R353Q polymorphism, guanine is substituted with adenine at the 353rd codon of the *FVII* gene. This missense replacement of arginine (R) by glutamine (Q) in this polymorphism has been reported to influence the factor VII levels [150]. Individuals who carry the Q allele carriers have been shown to have lower levels of Factor VII than those who carry the R allele. Nonetheless, the findings on the association between the R353 Q polymorphisms and CVR (thrombosis) are inconclusive [151]. Increased levels of factor VII are linked to thromboembolic disorders risk. A relationship between defects in the factor VII gene and CVD has been reported [114, 150, 151].

5. Conclusion

CVDs having a high prevalence and mortality rate globally need to be continually studied with the focus being risk prediction, prevention of disease as well as improving treatment strategies. This review supplements current evidence on the contribution of genetic polymorphisms in the pathophysiology of CVDs. Although the data from some of the early studies of these polymorphisms is conflicting, mainly because the study populations were small and not diverse enough, there are promising results in some of the CVR factors. It is therefore apparent that different polymorphisms should be studied in large sample sizes, diverse ethnicities and demographics. Genetic polymorphisms should be taken into consideration in the assessment of risk profiles for CVDs.

Acknowledgements

Financial support for this study was provided by Vaal University of Technology (VUT) and University of the Free State (UFS) in South Africa. The authors also wish to acknowledge team members of the CARE research group for their contribution to the study.

Conflict of interest

The authors declare no conflict of interest.

Author details

Joseph Musonda Chalwe[1*], Christa Grobler[1] and Wilna Oldewage-Theron[2,3]

1 Department of Health Sciences, Vaal University of Technology, Vanderbijlpark, South Africa

2 Department of Nutritional Sciences, Texas Tech University (TTU), Lubbock, TX, USA

3 Department of Sustainable Food Systems and Development, University of the Free State, Bloemfontein, South Africa

*Address all correspondence to: josephch@vut.ac.za; jheydot@gmail.com

IntechOpen

© 2021 The Author(s). Licensee IntechOpen. This chapter is distributed under the terms of the Creative Commons Attribution License (http://creativecommons.org/licenses/by/3.0), which permits unrestricted use, distribution, and reproduction in any medium, provided the original work is properly cited.

References

[1] WHO (2021) Cardiovascular diseases. Available from: https://www.who.int/news-room/fact-sheets/detail/cardiovascular-diseases-(cvds) [Accessed 2021-06-21]. World Health Organization

[2] ITO, F. (2021) Polyphenols can Potentially Prevent Atherosclerosis and Cardiovascular Disease by Modulating Macrophage Cholesterol Metabolism. Current Molecular Pharmacology, 14, 175-190.

[3] MILUTINOVIĆ, A., ŠUPUT, D. & ZORC-PLESKOVIČ, R. (2020) Pathogenesis of atherosclerosis in the tunica intima, media, and adventitia of coronary arteries: An updated review. Bosnian journal of basic medical sciences, 20, 21-30.

[4] NEWMAN, A. A. C., SERBULEA, V., BAYLIS, R. A., SHANKMAN, L. S., BRADLEY, X., ALENCAR, G. F., OWSIANY, K., DEATON, R. A., KARNEWAR, S., SHAMSUZZAMAN, S., SALAMON, A., REDDY, M. S., GUO, L., FINN, A., VIRMANI, R., CHEREPANOVA, O. A. & OWENS, G. K. (2021) Multiple cell types contribute to the atherosclerotic lesion fibrous cap by PDGFRÎ² and bioenergetic mechanisms. Nature Metabolism, 3, 166-181.

[5] QIAO, R., HUANG, X., QIN, Y., LI, Y., DAVIS, T. P., HAGEMEYER, C. E. & GAO, M. (2021) Recent advances in molecular imaging of atherosclerotic plaques and thrombosis. Nanoscale, 12, 8040-8064.

[6] ALKHALIL, M. & CHOUDHURY, R. P. (2018) Current concepts in atherosclerosis. Indian Journal of Thoracic and Cardiovascular Surgery, 34, 198-205.

[7] CINOKU, I. I., MAVRAGANI, C. P. & MOUTSOPOULOS, H. M. (2020) Atherosclerosis: Beyond the lipid storage hypothesis. The role of autoimmunity. *European Journal of Clinical Investigation,* 50, e13195.

[8] LIBBY, P., BURING, J. E., BADIMON, L., HANSSON, G. K., DEANFIELD, J., BITTENCOURT, M. S., TOKGÖZOĞLU, L. & LEWIS, E. F. (2019) Atherosclerosis. Nature Reviews Disease Primers, 5, 56.

[9] TYRRELL, D. J. & GOLDSTEIN, D. R. (2021) Ageing and atherosclerosis: vascular intrinsic and extrinsic factors and potential role of IL-6. Nature Reviews Cardiology, 18, 58-68.

[10] REA, I. M., GIBSON, D. S., MCGILLIGAN, V., MCNERLAN, S. E., ALEXANDER, H. D. & ROSS, O. A. (2018) Age and Age-Related Diseases: Role of Inflammation Triggers and Cytokines. *Frontiers in Immunology,* 9.

[11] Aruni, B. (2017) Environmental Determinants of Cardiovascular Disease. Circulation Research, 121, 162-180.

[12] SHABANA, N. A., SHAHID, S. U. & IRFAN, U. (2020) Genetic Contribution to Congenital Heart Disease (CHD). Pediatric Cardiology, 41, 12-23.

[13] PETRIE, J. R., GUZIK, T. J. & TOUYZ, R. M. (2018) Diabetes, Hypertension, and Cardiovascular Disease: Clinical Insights and Vascular Mechanisms. Canadian Journal of Cardiology, 34, 575-584.

[14] SYED, M. A., ALNUAIMI, A. S., ZAINEL, A. J. & A/QOTBA, H. A. (2019) Prevalence of non-communicable diseases by age, gender and nationality in publicly funded primary care settings in Qatar. *BMJ Nutrition, Prevention & Health,* bmjnph-2018-000014.

[15] VAN DER ENDE, M. Y., HARTMAN, M. H. T., HAGEMEIJER, Y., MEEMS, L. M. G., DE VRIES, H. S., STOLK, R. P., DE BOER, R. A., SIJTSMA, A., VAN

DER MEER, P., RIENSTRA, M. & VAN DER HARST, P. (2017) The LifeLines Cohort Study: Prevalence and treatment of cardiovascular disease and risk factors. International Journal of Cardiology, 228, 495-500.

[16] ANAND, S., BRADSHAW, C. & PRABHAKARAN, D. (2020) Prevention and management of CVD in LMICs: why do ethnicity, culture, and context matter? BMC Medicine, 18, 7.

[17] WHO (1988) The World Health Organization MONICA Project (monitoring trends and determinants in cardiovascular disease): a major international collaboration. WHO MONICA Project Principal Investigators. *Journal of Clinical Epidemiology,* 41, 105-114.

[18] EVANS, A., SALOMAA, V., KULATHINAL, S., ASPLUND, K., CAMBIEN, F., FERRARIO, M., PEROLA, M., PELTONEN, L., SHIELDS, D., TUNSTALL-PEDOE, H. & KUULASMAA, K. (2005) MORGAM (an international pooling of cardiovascular cohorts). International Journal of Epidemiology, 34, 21-27.

[19] Richards A. M. (2018) Future biomarkers in cardiology: my favourites. European Heart Journal Supplements, 20, G37-G44.

[20] CASTRO, A. R., SILVA, S. O. & SOARES, S. C. (2018) The Use of High Sensitivity C-Reactive Protein in Cardiovascular Disease Detection. *J Pharm Pharm Sci. 2018;21(1):496-503. doi: 10.18433/jpps29872.*

[21] ZIEGLER, L., GAJULAPURI, A., FRUMENTO, P., BONOMI, A., WALLÉN, H., FAIRE, U. D., ROSE-JOHN, S. & GIGANTE, B. (2019) Interleukin 6 trans-signalling and risk of future cardiovascular events. Cardiovascular Research, 115, 213-221.

[22] LAU, W. B., OHASHI, K., WANG, Y., OGAWA, H., MUROHARA, T., MA, X.-L. & OUCHI, N. (2017) Role of Adipokines in Cardiovascular Disease. Circulation Journal, 81, 920-928.

[23] PFEILER, S., WINKELS, H., KELM, M. & GERDES, N. (2019) IL-1 family cytokines in cardiovascular disease. Cytokine, 122, 154215.

[24] SHAHBAZI, H., MALEKNIA, M. & NOROOZI, S. (2021) Investigating the Association of IL-1beta IL-8 & IL 11 with Commonly used Cardiovascular Biomarkers (CK-MB & Troponin) in Patients with Myocardial Infarction (MI). Research Square.

[25] TABREZ, S., ALI, M., JABIR, N. R., FIROZ, C. K., ASHRAF, G. M., HINDAWI, S., DAMANHOURI, G. A. & NABIL ALAMA, M. (2017) A putative association of interleukin-10 promoter polymorphisms with cardiovascular disease. IUBMB Life, 69, 522-527.

[26] CAVALCANTE, J. E. A., DE SOUSA, E. L. H., De Oliveira Rodrigues, R., De Almeida Viana, G., DUARTE GADELHA, D., DE CARVALHO, M. M. D., SOUSA, D. L., SILVA, A. J. X., FILHO, R. R. B. X., FERNANDES, V. O. F., MONTENEGRO JUNIOR, R. M., DE SOUSA ALVES, R., MENESES, G. C., SAMPAIO, T. L. & QUEIROZ, M. G. R. (2020) Interleukin-18 promoter −137 G/C polymorphism (rs187238) is associated with biochemical markers of renal function and cardiovascular disease in type 2 diabetes patients *Clinical Biochemistry,* 80, 1-7.

[27] LANSER, L., PÖLZL, G., FUCHS, D., WEISS, G. & KURZ, K. (2019) Neopterin is Associated with Disease Severity and Outcome in Patients with Non-Ischaemic Heart Failure. Journal of Clinical Medicine, 8, 2230.

[28] ZHU, Y., LU, J.-M., YU, Z.-B., LI, D., WU, M.-Y., SHEN, P., LIN, H.-B., WANG, J.-B. & CHEN, K. (2019) Intra-individual variability of total cholesterol is associated with cardiovascular disease mortality: A

cohort study. Nutrition, Metabolism and Cardiovascular Diseases, 29, 1205-1213.

[29] FERENCE, B. A., GINSBERG, H. N., GRAHAM, I., RAY, K. K., PACKARD, C. J., BRUCKERT, E., HEGELE, R. A., KRAUSS, R. M., RAAL, F. J., SCHUNKERT, H., WATTS, G. F., BOREN, J., FAZIO, S., HORTON, J. D., MASANA, L., NICHOLLS, S. J., NORDESTGAARD, B. R. G., VAN DE SLUIS, B., TASKINEN, M.-R., TOKGÖZOGLU, L., LANDMESSER, U., LAUFS, U., WIKLUND, O., STOCK, J. K., CHAPMAN, M. J. & CATAPANO, A. L. (2017) Low-density lipoproteins cause atherosclerotic cardiovascular disease. 1. Evidence from genetic, epidemiologic, and clinical studies. A consensus statement from the European Atherosclerosis Society Consensus Panel. European Heart Journal, 38, 2459-2472.

[30] NICHOLLS, S. J. & NELSON, A. J. (2019) HDL and cardiovascular disease. Pathology, 51, 142-147.

[31] BOFFA, M. B. & KOSCHINSKY, M. L. (2019) Oxidized phospholipids as a unifying theory for lipoprotein(a) and cardiovascular disease. Nature Reviews Cardiology, 16, 305-318.

[32] SHAPIRO, M. D. & FAZIO, S. (2017) Apolipoprotein B-containing lipoproteins and atherosclerotic cardiovascular disease. *F1000Research*, 6, 134-134.

[33] Haji Aghajani, M., Madani Neishaboori, A., Ahmadzadeh, K., TOLOUI, A. & YOUSEFIFARD, M. (2021) The association between apolipoprotein A-1 plasma level and premature coronary artery disease: A systematic review and meta-analysis. *International Journal of Clinical Practice*, n/a, e14578.

[34] KOTUR-STEVULJEVIĆ, J., VEKIĆ, J., STEFANOVIĆ, A., ZELJKOVIĆ, A., NINIĆ, A., IVANIŠEVIĆ, J., MILJKOVIĆ, M., SOPIĆ, M., MUNJAS, J., MIHAJLOVIĆ, M., SPASIĆ, S., JELIĆ-IVANOVIĆ, Z. & SPASOJEVIĆ-KALIMANOVSKA, V. (2019) Paraoxonase 1 and atherosclerosis-related diseases. BioFactors, 46, 193-205.

[35] AGUIAR, C., DUARTE, R. & CARVALHO, D. (2019) New approach to diabetes care: From blood glucose to cardiovascular disease. Revista Portuguesa de Cardiologia (English Edition), 38, 53-63.

[36] ORMAZABAL, V., NAIR, S., ELFEKY, O., AGUAYO, C., SALOMON, C. & ZUÃ±IGA, F. A. (2018) Association between insulin resistance and the development of cardiovascular disease. Cardiovascular Diabetology, 17, 122.

[37] Li, S., Nemeth, I., Donnelly, L., Hapca, S., ZHOU, K. & PEARSON, E. R. (2019) Visit-to-Visit HbA1c Variability Is Associated With Cardiovascular Disease and Microvascular Complications in Patients With Newly Diagnosed Type 2 Diabetes. Diabetes Care, 43, 426-432.

[38] KYROU, I., TSANTARLIOTI, O., PANAGIOTAKOS, D. B., TSIGOS, C., GEORGOUSOPOULOU, E., CHRYSOHOOU, C., SKOUMAS, I., TOUSOULIS, D., STEFANADIS, C., PITSAVOS, C. & THE, A. S. G. (2017) Adiponectin circulating levels and 10-year (2002-2012) cardiovascular disease incidence: the ATTICA Study. Endocrine, 58, 542-552.

[39] KADOGLOU, N. P. E., BIDDULPH, J. P., RAFNSSON, S. B., TRIVELLA, M., NIHOYANNOPOULOS, P. & DEMAKAKOS, P. (2017) The association of ferritin with cardiovascular and all-cause mortality in community-dwellers: The English longitudinal study of ageing. PLOS ONE, 12, e0178994.

[40] POETSCH, M. S., STRANO, A. & GUAN, K. (2020) Role of Leptin in Cardiovascular Diseases. Frontiers in Endocrinology, 11.

[41] Ndrepepa G. (2019) Myeloperoxidase - A bridge linking

inflammation and oxidative stress with cardiovascular disease Clinica Chimica Acta, 493, 36-51.

[42] CHRYSANT, S. G. & CHRYSANT, G. S. (2018) The current status of homocysteine as a risk factor for cardiovascular disease: a mini review. Expert Review of Cardiovascular Therapy, 16, 559-565.

[43] LANGAN, R. C. & GOODBRED, A. J. (2017) Vitamin B12 Deficiency: Recognition and Management. Am Fam Physician. 2017 Sep 15;*96(6):384-389.*

[44] BASAK, T., GARG, G., BHARDWAJ, N., TANWAR, V., SETH, S., KARTHIKEYAN, G. & SENGUPTA, S. (2016) Low holo-transcobalamin levels are prevalent in vegetarians and is associated with coronary artery disease in Indian population. Biomarkers : biochemical indicators of exposure, response, and susceptibility to chemicals, 21, 1-5.

[45] YANG, S.-H., Du Y., Zhang Y., Li X.-L., LI, S., XU, R.-X., ZHU, C.-G., GUO, Y.-L., WU, N.-Q., QING, P., GAO, Y., CUI, C.-J., DONG, Q., SUN, J. & LI, J.-J. (2017) Serum fibrinogen and cardiovascular events in Chinese patients with type 2 diabetes and stable coronary artery disease: a prospective observational study. BMJ Open, 7, e015041.

[46] OLSON, N. C., RAFFIELD, L. M., LANGE, L. A., LANGE, E. M., LONGSTRETH JR, W. T., CHAUHAN, G., DEBETTE, S., SESHADRI, S., REINER, A. P. & TRACY, R. P. (2017) Associations of activated coagulation factor VII and factor VIIa-antithrombin levels with genome-wide polymorphisms and cardiovascular disease risk. Journal of Thrombosis and Haemostasis, 16, 19-30.

[47] RAFFIELD, L. M., Lu, A. T., Szeto, M. D., Little, A., GRINDE, K. E., SHAW, J., AUER, P. L., CUSHMAN, M., HORVATH, S., IRVIN, M. R., LANGE, E. M., LANGE, L. A., NICKERSON, D. A., THORNTON, T. A., WILSON, J. G., WHEELER, M. M., NHLBI TRANS-OMICS FOR PRECISION MEDICINE CONSORTIUM, T. H., HEMOSTASIS WORKING, G., ZAKAI, N. A. & REINER, A. P. (2020) Coagulation factor VIII: Relationship to cardiovascular disease risk and whole genome sequence and epigenome-wide analysis in African Americans. Journal of Thrombosis and Haemostasis, 18, 1335-1347.

[48] ZAKAI, N. A., MCCLURE, L. A., JUDD, S. E., KISSELA, B., HOWARD, G., SAFFORD, M. & CUSHMAN, M. (2017) D-dimer and the Risk of Stroke and Coronary Heart Disease. The REasons for Geographic and Racial Differences in Stroke (REGARDS) Study. *Journal of Thrombosis and Haemostasis,* 117, 618-624.

[49] CROLES, F. N., VAN LOON, J. E., DIPPEL, D. W. J., DE MAAT, M. P. M. & LEEBEEK, F. W. G. (2018) Antithrombin levels are associated with the risk of first and recurrent arterial thromboembolism at a young age. Atherosclerosis, 269, 144-150.

[50] CHICCO, D. & JURMAN, G. (2020) Machine learning can predict survival of patients with heart failure from serum creatinine and ejection fraction alone. BMC Medical Informatics and Decision Making, 20, 16.

[51] DIAZ, M. A. P., SANJURJO, S. C., CARO, J. L., CARRATALA, V. P., GARCIA, J. P., VARGAS, M. F., PAIS, P. A., FREIRE, S. Y. E., SECIN, A. R., ESCRIBANO, F. M., JIMENEZ, S. M., ROCA, G. R., ALLES, G. P., ESCOBAR, F. M., CARRASCO, E. C., IRISO, J. I., MENDOZA, L. G., BAZ, P., CRIADO, E. G. & VILLAR, J. M. (2018) Microalbuminuria and cardiovascular disease in hypertensive patients included in the Iberican Study. Journal of Hypertension, 36, e184.

[52] GARCIA-CARRETERO, R., VIGIL-MEDINA, L., BARQUERO-PEREZ, O., GOYA-ESTEBAN, R., MORA-JIMENEZ, I., SOGUERO-RUIZ, C. &

RAMOS-LOPEZ, J. (2017) Cystatin C as a predictor of cardiovascular outcomes in a hypertensive population. Journal of Human Hypertension, 31, 801-807.

[53] MARSTON, N. A., BONACA, M. P., JAROLIM, P., GOODRICH, E. L., BHATT, D. L., STEG, P. G., COHEN, M., STOREY, R. F., JOHANSON, P., WIVIOTT, S. D., BRAUNWALD, E., SABATINE, M. S. & MORROW, D. A. (2020) Clinical Application of High-Sensitivity Troponin Testing in the Atherosclerotic Cardiovascular Disease Framework of the Current Cholesterol Guidelines. JAMA Cardiology, 5, 1255-1262.

[54] LIZZY, M. B., YENTL, C. H., AEILKO, H. Z., BERT JAN VAN DEN, B. & GERT, A. V. M. (2020) CK (Creatine Kinase) Is Associated With Cardiovascular Hemodynamics. Hypertension, 76, 373-380.

[55] APOSTOLAKIS, M., ARMENI, E., BAKAS, P. & LAMBRINOUDAKI, I. (2018) Vitamin D and cardiovascular disease. Maturitas, 115, 1-22.

[56] WANG, Y., JIN, Y., WANG, Y., LI, L., LIAO, Y., ZHANG, Y. & YU, D. (2019) The effect of folic acid in patients with cardiovascular disease: A systematic review and meta-analysis. Medicine, 98, e17095-e17095.

[57] VARONA, J. F., ORTIZ-REGALÓN, R., SÁNCHEZ-VERA, I., LÓPEZ-MELGAR, B., GARCÍA-DURANGO, C., VÁZQUEZ, J. M. C., SOLÍS, J., FERNÁNDEZ-FRIERA, L. & VIDAL-VANACLOCHA, F. (2019) Soluble ICAM 1 and VCAM 1 Blood Levels Alert on Subclinical Atherosclerosis in Non Smokers with Asymptomatic Metabolic Syndrome. Archives of Medical Research, 50, 20-28.

[58] FEDELE, F., PUCCI, M. & SEVERINO, P. (2017) Genetic Polymorphisms and Ischemic Heart Disease. IN PARINE, N. R. (Ed.) *Genetic Polymorphisms.* Online, IntechOpen.

[59] FIATAL, S. & ÁDÁNY, R. (2017) Application of Single-Nucleotide Polymorphism-Related Risk Estimates in Identification of Increased Genetic Susceptibility to Cardiovascular Diseases: A Literature Review. *Frontiers in Public Health,* 5.

[60] JIA, Y., WEN, W., YANG, Y., HUANG, M., NING, Y., JIAO, X., LIU, S., QIN, Y. & ZHANG, M. (2021) The clinical role of combined serum C1q and hsCRP in predicting coronary artery disease. Clinical Biochemistry, 93, 50-58.

[61] NCBI (2021k) hs-CRP gene [Internet]. National Center for Biotechnology Information; 2004 – [cited 2021/09/1]. Available from: https://www.ncbi.nlm.nih.gov/gene/1401. *Bethesda (MD): National Library of Medicine (US).*

[62] ALI, S., Al-Azawi, R. & H.KZAR, H. (2020) Study the IL6 (C174G) Promoter SNP and Correlation with Physiological Growth Hormone and TNFA levels in Iraqi Subjects with Psoriasis. Systematic Reviews in Pharmacy, 11, 272-276.

[63] NCBI (2021c) Apo B gene [Internet]. National Center for Biotechnology Information; 2004 – [cited 2021/09/1]. Available from: https://www.ncbi.nlm.nih.gov/gene/338. *Bethesda (MD): National Library of Medicine (US).*

[64] JANG, D.-I., LEE, A. H., SHIN, H.-Y., SONG, H.-R., PARK, J.-H., KANG, T.-B., LEE, S.-R. & YANG, S.-H. (2021) The Role of Tumor Necrosis Factor Alpha (TNF-α) in Autoimmune Disease and Current TNF-α Inhibitors in Therapeutics *International journal of molecular sciences,* 22, 2719.

[65] NCBI (2021aa) TNF-α gene [Internet]. National Center for Biotechnology Information; 2004 – [cited 2021/09/1]. Available from: https://www.ncbi.nlm.nih.gov/

gene/7124. *Bethesda (MD): National Library of Medicine (US).*

[66] YU, S., XUE, M., YAN, Z., SONG, B., HONG, H. & GAO, X. (2021) Correlation between TNF- α −308 and +489 Gene Polymorphism and Acute Exacerbation of Chronic Obstructive Pulmonary Diseases. BioMed research international, 2021, 6661281-6661281.

[67] MAI, W. & LIAO, Y. (2020) Targeting IL-1β in the Treatment of Atherosclerosis. Frontiers in Immunology, 11.

[68] NCBI (2021m) IL-1 beta gene [Internet]. National Center for Biotechnology Information; 2004 – [cited 2021/09/1]. Available from: https://www.ncbi.nlm.nih.gov/gene/3553. *Bethesda (MD): National Library of Medicine (US).*

[69] Abu El-Asrar, A. M., Ahmad, A., Allegaert, E., SIDDIQUEI, M. M., GIKANDI, P. W., DE HERTOGH, G. & OPDENAKKER, G. (2020) Interleukin-11 Overexpression and M2 Macrophage Density are Associated with Angiogenic Activity in Proliferative Diabetic Retinopathy. Ocular Immunology and Inflammation, 28, 575-588.

[70] NCBI (2021p) IL-11-receptor antagonist gene [Internet]. National Center for Biotechnology Information; 2004 – [cited 2021/09/1]. Available from: https://www.ncbi.nlm.nih.gov/gene/3589. *Bethesda (MD): National Library of Medicine (US).*

[71] NCBI (2021o) IL-10 gene [Internet]. National Center for Biotechnology Information; 2004 – [cited 2021/09/1]. Available from: https://www.ncbi.nlm.nih.gov/gene/3586. *Bethesda (MD): National Library of Medicine (US).*

[72] SHIFRISA, I., DUDARA, I., DRIYANSKA, V., HONCHARB, Y. & SAVCHENKOB, V. (2021) Comorbidity status and interleukin-10 levels in end-stage renal disease patients treated with hemodialysis. Polish Medical Journal, 49, 182-186.

[73] FORMANOWICZ, D., RYBARCZYK, A., RADOM, M., TANAS, K. & FORMANOWICZ, P. (2020) A Stochastic Petri Net-Based Model of the Involvement of Interleukin 18 in Atherosclerosis. International journal of molecular sciences, 21, 8574.

[74] MIZUTA, M., SHIMIZU, M., INOUE, N., IKAWA, Y., NAKAGISHI, Y., YASUOKA, R., IWATA, N. & YACHIE, A. (2021) Clinical significance of interleukin-18 for the diagnosis and prediction of disease course in systemic juvenile idiopathic arthritis. Rheumatology, 60, 2421-2426.

[75] NCBI (2021q) IL-18 gene [Internet]. National Center for Biotechnology Information; 2004 – [cited 2021/09/1]. Available from:. *Bethesda (MD): National Library of Medicine (US).*

[76] Colette Daubner, S. & Lanzas, R. O. (2018) Pteridines. *Reference Module in Biomedical Sciences.* Elsevier.

[77] VARGAS-ALARCON, G., PEREZ-MENDEZ, O., RAMIREZ-BELLO, J., POSADAS-SANCHEZ, R., GONZALEZ-PACHECO, H., ESCOBEDO, G., NIETO-LIMA, B., CARREON-TORRES, E. & FRAGOSO, J. M. (2020) The c.*52 A/G and c.*773 A/G Genetic Variants in the UTR'3 of the LDLR Gene Are Associated with the Risk of Acute Coronary Syndrome and Lower Plasma HDL-Cholesterol Concentration. *Biomolecules,* 10, 1381.

[78] NCBI (2021s) LDLR gene [Internet]. National Center for Biotechnology Information; 2004 – [cited 2021/09/1]. Available from: https://www.ncbi.nlm.nih.gov/gene/3949. *Bethesda (MD): National Library of Medicine (US).*

[79] REESKAMP, L. F., BALVERS, M., PETER, J., VAN DE KERKHOF, L., KLAAIJSEN, L. N., MOTAZACKER, M.

M., GREFHORST, A., VAN RIEL, N. A. W., HOVINGH, G. K., DEFESCHE, J. C. & ZUURBIER, L. (2021) Intronic variant screening with targeted next-generation sequencing reveals first pseudoexon in LDLR in familial hypercholesterolemia *Atherosclerosis,* 321, 14-20.

[80] LIU, Y., WANG, W., SONG, J., ZHANG, K., XU, B., LI, P., SHAO, C., YANG, M., CHEN, J. & TANG, Y.-D. (2021) Association Between Lipoprotein(a) and Peri-procedural Myocardial Infarction in Patients With Diabetes Mellitus Who Underwent Percutaneous Coronary Intervention. Frontiers in endocrinology, 11, 603922-603922.

[81] NCBI (2021u) Lp-(a) gene [Internet]. National Center for Biotechnology Information; 2004 – [cited 2021/09/1]. Available from: https://www.ncbi.nlm.nih.gov/gene/4018. *Bethesda (MD): National Library of Medicine (US).*

[82] SAID, M. A., MING WAI, Y. Yordi, J. V. D. V., JAN WALTER, B., ROBIN, P. F. D., SANNI, R., SAMULI, R., PRADEEP, N., LUIS EDUARDO, J.-O., NIEK, V. & HARST, P. V. D. (2021) Genome-Wide Association Study and Identification of a Protective Missense Variant on Lipoprotein(a) Concentration. Arteriosclerosis, Thrombosis, and Vascular Biology, 41, 1792-1800.

[83] GIAMMANCO, A., SPINA, R., FAYER, F., BARBAGALLO, C. M., NOTO, D., CEFALU, A. B. & AVERNA, M. R. (2020) Lack of phenotypic additive effect of familial defective apolipoprotein B3531 in familial hypercholesterolaemia. Internal Medicine Journal, 51, 585-590.

[84] CUI, G., TIAN, M., Hu, S., Wang, Y. & WANG, D. W. (2020) Identifying functional non-coding variants in APOA5/A4/C3/A1 gene cluster associated with coronary heart disease. Journal of Molecular and Cellular Cardiology, 144, 54-62.

[85] NCBI (2021b) Apo A-I gene [Internet]. National Center for Biotechnology Information; 2004 – [cited 2021/09/1]. Available from: https://www.ncbi.nlm.nih.gov/gene/335. *Bethesda (MD): National Library of Medicine (US).*

[86] ASHIQ, S. & ASHIQ, K. (2021) The Role of Paraoxonase 1 (PON1) Gene Polymorphisms in Coronary Artery Disease: A Systematic Review and Meta-Analysis. Biochemical Genetics, 59, 919-939.

[87] NCBI (2021x) PON1 gene [Internet]. National Center for Biotechnology Information; 2004 – [cited 2021/09/1]. Available from: https://www.ncbi.nlm.nih.gov/gene/5444. *Bethesda (MD): National Library of Medicine (US).*

[88] IWANICKA, J., IWANICKI, T., NIEMIEC, P., BALCERZYK, A., KRAUZE, J., GÓRCZYŃSKA-KOSIORZ, S., OCHALSKA-TYKA, A., GRZESZCZAK, W. & ŻAK, I. (2018) Relationship between CETP gene polymorphisms with coronary artery disease in Polish population. Molecular Biology Reports, 45, 1929-1935.

[89] NCBI (2021d) CETP gene [Internet]. National Center for Biotechnology Information; 2004 – [cited 2021/08/17]. Available from: https://www.ncbi.nlm.nih.gov/gene/1071. *Bethesda (MD): National Library of Medicine (US).*

[90] LIUTKEVICIENE, R., VILKEVICIUTE, A., STRELECKIENE, G., KRIAUCIUNIENE, L., CHALECKIS, R. & DELTUVA, V. P. (2017) Associations of cholesteryl ester transfer protein (CETP) gene variants with predisposition to age-related macular degeneration. Gene, 636, 30-35.

[91] Millwood, I. Y., Bennett, D. A., Holmes, M. V., BOXALL, R., GUO, Y., BIAN, Z., YANG, L., SANSOME, S., CHEN, Y., DU, H., YU, C., HACKER,

A., REILLY, D. F., TAN, Y., HILL, M. R., CHEN, J., PETO, R., SHEN, H., COLLINS, R., CLARKE, R., LI, L., WALTERS, R. G., CHEN, Z. & FOR THE CHINA KADOORIE BIOBANK COLLABORATIVE, G. (2018) Association of CETP Gene Variants With Risk for Vascular and Nonvascular Diseases Among Chinese Adults. JAMA Cardiology, 3, 34-43.

[92] ESTEVES, J. V., YONAMINE, C. Y. & MACHADO, U. F. (2020) *SLC2A4 expression and its epigenetic regulation as biomarkers for insulin resistance treatment in diabetes mellitus*, Biomark Med. 2020 Apr;14(6):413-416. doi: 10.2217/bmm-2019-0481. Epub 2020 Apr 6.

[93] NCBI (2021j) GLUT4 gene (SLC2A4) [Internet]. National Center for Biotechnology Information; 2004 – [cited 2021/09/1]. Available from: https://www.ncbi.nlm.nih.gov/gene/6517. *Bethesda (MD): National Library of Medicine (US)*.

[94] WANG, H., SAINT-MARTIN, C., Xu, J., Ding, L., WANG, R., FENG, W., LIU, M., SHU, H., FAN, Z., HAATAJA, L., ARVAN, P., BELLANNE-CHANTELOT, C., CUI, J. & HUANG, Y. (2020a) Biological behaviors of mutant proinsulin contribute to the phenotypic spectrum of diabetes associated with insulin gene mutations. Molecular and cellular endocrinology, 518, 111025-111025.

[95] NCBI (2021r) INS gene [Internet]. National Center for Biotechnology Information; 2004 – [cited 2021/09/1]. Available from: https://www.ncbi.nlm.nih.gov/gene/3630. *Bethesda (MD): National Library of Medicine (US)*.

[96] ALTAWALLBEH, G., KHABOUR, O. F., ALFAQIH, M. A., ABBOUD, M. M., GHARIBEH, M. & MOHAMMED, N. A. (2021) Association of RETN +299(G>A) polymorphism with type two diabetes mellitus. Acta Biochimica Polonica, 7, 77-81.

[97] NCBI (2021y) Resistin (RETN) gene [Internet]. National Center for Biotechnology Information; 2004 – [cited 2021/09/1]. Available from: https://www.ncbi.nlm.nih.gov/gene/56729. *Bethesda (MD): National Library of Medicine (US)*.

[98] RUBIO-CHAVEZ, L. A., ROSALES-GOMEZ, R. C., RUBIO-CHAVEZ, K. L., RAMOS-NUNEZ, J. L., GARCIA-COBIAN, T. A., CAMARGO-HERNANDEZ, G., SANCHEZ-CORONA, J. & GUTIERREZ-RUBIO, S. A. (2020) The rs822396 Polymorphism of the ADIPOQ Gene Is Associated with Anthropometric, Clinical, and Biochemical Alterations Related to the Metabolic Syndrome in the Mexican Population. Metabolic Syndrome and Related Disorders, 18, 243-250.

[99] NCBI (2021a) ADIPOQ gene [Internet]. National Center for Biotechnology Information; 2004 – [cited 2021/09/1]. Available from: https://www.ncbi.nlm.nih.gov/gene/9370. *Bethesda (MD): National Library of Medicine (US)*.

[100] HUANG, H., QIU, Y., HUANG, G., ZHOU, X., ZHOU, X. & LUO, W. (2019) Value of Ferritin Heavy Chain (FTH1) Expression in Diagnosis and Prognosis of Renal Cell Carcinoma. Medical science monitor: international medical journal of experimental and clinical research, 25, 3700-3715.

[101] NCBI (2021i) FTH1 gene [Internet]. National Center for Biotechnology Information; 2004 – [cited 2021/09/1]. Available from: https://www.ncbi.nlm.nih.gov/gene/2495. *Bethesda (MD): National Library of Medicine (US)*

[102] KIERNAN, K. & MACIVER, N. J. (2021) The Role of the Adipokine Leptin in Immune Cell Function in Health and Disease. Frontiers in immunology, 11, 622468-622468.

[103] NCBI (2021t) Leptin (LEP) gene [Internet]. National Center for Biotechnology Information; 2004 – [cited 2021/09/1]. Available from: https://www.ncbi.nlm.nih.gov/gene/3952. *Bethesda (MD): National Library of Medicine (US).*

[104] WANG, P., CHENG, M., WANG, P., XIONG, L., ZENG, Y., TU, X., ZHANG, R., XIA, Y., WU, G., WANG, Q., CHENG, X. & XU, C. (2020b) SNP rs2243828 in MPO associated with myeloperoxidase level and atrial fibrillation risk in Chinese Han population. Journal of cellular and molecular medicine, 24, 10263-10266.

[105] NCBI (2021w) Myeloperoxidase (MPO) gene [Internet]. National Center for Biotechnology Information; 2004 – [cited 2021/09/1]. Available from: https://www.ncbi.nlm.nih.gov/gene/4353. *Bethesda (MD): National Library of Medicine (US).*

[106] WANG, W.-M. & JIN, H.-Z. (2017) Homocysteine: A Potential Common Route for Cardiovascular Risk and DNA Methylation in Psoriasis. Chinese medical journal, 130, 1980-1986.

[107] HUANG, X., ZHAO, Q., Li, D., Ren, B., Yue, L., Shi, F., WANG, X., ZHENG, C., CHEN, X., ZHANG, C. & ZHANG, W. (2020) Association between gene promoter methylation of the one-carbon metabolism pathway and serum folate among patients with hyperhomocysteinemia. European Journal of Clinical Nutrition, 74, 1677-1684.

[108] NCBI (2021v) MTHFR gene [Internet]. National Center for Biotechnology Information; 2004 – [cited 2021/08/17]. Available from: https://www.ncbi.nlm.nih.gov/gene/4524. *Bethesda (MD): National Library of Medicine (US).*

[109] ENGIN, K., OZGE, B., ELIF, G., SUZAN, S., YESIM, O., SELIME, O. & RANA, I. (2020) Transcobalamin II deficiency in twins with a novel variant in the TCN2 gene: case report and review of literature. Journal of Pediatric Endocrinology and Metabolism, 33, 1487-1499.

[110] NCBI (2021ab) Transcobalamin (TCN2) gene [Internet]. National Center for Biotechnology Information; 2004 – [cited 2021/09/1]. Available from: https://www.ncbi.nlm.nih.gov/gene/6948. *Bethesda (MD): National Library of Medicine (US).*

[111] NAPOLITANO, M., SIRAGUSA, S. & MARIANI, G. (2017) Factor VII Deficiency: Clinical Phenotype, Genotype and Therapy. Journal of Clinical Medicine, 6, 38.

[112] Quintavalle, G., Riccardi, F., Rivolta, G. F., MARTORANA, D., DI PERNA, C., PERCESEPE, A., TAGLIAFERRI, A. & ON BEHALF OF THE AD-HOC STUDY, G. (2017) F7 gene variants modulate protein levels in a large cohort of patients with factor VII deficiency. Journal of Thrombosis and Haemostasis, 117, 1455-1464.

[113] Li, F., Hu, S., Zhou, X., Mei, X. & ZHOU, Y. (2020) Association Between R353Q (rs6046) Polymorphism in Factor VII with Coronary Heart Disease A Meta-Analysis. International Heart Journal, 61, 641-650.

[114] NCBI (2021g) Factor VII gene [Internet]. National Center for Biotechnology Information; 2004 – [cited 2021/08/17]. Available from: https://www.ncbi.nlm.nih.gov/gene/2155. *Bethesda (MD): National Library of Medicine (US).*

[115] MOSAAD, R. M., AMR, K. S., RABIE, E. A., MOSTAFA, N. O., HABIB, S. A. & EL-KAMAH, G. Y. (2021) Genomic alterations in the F8 gene correlating with severe hemophilia A in Egyptian patients. Molecular genetics & genomic medicine, 9, e1575-e1575.

[116] NCBI (2021h) Factor VIII gene [Internet]. National Center for

Biotechnology Information; 2004 – [cited 2021/09/1]. Available from: https://www.ncbi.nlm.nih.gov/gene/2157. *Bethesda (MD): National Library of Medicine (US)*.

[117] ZHANG, F., GUI, Y., LU, Y., LIU, D., CHEN, H., QIN, X. & LI, S. (2020) Novel SERPINC1 missense mutation (Cys462Tyr) causes disruption of the 279Cys-462Cys disulfide bond and leads to type I hereditary antithrombin deficiency. Clinical Biochemistry, 85, 38-42.

[118] NCBI (2021z) SERPINC1 gene [Internet]. National Center for Biotechnology Information; 2004 – [cited 2021/09/1]. Available from: https://www.ncbi.nlm.nih.gov/gene/462. *Bethesda (MD): National Library of Medicine (US)*.

[119] NCBI (2021f) Cystatin 3 (CST3) gene [Internet]. National Center for Biotechnology Information; 2004 – [cited 2021/09/1]. Available from: https://www.ncbi.nlm.nih.gov/gene/1471. *Bethesda (MD): National Library of Medicine (US)*.

[120] XIONG, H., WANG, L., JIN, F., ZHANG, B., WANG, X., CHANG, X. & ZHAO, L.-P. (2021) Association of cystatin C with coronary artery calcification in patients undergoing multidetector computed tomography. Medicine, 100, e26761-e26761.

[121] SUGIURA, T., DOHI, Y., TAKASE, H., FUJII, S., SEO, Y. & OHTE, N. (2020) Relationship of pulmonary function with myocardial microdamage and oxidative stress in the Japanese population without a history of cardiopulmonary disease. Medicine, 99, e21945-e21945.

[122] NCBI (2021ac) Troponin I3 (TNNI3) gene [Internet]. National Center for Biotechnology Information; 2004 – [cited 2021/09/1]. Available from: https://www.ncbi.nlm.nih.gov/gene?Db=gene&Cmd=DetailsSearch&Term=7137. *Bethesda (MD): National Library of Medicine (US)*.

[123] HAN, S., Xu, H., Zheng, J., Sun, J., Feng, X., WANG, Y., YE, W., KE, Q., REN, Y., YAO, S., ZHANG, S., CHEN, J., GRIGGS, R. C., ZHAO, Z., QI, M. & GATHERIDGE, M. A. (2020) Population-Wide Duchenne Muscular Dystrophy Carrier Detection by CK and Molecular Testing. BioMed research international, 2020, 8396429-8396429.

[124] NCBI (2021e) Creatine Kinase, M-Type (CKM) gene [Internet]. National Center for Biotechnology Information; 2004 – [cited 2021/09/1]. Available from: https://www.ncbi.nlm.nih.gov/gene/1158. *Bethesda (MD): National Library of Medicine (US)*

[125] NCBI (2021ae) Vitamin D receptor (VDR) gene [Internet]. National Center for Biotechnology Information; 2004 – [cited 2021/09/1]. Available from: https://www.ncbi.nlm.nih.gov/gene/7421. *Bethesda (MD): National Library of Medicine (US)*.

[126] PROTYUSHA, G. & SUNDHARAM, B. (2021) Analysis of the association between polymorphisms in Vitamin D receptor gene and dental caries. Indian Journal of Dental Research, 32, 3-7.

[127] NCBI (2021l) ICAM-1 gene [Internet]. National Center for Biotechnology Information; 2004 – [cited 2021/09/1]. Available from: https://www.ncbi.nlm.nih.gov/gene/3383. *Bethesda (MD): National Library of Medicine (US)*.

[128] TAFTAF, R., LIU, X., SINGH, S., JIA, Y., DASHZEVEG, N. K., HOFFMANN, A. D., EL-SHENNAWY, L., RAMOS, E. K., ADORNO-CRUZ, V., SCHUSTER, E. J., SCHOLTEN, D., PATEL, D., ZHANG, Y., DAVIS, A. A., REDUZZI, C., CAO, Y., D'AMICO, P., SHEN, Y., CRISTOFANILLI, M., MULLER, W. A., VARADAN, V. & LIU, H. (2021) ICAM1 initiates CTC cluster formation and trans-endothelial migration in lung metastasis of breast cancer. Nature communications, 12, 4867-4867.

[129] NCBI (2021ad) VCAM-1 gene [Internet]. National Center for Biotechnology Information; 2004 – [cited 2021/09/1]. Available from: https://www.ncbi.nlm.nih.gov/gene/7412. *Bethesda (MD): National Library of Medicine (US).*

[130] SALEM, H. R. & ZAHRAN, E. S. (2021) Vascular cell adhesion molecule-1 in rheumatoid arthritis patients. Relation to disease activity, oxidative stress, and systemic inflammation, 42, 620-628.

[131] JIHONG, Z. & SHAOKUN, W. (2019) MTHFR (C677T, A1298C) and MTRR (A66G) polymorphisms associated with the risk of megaloblastic anemia in China. *Research Square*, 1-18.

[132] BLAUW, L. L., NOORDAM, R., SOIDINSALO, S., BLAUW, C. A., LI-GAO, R., MUTSERT, R. D., BERBÉE, J. F. P., WANG, Y., HEEMST, D. V., ROSENDAAL, F. R., JUKEMA, J. W., MOOK-KANAMORI, D. O., WÜRTZ, P., DIJK, K. W. V. & RENSEN, P. C. N. (2018) Mendelian randomization reveals unexpected effects of CETP on the lipoprotein profile. European Journal of Human Genetics, 27, 422-431.

[133] BORDONI, L., SAMULAK, J. J., SAWICKA, A. K., PELIKANT-MALECKA, I., RADULSKA, A., LEWICKI, L., KALINOWSKI, L., GABBIANELLI, R. & OLEK, R. A. (2020) Trimethylamine N-oxide and the reverse cholesterol transport in cardiovascular disease: a cross-sectional study. Scientific Reports, 10, 18675.

[134] ZHAO, H., ZHAO, R., HU, S. & RONG, J. (2020) Gene polymorphism associated with angiotensinogen (M235T), endothelial lipase (584C/T) and susceptibility to coronary artery disease: a meta-analysis. *Bioscience Reports,* 40.

[135] ZHANG, P., WU, X., LI, G., HE, Q., DAI, H., AI, C. & SHI, J. (2017) Tumor necrosis factor-alpha gene polymorphisms and susceptibility to ischemic heart disease: A systematic review and meta-analysis. Medicine, 96, e6569-e6569.

[136] DENG, S.-J., SHEN, Y., Gu, H.-M., Guo, S., WU, S.-R. & ZHANG, D.-W. (2020) The role of the C-terminal domain of PCSK9 and SEC24 isoforms in PCSK9 secretion. Biochimica et Biophysica Acta (BBA) - Molecular and Cell Biology of Lipids, 1865, 158660.

[137] GHOLAMALIZADEH, M., Mirzaei Dahka, S., Vahid, F., BOURBOUR, F., BADELI, M., JAVADIKOOSHESH, S., MOSAVI JARRAHI, S. A., AKBARI, M. E., AZIZI TABESH, G., MONTAZERI, F., HASSANPOUR, A. & DOAEI, S. (2020) Does the rs9939609 FTO gene polymorphism affect fat percentage? A meta-analysis. *Archives of Physiology and Biochemistry*, 1-5.

[138] NCBI (2021n) IL-6 gene [Internet]. National Center for Biotechnology Information; 2004 – [cited 2021/08/17]. Available from: https://www.ncbi.nlm.nih.gov/gene/3569. *Bethesda (MD): National Library of Medicine (US).*

[139] YUEPENG, J., ZHAO, X., ZHAO, Y. & LI, L. (2019) Gene polymorphism associated with TNF-α (G308A) IL-6 (C174G) and susceptibility to coronary atherosclerotic heart disease. Medicine, 98, e13813-e13813.

[140] BARARTABAR, Z., NIKZAMIR, A., SIRATI-SABET, M., AGHAMOHAMMADI, E., CHALESHI, V., ROSTAMI NEJAD, M., ASADZADEH-AGHDAEI, H. & REZA ZALI, M. (2018) The relationship between 174 G/C and −572 G/C of IL-6 gene polymorphisms and susceptibility of celiac disease in the Iranian population. Przeglad gastroenterologiczny, 13, 293-298.

[141] BEDAIR, R. N., MAGOUR, G. M., OODA, S. A., AMAR, E. M. & AWAD,

A. M. (2021) Insulin receptor substrate-1 G972R single nucleotide polymorphism in Egyptian patients with chronic hepatitis C virus infection and type 2 diabetes mellitus. Egyptian Liver Journal, 11, 2.

[142] SHAKERI, H., KHOSHI, A., Kaffash Bajestani, M., Farahi, A., JAVADZADEH, M. S., HOSSEINI, Z. & MOHAMMADI, R. (2019) ASSOCIATION OF IRS1 GLY971ARG GENE POLYMORPHISM WITH INSULIN RESISTANCE IN IRANIAN NEWLY DIAGNOSED DIABETIC ADULTS. *Acta endocrinologica (Bucharest, Romania : 2005)*, 15, 317-322.

[143] GORSKA, A., WOLEK, M., CZERNY, B. A., UZAR, I., SEREMAK-MROZIKIEWICZ, A., OLBROMSKI, P., BARANIAK, J., KANIA-DOBROWOLSKA, M. G., SIENKO, M. & BOGACZ, A. (2020) Polymorphism analysis of the Gly972Arg IRS-1 and Gly1057Asp IRS-2 genes in obese pregnant women. Reproductive Biology, 20, 365-370.

[144] SYAHRUL, Wibowo, S., Haryana, S. M., Astuti, I. & Nurwidya, F. (2018) The role of insulin receptor substrate 1 gene polymorphism Gly972Arg as a risk factor for ischemic stroke among Indonesian subjects. BMC Research Notes, 11, 718.

[145] ABOOD, E. S., NASER, M. S. & NASER, R. J. (2021) MTHFR 677 C< T and 1298 A>C polymorphisms increases the risk of recurrent abortion in the Iraqi woman. Research Square, 1-11.

[146] Al-Batayneh, K. M., Zoubi, M. S. A., Shehab, M., AL-TRAD, B., BODOOR, K., KHATEEB, W. A., ALJABALI, A. A. A., HAMAD, M. A. & EATON, G. (2018) Association between MTHFR 677C>T Polymorphism and Vitamin B12 Deficiency: A Case-control Study. Journal of medical biochemistry, 37, 141-147.

[147] ANTONAROS, F., OLIVUCCI, G., CICCHINI, E., RAMACIERI, G., PELLERI, M. C., VITALE, L., STRIPPOLI, P., LOCATELLI, C., COCCHI, G., PIOVESAN, A. & CARACAUSI, M. (2019) MTHFR C677T polymorphism analysis: A simple, effective restriction enzyme-based method improving previous protocols. Molecular genetics & genomic medicine, 7, e628-e628.

[148] INCE, F. D., ATAY, A., KOSEOGLU, M. H., ELLIDAG, H. Y., YESIL, M. & DEVECI, E. (2016) The Severity of Coronary Artery Disease and Methylenetetrahydrofolate Reductase (MTHFR) Enzyme Gene Polymorphism. International Cardiovascular Research Journal, 10, e9805.

[149] SHIVKAR, R. R., GAWADE, G. C., PADWAL, M. K., DIWAN, A. G., MAHAJAN, S. A. & KADAM, C. Y. (2021) Association of MTHFR C677T (rs1801133) and A1298C (rs1801131) Polymorphisms with Serum Homocysteine, Folate and Vitamin B12 in Patients with Young Coronary Artery Disease. Indian Journal of Clinical Biochemistry.

[150] HUANG, H., LONG, W., ZHAO, W., ZOU, L., SONG, Y., ZUO, J. & YANG, Z. (2018) Polymorphism of R353Q (rs6046) in factor VII and the risk of myocardial infarction: A systematic review and meta-analysis. Medicine, 97, e12566-e12566.

[151] AZZAM, H., El-Farahaty, R. M., Abousamra, N. K., ELWAKEEL, H., SAKR, S., HELMY, A. & KHASHABA, E. (2017) Contribution of coagulation factor VII R353Q polymorphism to the risk of thrombotic disorders development (venous and arterial): A case-control study *Egyptian Journal of Medical Human Genetics*, 18, 275-279.

Chapter 4

Risk Factors for Cardiovascular Diseases in Aircrew

Nathan B. Buila, Gilbert K. Kabanda, Elysee M-C. Munyoka, Jean-Marc B. Bantu and Jean René M'Buyamba-Kabangu

Abstract

The relation of atherosclerotic cardiovascular disease (ASCVD) to not only traditional but also new and emergent risk factors has been assessed in aircrew. Total flight hours (TFH), high altitude and weightlessness exposure have been accounted among traditional risk factors for CVD among the aircrew. The risk factors do not perform in loneliness. To predict the 10 years global CV risk, several scores are being applied either based on traditional CVD risk factors only or also including new and emergent risk factors. To prevent aircrew from developing CVD, one should focus on the control of behavioral and metabolic risks as well as the polymorphe treatment of high CV risk individuals.

Keywords: Cardiovascular risk factors, Screening, Aircre

1. Introduction

Aircrew represent a particular group among " high cardiovascular disease (CVD) risk individuals". In addition to common life strain, aircrew face typical stress such as repeatedly proficiency simulator checks, intermittent medical exams and total flight hour obligations, employer pressure, responsibility, and scheduled accomplishment. These factors may lead to CVD, either directly or indirectly. They interact with traditional risk factors (genetic risk factors: aging, gender, ethnicity, chromosomes, HLA, genes, inflight incapacitation) and behavioral risk factors (inactivity, alcohol drinking, smoking, unhealthy diet) and emerging cardiovascular risk factors. The consequence is cardiovascular remodeling triggered by oxidative stress, inflammation and endothelial dysfunction. Unexpected in-flight medical incapacitation or distraction of a pilot may result in aviation accident, which is of public interest, harming himself, aircrafts, passengers and environment. Notwithstanding progress in prevention and early disease intervention, ischemic events secondary to coronary artery disease (CAD) remains among the commonest causes of unheralded acute incapacitation in the Western population. Thus, aeromedical providers should help aircrew to prevent CVD. It is essential to assess and stabilize the patient, control risk factors and optimize pharmacological treatments. Controlling weight and managing obesity, providing healthy diet and promoting physical activity, and educating aircrew and instituting home-based care monitoring is an important tool to preventing CVD. Aircrew with CVD are at high-risk and require a multifaceted and multidisciplinary intervention that should be started as soon as possible.

IntechOpen

The health of aircrew is an imperative requirement for safe travels of millions of people worldwide. The presence or development of CVD in aircrew, with the risk of potential clinical manifestations, continues to be a major concern to aviation medical practitioners. Despite the rigorously medical screen of pilots compared with several other professions, the presence of multi-crew environment, and the cockpit resource management with incapacitation training, acute coronary artery events remain an important cause of in-flight incapacitation or distraction ending in aircraft accidents and fatalities [1]. Few, if any, aircrew involved in accidents and incidents suffer from antecedent symptomatic coronary disease. Cardiovascular incapacitation of a pilot though rare event represents a seriously potential threat for flight safety [2]. In addition, CVDs linked to unexpected in-flight medical incapacitation or impairment account for half of human factor-related causes of aviation accidents [1]. In military operation, using single-pilot, high-performance aircraft, and even in dual-pilot, cardiac events were found to be second cause of aircraft accidents due to acute incapacitation [3].

From 1962 to 2015, Gray et al. listed 10 accidents and incidents in commercial passenger flights related to coronary artery events which concerned either the commandant or the first officer and resulted in 240 fatalities [4]. Moreover, 10 out of the 98 in-flight medical events addressed by the Australian Transport Safety Bureau (ATSB) between 1 January 1975 and 31 March 2006, consisted of heart attack explaining the high-observed mortality rate [5]. Autopsy studies of young military personnel and aircrew have demonstrated atherosclerosis as a common finding, including cases of severe disease and aeromedically disqualifying findings [6–8].

2. Epidemiology of risk factors for cardiovascular disease in aircrew

2.1 Traditional risk factors for cardiovascular disease in aircrew

Several studies mentioned the established risk factors for CVD continuum including hypertension, type-2 diabetes, dyslipidemia, smoking, overweight and mainly abdominal adiposity, physical inactivity and Mets [9]. Recent data suggest disturbing increases in the prevalence of these risk factors for CVD (**Figure 1**) [10].

2.1.1 Hypertension

Worldwide, hypertension is the leading etiology of morbidity and mortality [11, 12]. Hypertension is the first issue for pilots to secure their medical certificate [1, 13]. Through complications such as myocardial infarction, stroke, renal failure and death, hypertension constitutes a risk of in-flight incapacitation. In-flight CV events are believed to be scarce although allegation of in-flight CV incapacitation misdiagnosis has once been put forth [14]. Exposure to flight stress could be listed as a plausible explanation as weighted by total flight time at baseline. Indeed, considering the responsibility to fly the plane, flight crew is exposed to chronic stress that might trigger both hypothalamo-pituitary- adrenocortical and sympatho-adreno-medullary pathways to raise arterial blood pressure. In addition, it has been reported that chronic stress could lead to hypertension, which is triggered by angiotensin II through either lymphocyte T activation or vascular inflammation.

2.1.2 Types-2 diabetes

Type-2 diabetes either through chronic complications (heart disease, hypertension, and stroke) or acute complications (hypoglycemia or hyperglycemia episodes)

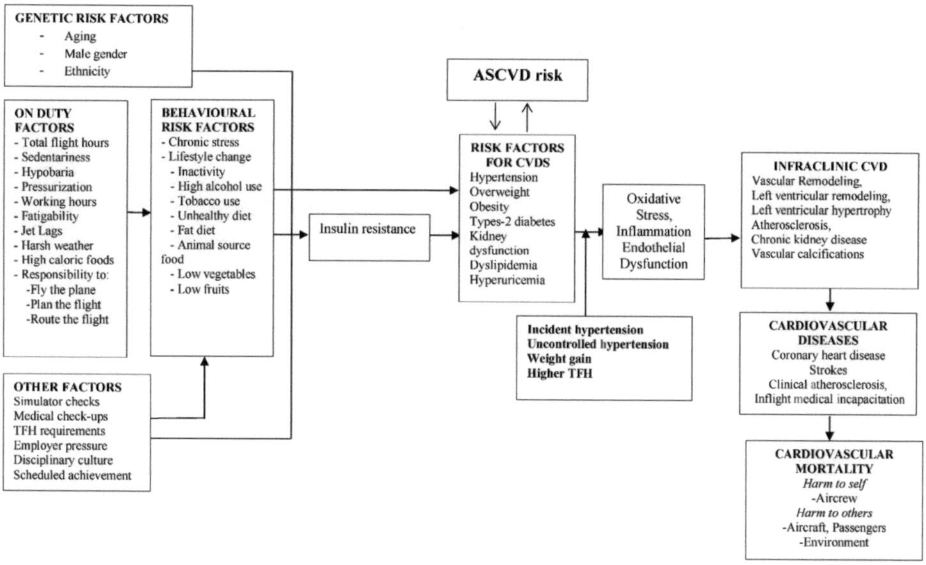

Figure 1.
Relationship between risk factors and CVD among aircrew. ASCVD: atherosclerotic cardiovascular disease; CVD: cardiovascular disease; TFH: total flight hours.

can grievously compromise flight safety and harm not only the aircrew himself but also the passengers, the aircraft, and the environment [15]. The relationship between blood glucose control and the establishment of CVD in diabetes remains a matter of controversy. Whilst several glucose-lowering trials in diabetes showed significant reduction in microvascular complications, they systematically failed to achieve significantly in macrovascular complications. Still, it should be mentioned that some systematic reviews and meta-analysis have recommended that efforts to improve blood glucose lower the incidence of CVD [16].

2.1.3 Smoking

Smoking has long been considered as the major risk factor for the establishment of CVD. Tobacco use, the single largest preventable cause of CV morbidity, is responsible for 10% of all of CVDs and doubles the 10-y mortality rate [17]. Worldwide, nearly a billion people are smokers and newly smokers are men from low- and middle-income countries (LMICs). Smoking delirious effect is dose related with no safe limit observed. It has been shown that passive smoking produces noticeable interferences in the normal autonomic nervous system functioning characterized by increased sympathetic drive and reduced HR variability (HRV) and parasympathetic modulation.

2.1.4 Overweight/obesity

Obesity, a significant determinant of CVDs, is extensively related to hypertension even if the exact mechanisms remain not totally unraveled [18]. This relation should now focus on weight variation across time along with visceral or intra-abdominal fat that is likely linked to the insulin resistance syndrome, an indicator of generalized metabolic disorder [18]. Obesity interacts with aviation duties. In fact, not only does obesity increase the risk of sudden CV incapacitation, but the risk of sudden and subtle incapacitation consequential to sleep apnea and the risk of pulmonary embolus do [19]. On the other hand, obesity can jeopardize the egress of aircraft in emergency [19]. The current results demonstrated that short term commercial flying significantly altered cardiovascular function including the reduction of parasympathetic modulations. Further, greater physical fitness and lower body fat composition were associated with greater cardiac autonomic control for passengers during flights. Enhanced physical fitness and leaner body composition may enable passengers to cope better with the cardiovascular stress and high allostatic load associated with air travel for enhanced passenger well-being [20]. In an observational cross-sectional study among Brazilian pilots, Palmeira found that more than half of and nearly a quart pilots were overweighed and obese, respectively. These authors concluded that overweight and obesity among the commercial airline pilots was high and represents a serious health problem in this population [21].

2.1.5 Physical inactivity

The lack of physical activity has contributed increasingly to overweight and obesity in young persons and adults. Physical activity is significant for primary and secondary prevention as well notwithstanding of BMI. Aircrew have little physical activity and eat higher caloric foods away from home at unscheduled time intervals [21]. Physical inactivity and unhealthy diet are responsible of raised BP, increased blood glucose, increased blood lipids, and overweight and obesity.

2.1.6 Total flight hours

The relationship between higher TFH and ASCVD risk in pilots have been established [22] as well as how TFH expresses the likelihood of crash involvement significantly compared with aging, which encompasses a conflict between decreasing cognitive functions that jeopardizes flight safety and increasing flying expertise that enhances fight safety [23]. Similarly, having 5,000 tfh or more protects against crash involvement but this protection levels off at a threshold of 10,000 tfh [23]. Likewise, inverse nonlinear relationship has been found between crash involvement and total flight time [23].

2.1.7 High altitude exposure

Pilots have to cope with stress due to 6,000 to 8,000 feet pressurized environment, and working hours [21]. It is known that the increase of BP with high altitude exposure 3000 m above sea level (asl) [24]. The explanation among several is the sympathetic activation (increased BP, HR, cardiac output, myocardial twist) through peripheral chemoreceptor [24]. Individuals with grade 2 hypertension and increased ASCVD risk should check their BP values before and during HA (>2500 m) exposure. Individuals with grade 1 hypertension may reach very HA (>4000 m) with adequate medical therapy; uncontrolled severe hypertensive individuals (grade 3) should avoid exposure to very HA [24]. At HA, left ventricular experiences changes such as an increase of systolic function with elevated sphericity index, but a decrease of diastolic function [25, 26]. Moreover, HA exposure may increase risk of cerebral ischemia for individuals with antecedent of ischemic stroke [26–28]. Background contributors are increased hematocrit and greater blood viscosity. HA exposure increases risk of hemorrhagic stroke in those with cerebral aneurysms and arterial/venous malformation [29]. HA may be at benefit for arrhythmia [24]. High altitude less than 4000 m does not affect pacing and implantable cardioverter devices [30].

At sea level, barometric pressure is 760 mmHg, and air has a partial pressure of oxygen (PO_2) of 160 mmHg. Airline flight usually cruises at altitudes of 9,150–13,000 m (30–40,000 feet) asl where the atmospheric PO_2 is usually ≤38 mmHg, which would normally result in a lethal level of airway (alveolar) hypoxia. Aircraft cabins are therefore environmentally modified (pressurized) to atmospheric pressures of 1,530–2,440 m (5,000–8,000 feet) asl [24].

2.1.8 Weightlessness exposure

Microgravity is a concern as it affects the entire body's systems, especially the cardiovascular system. Even with very short-duration exposure to microgravity, the cardiovascular system meets the return to gravity with CV deconditioning [24].

2.2 New and emergent risk factors for cardiovascular in aircrew

Atherosclerotic cardiovascular disease (ASCVD) starts at a very young age and progresses over time allowing sufficient time for screening and early detection of the condition. Because CVD often appears in individuals with lower CVD risk, some other markers should be able to provide added information about individual's risk, above and beyond the traditional risk factors at baseline. Among them are hs-CRP, intima-media thickness (CIMT), LVH, faster HR, kidney dysfunction, carotid ankle-brachial index (ABI), coronary artery calcium (CAC) score, cardio-respiratory fitness, apolipoprotein B (ApoB), micro-albuminuria, and genetic risk markers.

2.2.1 Fast resting heart rate

Several clinical and epidemiological reports have suggested that fast resting HR, as a marker of sympathetic nervous system and RAS overactivity, not only is a powerful independent predictor of CVD, but also of all-cause mortality. Resting faster HR could be associated, through oxidative stress and subsequent inflammation, with development of atherosclerosis, progression of heart failure, and enhancement of myocardial ischemia or infarction [31]. In a cross-sectional study of Congolese aircrew from both African and Caucasian origin, the proportion of subjects with a faster resting HR was of the same magnitude as the 6.8% observed in a normative sample from the First U.S. National Health and Nutrition Examination Survey (NHANES) I data [32]. It was nearly five times more frequent in flight than in cabin crew.

2.2.2 Left ventricular hypertrophy

LVH is an independent predictor of morbidity and mortality including disabling events such as sudden death, myocardial infarction and stroke. Echo-based LVH is a well-established predictor of CV morbidity and mortality in either the general population or high-risk groups. LVH has been found to be the most powerful risk factor for sudden death, ventricular arrhythmias, myocardial ischemia, CHD, and congestive heart failure. LVH regression due to treatment of hypertension predicts an improved prognosis. Abnormal LV geometry in hypertensive patients is frequently associated with diastolic dysfunction, which can be further evaluated, by a combination of transmitral flow and tissue Doppler studies. Aging–associated vascular remodeling and insulin resistance with subsequent constellation of multiple CVD risk factors might have led to LVH [33] with elevated 10-year global cardiovascular risk as observed in our airmen. Insulin resistance and subsequent hyperinsulinemia have been reported to activate the sympathetic nervous and the renin angiotensin systems resulting in endothelial dysfunction. With reference to

Laplace's law, high blood pressure and obesity could trigger cardiac remodeling through hemodynamic and humoral mechanisms and the thickening of cardiac wall may occur through collagen deposits. It has been reported that moderate to severe LVH, of mainly concentric geometric subtype is a common finding among aircrew with age, subclinical atherosclerosis and components of the MetS as its main associated CV risk factors [34].

2.2.3 Intima media thickness

The determination of cIMT in individual CV risk stratification and target organ appears in recent hypertension guidelines because of pathological IMT consistency related to future cardiovascular events.

2.2.4 Kidney dysfunction

Chronic kidney disease (CKD) stands as a global public health problem in HICs as well as in LMICs. In the USA, the third National Health and Nutrition Examination Survey (NHANES III) estimated that the prevalence of CKD has risen from 11% between 1988 and 1994 up to 13% between 1999 and 2004 [35, 36]. In a systematic review and a meta-analysis from 21 medium- and high-quality studies, Stanifer found 13.9% overall prevalence of CKD in SSA [37].

2.2.5 High sensitivity C-reactive protein

Hs-CRP is a marker of inflammation and endothelial dysfunction and subsequent atherosclerosis. It is produced by hepatocytes in response to circulating cytokines, particularly IL-6.18. It is also a robust downstream marker of inflammation, although unlikely to have a causative role in CVD. Consequently, the relationship between elevated hs-CRP and ASCVD risk remains a matter of controversy. The merit of hs-CRP use is because it does require neither sophisticated equipment nor particular operator skills, especially in developing countries. The hs-CRP, which is incorporated in the Reynolds score, may provide supplemental predictive capacity compared with the FRS [38]. Moreover, the 2013 ACC/AHA guidelines on the assessment of CV risk recommend hs-PCR in men (>50 y) and in women (>60 y) at intermediate risk, which are qualified for lipid lowering drugs [39]. In this regard, many studies reported a robust association of hs-CRP with numerous traditional risk factors for CHD such as obesity, diabetes, physical inactivity, smoking, and alcohol use [40–42]. Other studies highlighted the modest relationship between hs-CRP and CVD, because of its variability among age, gender (higher magnitude in men), and ethnicity (higher magnitude in African Americans vs. Caucasians) [43, 44]. A study comprised of aircrew from both African and Caucasian origin reported a net reclassified global ASCVD risk based on 2018 ESC/ESH guidelines chiefly in intermediate risk hypertensive individuals [40].

2.2.6 Coronary artery calcium

Coronary artery calcium (CAC) a powerful novel risk indicator for ASCVD risk. It is linked with an enhanced risk to develop harmful cardiovascular events independently of clinical markers and inflammatory biomarkers [45]. Conversely, a calcium artery score of 0 has a strong negative predictive value for the development of coronary artery diseases (CAD).

2.2.7 Genetic risk scores

Genetic risk scores have been proposed because of the association between loci or genes and higher ASCVD risk. The advantage of genetic biomarkers on other biomarkers is that they exist at birth and can be determined even in antenatal period. But, gene–environment interactions can sometimes be responsible for development of disease states. Furthermore, using new variables such as genetic markers may enhance CV prediction even if this possibility remains questionable [46]. In a post-hoc meta-analyze of six systematic reviews on effect of ASCVD risk estimate in primary prevention, Collins et al. reported that there was no evidence that the potential use of ASCVD risk estimate leads to decreasing in CVD morbidity and mortality due to the deficient quality of systematic reviews.

3. Global cardiovascular risk estimate in aircrew

3.1 Global cardiovascular risk estimate using traditional risk factors

Given that risk factors for CVDs do not act in isolation, quantification of risk is an important part of the risk stratification process. The prediction of an individual's ASCVD risk over a one 10-y period traditionally involves assessment of CVD risk factors such as age, gender, baseline levels of systolic and diastolic BP, serum cholesterol, smoking status and history of diabetes. Published in 1998 [47] and modified in 2002 [48], the Framingham risk score (FRS) derived from the Framingham Heart Study (FHS) which is broadly granted as the pioneering longitudinal cohort study [49, 50]. FHS chart, a risk prediction model, assigns weight (points) to traditional risk factors for ASCVD such as age, total cholesterol (TC), high-density lipoprotein cholesterol (HDL-c), treated or untreated SBP (yes or no), smoking status (yes or no), and type-2 diabetes (yes or no). This FHS chart produces an estimate (or risk) of developing CVD or a component of CVD (such as stroke, peripheral vascular disease, or heart failure) over a fixed time, for example, the next 10 years [50]. Also, Framingham investigators presented heart /vascular age which is the age that corresponds to a person with normal risk factors and the same 10-year CV risk stating that low 10-year risk can cohabit with a vascular age higher than the chronological one [51]. FHS chart has been broadly utilized for clinical guidelines [52], transported, and validated in several non-Framingham settings [53].

Besides the Framingham estimate functions, other significant risk functions such as the European Systematic Coronary Risk Evaluation (SCORE) function, the Prospective Cardiovascular Münster (PROCAM) function [53], the QRISK [54, 55] algorithms, the Reynolds risk score [56, 57], the Multi Ethnic Study of Atherosclerosis (MESA) algorithms may be used [58]. The final objective of all these ASCVD risk prediction models should be to improve clinical guidelines in detecting silent and undiagnosed CVD. Nevertheless, there are some caveats to using these risk factors alone in a model as prognostic tools for CVD risk prediction. Most of these risk equations have been constructed with data from Western populations, are generally population-specific, and may not be safely extrapolated to other populations. One must consider the fact that the calculated risk does not mean the occurrence of event in any specific individual but rather in 100 individuals with identical features.

For aviation personnel, rigorous medical scrutiny leads to the exclusion of those with evident CVDs at either initial or renewal of their medical licenses [2]. CVD events are often silent or may present without warning. All the licensed aviation personnel undergo CV assessment including electrocardiogram (ECG), echocardiography, and lipid profile at initial. An ECG can be done at renewal as appropriate.

Several Civil Aviation Authorities (CAA) highly recommend aircrew, chiefly those aged 40 years or more, to periodically be screened for cardiovascular risk using suitable risk investigative tools that comprise family history and non-fatal and fatal end points, and a resting ECG. For most aircrew, the Reynold's risk equation provides a reasonably well-calibrated risk estimate, which includes family history [57]. The assessment and management of aeromedical risk continue to be a balancing act between practicality, risk tolerance and the advances of diagnostic medicine. The risk, which can be considered as a minimum objective for a large public transport aircraft due to medical causes, lies in the region of 10^{-8} and 10^{-9} per hour or per flight as appropriate.

A single risk matrix cannot reflect the operational impact of a medical event for all aircrew roles. To reflect the operational impact of a medical event incorporating aircrew role, a series of risk matrices that reflect the varying operational risk pertinent to specific aircrew role (the third dimension) is required. This led Gray et al. to develop a three-sized risk matrix, which embodies discrete aircrew duties: (i) aircrew with direct control over the aircraft (ie, pilot, copilot), (ii) aircrew personnel with input to navigation or engine/mechanical systems (ie, navigator, FEs), and (iii) aircrew responsible for passenger or cargo (ie, loadmasters, cabin crew) [4]. Although technically, air traffic controllers (ATCs) are not considered crews, they are considered to have an attributable risk similar to that of pilots.

Thus, ICAO asks stakeholder countries to use ASCVD estimate scores in aeromedical risk assessment to help alleviating morbidity and mortality in aeronautical setting. For example, the New Zealand Guideline Group (NZGG) adjusted [59], updated [60], and even assessed [61] the Framingham ASCVD estimate tools. In a matched case–control study accounting Oceania- based airline pilots using the NZGG adjusted Framingham score, Wirawan posited the NZGG score had low sensitivity and thus missed to predict 47% of the CV events [62].

3.2 Global cardiovascular risk estimate using new and emergent risk factors

Risk in CVD is still assessed chiefly by clinical features such as age, hypertension, diabetes mellitus, hyperlipidemia, and family history. Nonetheless, biochemical, cellular, and imaging frameworks are firmly allowing for increasingly improved risk assessment.

Aircrew undergo various investigations to assess cardiovascular risk that are anatomical (Cardiac CT, cardiac MR or invasive coronary angiography, transthoracic and transesophageal echocardiography), physiological (Myocardial perfusion imaging, including perfusion MRI, myocardial perfusion scintigraphy [MPS], both single photon emission CT [SPECT] and positron emission tomography [PET]), stress echocardiogram (with either physiological or pharmacological stress) and fractional flow reserve (FFR) and Clinical (Exercise stress ECG test, CAC scoring). Exercise stress ECG test is not recommended as a solely investigative tool for assessment of significant CAD in aircrew [63]. It is relevant to note that the negative predictive value (NPV) of the CCT for the detection of CHD is almost 100%, which implies that a negative scanner is very reassuring at least for the next 35 years [64].

To comply with the approach of the ICAO, it is recommended to CAAs to hold an inventory of the effective of aircrew to monitor their careers and health, their accidents and impairments [65]. Even for private aircrew, there are concerns, which imply that some degree of restriction must be applied. On the other hand, several CAAs prohibit pilots aged 65y or older from flying on commercial flight operations even if this remains debatable [63]. The so-called "age-65 rule" is of concerns about the potential deleterious effects of aging on pilots' safety performance [66].

Aircrew with elevated cardiovascular risk established on inceptive screening should go through intensified screening that includes ancillary, to name but a few, stress ECG, CAC scoring solely, or combined with a CT coronary angiogram (CTCA) investigation, and vascular ultrasound imaging (VUI). Second-line investigative risk tools for CAD assessment comprise functional imaging, and invasive coronary angiography (ICA). Emerging technologies comprise CMR for plaque imaging and FFR that is a technique traditionally used as an adjunct to ICA to measure pressure differences across coronary stenosis.

Exercise stress ECG provides useful risk-stratification information including aerobic fitness, BP response and arrhythmia assessment, which may be incorporated in intensified screening. The use of routine exercise stress testing as a sole screening tool for CAD is not supported by evidence and is not recommended. Exercise stress tests are limited in their ability to detect potentially flow-limiting CAD and to predict future cardiovascular events. Because of its restricted sensitivity and specificity, exercise stress ECG has a flaw as screening test for coronary atherosclerosis. Moreover, because of its very low PPV for future coronary events, stress ECG should be discouraged as a stand-alone tool to determine aeromedically significant CAD.

The Astro-CHARM tool is the first integrated ASCVD risk calculator to incorporate risk factors, including hs-CRP, family history, and CAC data. It improves risk prediction in comparison with traditional risk factor equations and could be useful in risk-based decision making for cardiovascular disease prevention in the middle-aged general population.

Ultrasound imaging of the carotid and femoral arteries provides easily accessible visualization of vascular anatomy without radiation. cIMT and carotid and femoral artery plaque, have been evaluated as markers for cardiac disease and stroke risk. Several prospective studies have shown that the presence of carotid and femoral bifurcation plaques is associated with future cardiovascular events, independent of other risk factors. Guidelines support the use of carotid artery ultrasound in the cardiovascular risk assessment of asymptomatic aircrew at intermediate risk.

To identify aeromedically significant CAD, physiological imaging such as stress echo, perfusion MRI or myocardial perfusion scintigraphy (MPS) has limited utility and is not recommended as the sole secondary investigation for aircrew considered to be at high cardiovascular risk as it may overlook aeromedically significant (aggregate) stenosis. ICA should be reserved for those aircrew who are deemed at high risk for significant CAD or where accurate delineation of percentage coronary stenosis is required. ICA currently remains the gold standard for anatomical imaging of coronary arteries. This is because the spatial resolution of ICA is superior to that of CTCA. CTCA is less accurate than ICA for quantifying luminal stenosis. The threshold for initiating enhanced screening of aircrew with increased estimated risk for a coronary event is an organizational decision.

4. Preventing cardiovascular disease

Aircrew retirement age is increasing and the burden of subclinical, but potentially significant, coronary artery atherosclerosis is unknown in pilots above age 40 [20]. Prevention of CVD in aircrew may be even more problematic than in the general population. The control of CVD should focus on the reduction of behavioral risks (salt, tobacco, alcohol, physical inactivity) and metabolic risks (high BP, diabetes mellitus, and obesity), and on multidrug therapy for treatment of individuals at high risk of heart attack and stroke based on these risks. Preventive initiatives should make it easier for healthy aircrew to stay healthy, and for those with established CVD or at high risk for CVD to modify their behavior [67]. To prevent the onset of CVD in aircrew, many avenues including healthier lifestyle such as regular physical activity, healthier diet, weight loss, moderate alcohol consumption, and smoking cessation, and the control risk factors can be considered.

Regular physical activity lowers the risk of CVD, improves endothelial and platelet function, and diminishes insulin resistance [68]. In fact, regular physical activity corrects raised BP and lipid profile, increases the level of HDL but lowers that of TC and LDL-c [68–70]. NICE guidelines recommend 150 minutes of moderate intensity aerobic activity per week, or 75 minutes of vigorous aerobic activity. Whilst NICE give only a consensus recommendation regarding the utility of exercise as primary prevention, guidelines from the AHA and ESC give class 1A recommendations with almost identical prescriptions, referring to a solid and consensual body of evidence [17, 71]. It has been reported in a recent cross-sectional study including 22 physically active men, exempt from CVD, that particular features of physical fitness such as aerobic capacity were associated with better cardiovascular control (HRV and BP) during flights. These authors encouraged future studies to investigate the role of physical fitness in reducing the flight-induced stress and related cardiac autonomic alterations for the general population [20].

Diet represents the most significant modifiable factor in the primary prevention of CVD. There is evidence that eating fruit and vegetables have been found to have compelling cardiovascular effects [69]. Epidemiological evidence shows that a diet low in fruits is the third most important risk factor of CVDs following high BP and cigarette smoking, accounting for more than 5 million deaths worldwide in 2010 [72]. The mechanisms of action mainly included the modulation of molecular events and signaling pathways associated with correcting endothelial dysfunction, reducing disorders in lipids metabolism, anti-hypertension, suppressing platelet's function, alleviating I/R injury, inhibiting thrombosis, reducing oxidative stress, and inhibiting inflammation responses [73]. Several studies have highlighted the impact of high-potassium diet on high BP, singularly in the presence of high dietary sodium, using the inward-rectifying potassium (K_{ir}) [74].

There is evidence that modest weight loss (e.g., 5–10%) can reduce CVD risk profile even when the patient remains in the obese range [75, 76]. Modest weight loss has been linked with an improvement in fasting glycaemia, glycosylated hemoglobin (HBA1c), and systolic and diastolic BP and plasma lipid profile (TG, TC, and LDL-c) [77]. Moreover, weight loss can also improve the efficacy of antihypertensive medications. Weight loss should employ a multidisciplinary approach that includes dietary advice, regular exercise, and motivational counseling [17, 78]. Weight loss can also be promoted by anti-obesity drugs and, to a greater degree, bariatric surgery, which appears to decrease CV risk in severely obese patients [79]. There are moves to suggest that, alongside reduction in BMI, reduction in WC as a proxy for reductions in visceral adiposity should become an important target for amelioration of CVD risk.

Four decades ago, epidemiological studies showed the historically J-shaped curve between alcohol consumption and cardiovascular risk [80, 81]. Recently, both cohort studies and meta-analyses corroborated the robustness of the mentioned relationship [82]. These authors argued that abstinence is associated with an increase in cardiovascular risk compared to light drinking and low levels of alcohol consumption associated with a lower level of CHD. Similarly, INTERHEART, NICE, and ACC studies showed moderate to light alcohol use was linked with preventing CVD. Contrastingly, through a large mendelian randomization meta-analysis, Holmes et al. showed that reduction in alcohol intake is linked with reduction in CVD risk even in light-moderate drinkers [83]. It is on this basis that the ESC guidelines recommend no safe level of alcohol intake [84].

Smoking cessation is strongly recommended by all guidelines and smoker is likely to use nicotine replacement therapy (NRT), bupropion (a norepinephrine dopamine reuptake inhibitor) and particularly varenicline (a partial nicotine receptor agonist). Evidence suggests the use of NRT outweigh its cardiovascular risks whilst the use of E-cigarettes are still controversial [85].

Lowering BP to an optimal level (<130/80 mmHg) has been found to significantly reduce the risk of CVD [86]. Best proven non pharmacologic Interventions for prevention and treatment of hypertension that are weight loss, health diet, lower intake of dietary $Na+$, enhanced intake of dietary $K+$, physical exercise, and moderate alcohol intake approximately impact on SBP by 5, 11, 6, 5, 5, and 4 mmHg, respectively. Specific BP lowering drugs include calcium blockers, diuretics, ACEI, ARBS, and beta-blockers [84]. Medical practitioners are advised to avoid pharmacological inertia characterized by negligence of medical providers to initiate or intensify pharmacological therapy as stated by guidelines [84].

The overall strategy toward risk management for type-2 diabetes patients should focus on BP and lipid control to lower the leading complications of diabetes. Diabetes is treated with diet, exercise, and some antidiabetic medications [87]. Lowering cholesterol by means of drugs such as statins alone or associated with either ezetimibe or anti-proprotein convertase subtilisin/kexin type 9 (PCSK9) monoclonal antibodies (mAbs), has been found to reduce ASCVD risk; however, lipid-lowering diet and physical exercise are also important [88].

In aircrew with heart failure, medications should include B-adrenergic blockers, ACEIs, and more recently Ivabradine and/or sacubitril/ valsartan combination, when appropriate. Implantable cardioverter defibrillators and/or resynchronization should be associated. Exercise training is usually indicated based on the patient response to applied exercise protocols. In patients with CKD, risk factors such as hypertension, type-2 diabetes, and obesity should be controlled [89].

Traditional herbal remedies should be avoided for numerous riveting studies showed their toxicity even if histological and toxicological studies are needed to validate this causal relationship [89]. Antihypertensive treatment reverses myocardial hypertrophy, and additionally reduces repolarization time and its dispersion, the incidence and the severity of ventricular arrhythmia, and the risk of cardiovascular events.

Flight crew represent a high CVD risk subgroup requiring development of a comprehensive prevention and care program to mitigate the elevated risk and improve their quality of life and performance.

Author details

Nathan B. Buila[1]*, Gilbert K. Kabanda[2], Elysee M-C. Munyoka[3], Jean-Marc B. Bantu[4] and Jean René M'Buyamba-Kabangu[2]

1 Cardiology Division, Department of Internal Medicine, University of Kinshasa Hospital, University of Kinshasa, Kinshasa, Democratic Republic of the Congo

2 Hypertension Unit, Cardiology Division, Department of Internal Medicine, University of Kinshasa Hospital, University of Kinshasa, Kinshasa, Democratic Republic of the Congo

3 Papavest Medical, Brussels, Belgium

4 Free University of Brussels, Brussels, Belgium

*Address all correspondence to: drnathanbuila@gmail.com

IntechOpen

© 2021 The Author(s). Licensee IntechOpen. This chapter is distributed under the terms of the Creative Commons Attribution License (http://creativecommons.org/licenses/by/3.0), which permits unrestricted use, distribution, and reproduction in any medium, provided the original work is properly cited.

References

[1] DeJohn CA, Wolbrink AM, Larcher JG. In-flight medical incapacitation and impairment of airline pilots. Aviat Space Environ Med. 2006;77(10):1077-1079.

[2] Taneja N, Wiegmann DA. Prevalence of cardiovascular abnormalities in pilots involved in fatal general aviation airplane accidents. Aviat Space Environ Med. 2002;73(10):1025-1030.

[3] DeJohn CA, Mills WD, Hathaway W, Larcher J. Cardiac Inflight Incapacitations of U.S. Airline Pilots: 1995-2015. Aerosp Med Hum Perform. 2018;89(9):837-841.

[4] Gray G, Davenport ED, Bron D, Rienks R, d'Arcy J, Guettler N, et al. The challenge of asymptomatic coronary artery disease in aircrew; detecting plaque before the accident. Heart (British Cardiac Society). 2019;105 (Suppl 1):s17-s24.

[5] Newman B. Pilot Incapacitation: Analysis of Medical Conditions Affecting Pilots Involved in Accidents and Incidents. ATSB TRANSPORT SAFETY REPORT. 2007;Aviation Research and Analysis Report - B2006/0170

[6] Enos WF, Holmes RH, Beyer J. CORONARY DISEASE AMONG UNITED STATES SOLDIERS KILLED IN ACTION IN KOREA: PRELIMINARY REPORT. Journal of the American Medical Association. 1953;152(12): 1090-1093.

[7] Mason KT. Military Flying and Aeromedical Evaluation of Cardiac Arrhythmias. 1994.

[8] Webber BJ, Seguin PG, Burnett DG, Clark LL, Otto JL. Prevalence of and risk factors for autopsy-determined atherosclerosis among US service members, 2001-2011. Jama. 2012;308(24):2577-2583.

[9] O'Rourke MF, Safar ME, Dzau V. The Cardiovascular Continuum extended: Aging effects on the aorta and microvasculature. Vascular Medicine. 2010;15(6):461-468.

[10] Roth GA, Johnson C, Abajobir A, Abd-Allah F, Abera SF, Abyu G, et al. Global, Regional, and National Burden of Cardiovascular Diseases for 10 Causes, 1990 to 2015. J Am Coll Cardiol. 2017;70(1):1-25.

[11] Buila NB, Ngoyi GN, Bayauli PM, Katamba FK, Lubenga YN, Kazadi SM, et al. Analysis of blood pressure and selected cardiovascular risk factors in the Democratic Republic of the Congo: the May Measurement Month 2018 results. Eur Heart J Suppl. 2020; 22(Suppl H):H50-H2.

[12] M'Buyamba-Kabangu J-R, Katamba FK, Ntambwe ML, Ngoyi GN, Tshiswaka TM, Bayauli PM, et al. May Measurement Month 2019: an analysis of blood pressure screening results from the Democratic Republic of the Congo. European Heart Journal Supplements. 2021;23(Supplement_B):B52-B4.

[13] Buila NB KG, Bantu J-MB, Ngoyi GN, Mvunzi TS, Otshudi NO, et al. Hypertension and Associated Cardiometabolic Risk Factors among Civilian Aircrew. Ann Afr Med. 2019;12, n° 3.

[14] Ekstrand K, Boström PA, Arborelius M, Nilsson JA, Lindell SE. Cardiovascular risk factors in commercial flight aircrew officers compared with those in the general population. Angiology. 1996;47(11): 1089-1094.

[15] Junttila IS, Vuorio A, Budowle B, Laukkala T, Sajantila A. Challenges in investigation of diabetes-related aviation fatalities-an analysis of 1491 subsequent aviation fatalities in USA

during 2011-2016. Int J Legal Med. 2018;132(6):1713-1718.

[16] Conget I, Giménez M. Glucose control and cardiovascular disease: is it important? No. Diabetes Care. 2009;32 Suppl 2(Suppl 2):S334-S6.

[17] Piepoli MF, Hoes AW, Agewall S, Albus C, Brotons C, Catapano AL, et al. 2016 European Guidelines on cardiovascular disease prevention in clinical practice: The Sixth Joint Task Force of the European Society of Cardiology and Other Societies on Cardiovascular Disease Prevention in Clinical Practice (constituted by representatives of 10 societies and by invited experts)Developed with the special contribution of the European Association for Cardiovascular Prevention & Rehabilitation (EACPR). Eur Heart J. 2016;37(29):2315-81.

[18] Jiang SZ, Lu W, Zong XF, Ruan HY, Liu Y. Obesity and hypertension. Exp Ther Med. 2016;12(4):2395-2399.

[19] Ghiasi F, Ahmadpoor A, Amra B. Relationship between obstructive sleep apnea and 30-day mortality among patients with pulmonary embolism. J Res Med Sci. 2015;20(7):662-667.

[20] Oliveira-Silva I, Leicht AS, Moraes MR, Simões HG, Del Rosso S, Córdova C, et al. Heart Rate and Cardiovascular Responses to Commercial Flights: Relationships with Physical Fitness. Front Physiol. 2016;7:648-.

[21] de Souza Palmeira ML, Cristina Marqueze E. Excess weight in regular aviation pilots associated with work and sleep characteristics. Sleep Sci. 2016;9(4):266-271.

[22] Buila NB BJ-M, Kabanda GK, Bayauli PM, Nkodila AN, Lepira FB, et al. Atherosclerotic Cardiovascular Disease Short-Term Risk Estimate among Civilian Licensed Aircrew. World Journal of Cardiovascular Diseases. 2019;09:92-108.

[23] Li G, Baker SP, Grabowski JG, Qiang Y, McCarthy ML, Rebok GW. Age, flight experience, and risk of crash involvement in a cohort of professional pilots. Am J Epidemiol. 2003;157(10): 874-880.

[24] Parati G, Agostoni P, Basnyat B, Bilo G, Brugger H, Coca A, et al. Clinical recommendations for high altitude exposure of individuals with pre-existing cardiovascular conditions: A joint statement by the European Society of Cardiology, the Council on Hypertension of the European Society of Cardiology, the European Society of Hypertension, the International Society of Mountain Medicine, the Italian Society of Hypertension and the Italian Society of Mountain Medicine. European heart journal. 2018;39(17): 1546-54.

[25] Osculati G, Revera M, Branzi G, Faini A, Malfatto G, Bilo G, et al. Effects of hypobaric hypoxia exposure at high altitude on left ventricular twist in healthy subjects: data from HIGHCARE study on Mount Everest. European Heart Journal - Cardiovascular Imaging. 2015;17(6):635-643.

[26] Caravita S FA, Bilo G, Revera M, Giuliano A, Gregorini F, et al. Ischemic changes in exercise ECG in a hypertensive subject acutely exposed to high altitude. Possible role of a high-altitude induced imbalance in myocardial oxygen supply-demand. Int J Cardiol 2014;171(3):e100-2.

[27] Clarke C. Acute mountain sickness: medical problems associated with acute and subacute exposure to hypobaric hypoxia. Postgrad Med J. 2006;82(973):748-753.

[28] Le Roux G, Larmignat P, Marchal M, Richalet JP. Haemostasis at high altitude. Int J Sports Med. 1992;13 Suppl 1:S49-S51.

[29] Wilson MH, Newman S, Imray CH. The cerebral effects of ascent to high altitudes. Lancet Neurol. 2009;8(2): 175-191.

[30] Weilenmann D, Duru F, Schönbeck M, Schenk B, Zwicky P, Russi EW, et al. Influence of acute exposure to high altitude and hypoxemia on ventricular stimulation thresholds in pacemaker patients. Pacing Clin Electrophysiol. 2000;23 (4 Pt 1):512-515.

[31] Fox K, Borer JS, Camm AJ, Danchin N, Ferrari R, Lopez Sendon JL, et al. Resting heart rate in cardiovascular disease. J Am Coll Cardiol. 2007;50(9): 823-830.

[32] Ostchega Y, Porter KS, Hughes J, Dillon CF, Nwankwo T. Resting pulse rate reference data for children, adolescents, and adults: United States, 1999-2008. Natl Health Stat Report. 2011(41):1-16.

[33] Mehta SK, Rame JE, Khera A, Murphy SA, Canham RM, Peshock RM, et al. Left ventricular hypertrophy, subclinical atherosclerosis, and inflammation. Hypertension. 2007;49(6):1385-1391.

[34] Buila N, Ngoyi G, Lubenga Y, Bantu J-M, Mvunzi T, Kabanda G, et al. Left ventricular hypertrophy and linked cardiovascular risk factors among Congolese licensed civilian aircrew. Journal of Epidemiological Research. 2020;5:28.

[35] Coresh J, Astor BC, Greene T, Eknoyan G, Levey AS. Prevalence of chronic kidney disease and decreased kidney function in the adult US population: Third National Health and Nutrition Examination Survey. Am J Kidney Dis. 2003;41(1):1-12.

[36] Coresh J, Selvin E, Stevens LA, Manzi J, Kusek JW, Eggers P, et al. Prevalence of chronic kidney disease in the United States. Jama. 2007;298(17): 2038-2047.

[37] Stanifer JW, Jing B, Tolan S, Helmke N, Mukerjee R, Naicker S, et al. The epidemiology of chronic kidney disease in sub-Saharan Africa: a systematic review and meta-analysis. Lancet Glob Health. 2014;2(3): e174-81.

[38] Cook NR, Paynter NP, Eaton CB, Manson JE, Martin LW, Robinson JG, et al. Comparison of the Framingham and Reynolds Risk scores for global cardiovascular risk prediction in the multiethnic Women's Health Initiative. Circulation. 2012;125(14):1748-1S11.

[39] Goff DC, Jr., Lloyd-Jones DM, Bennett G, Coady S, D'Agostino RB, Gibbons R, et al. 2013 ACC/AHA guideline on the assessment of cardiovascular risk: a report of the American College of Cardiology/ American Heart Association Task Force on Practice Guidelines. Circulation. 2014;129(25 Suppl 2):S49-S73.

[40] Buila NB, Ntambwe ML, Mupepe DM, Lubenga YN, Bantu JB, Mvunzi TS, et al. The Impact of hs-CRP on Cardiovascular Risk Stratification in Pilots and Air Traffic Controllers. Aerosp Med Hum Perform. 2020;91(11):886-891.

[41] Yü TF, Berger L, Dorph DJ, Smith H. Renal function in gout. V. Factors influencing the renal hemodynamics. Am J Med. 1979;67(5):766-771.

[42] Chen PC, Chien KL, Hsu HC, Su TC, Sung FC, Lee YT. Metabolic syndrome and C-reactive protein in stroke prediction: a prospective study in Taiwan. Metabolism. 2009;58(6): 772-778.

[43] DeGoma EM, French B, Dunbar RL, Allison MA, Mohler ER, 3rd, Budoff MJ. Intraindividual variability of C-reactive protein: the Multi-Ethnic Study of

Atherosclerosis. Atherosclerosis. 2012;224(1):274-279.

[44] Matthews KA, Sowers MF, Derby CA, Stein E, Miracle-McMahill H, Crawford SL, et al. Ethnic differences in cardiovascular risk factor burden among middle-aged women: Study of Women's Health Across the Nation (SWAN). Am Heart J. 2005;149(6):1066-1073.

[45] Jenny NS, Brown ER, Detrano R, Folsom AR, Saad MF, Shea S, et al. Associations of inflammatory markers with coronary artery calcification: results from the Multi-Ethnic Study of Atherosclerosis. Atherosclerosis. 2010;209(1):226-229.

[46] Knowles JW, Ashley EA. Cardiovascular disease: The rise of the genetic risk score. PLoS Med. 2018;15(3):e1002546.

[47] Wilson PW, D'Agostino RB, Levy D, Belanger AM, Silbershatz H, Kannel WB. Prediction of coronary heart disease using risk factor categories. Circulation. 1998;97(18):1837-1847.

[48] National Cholesterol Education Program (NCEP) Expert Panel on Detection E, and Treatment of High Blood Cholesterol in Adults (Adult Treatment Panel III). Third Report. Circulation. 2002;106(25):3143-421.

[49] Culleton BF, Larson MG, Kannel WB, Levy D. Serum uric acid and risk for cardiovascular disease and death: the Framingham Heart Study. Ann Intern Med. 1999;131(1):7-13.

[50] D'Agostino RB, Sr., Grundy S, Sullivan LM, Wilson P. Validation of the Framingham coronary heart disease prediction scores: results of a multiple ethnic groups investigation. Jama. 2001;286(2):180-187.

[51] D'Agostino RB, Sr., Vasan RS, Pencina MJ, Wolf PA, Cobain M, Massaro JM, et al. General cardiovascular risk profile for use in primary care: the Framingham Heart Study. Circulation. 2008;117(6):743-753.

[52] D'Agostino RB, Sr., Pencina MJ, Massaro JM, Coady S. Cardiovascular Disease Risk Assessment: Insights from Framingham. Glob Heart. 2013;8(1):11-23.

[53] Assmann G, Cullen P, Schulte H. Simple Scoring Scheme for Calculating the Risk of Acute Coronary Events Based on the 10-Year Follow-Up of the Prospective Cardiovascular Münster (PROCAM) Study. Circulation. 2002;105(3):310-315.

[54] Hippisley-Cox J, Coupland C, Vinogradova Y, Robson J, May M, Brindle P. Derivation and validation of QRISK, a new cardiovascular disease risk score for the United Kingdom: prospective open cohort study. BMJ. 2007;335(7611):136-.

[55] Hippisley-Cox J, Coupland C, Vinogradova Y, Robson J, Minhas R, Sheikh A, et al. Predicting cardiovascular risk in England and Wales: prospective derivation and validation of QRISK2. BMJ. 2008;336(7659):1475-1482.

[56] Ridker PM, Paynter NP, Rifai N, Gaziano JM, Cook NR. C-reactive protein and parental history improve global cardiovascular risk prediction: the Reynolds Risk Score for men. Circulation. 2008;118(22):2243-51, 4p following 51.

[57] Ridker PM, Buring JE, Rifai N, Cook NR. Development and validation of improved algorithms for the assessment of global cardiovascular risk in women: the Reynolds Risk Score. Jama. 2007;297(6):611-619.

[58] Yang X, Li J, Hu D, Chen J, Li Y, Huang J, et al. Predicting the 10-Year Risks of Atherosclerotic Cardiovascular

Disease in Chinese Population. Circulation. 2016;134(19):1430-1440.

[59] CAA NZ. CAA medical information sheet: cardiovascular risk. Wellington, New Zealand: Civil Aviation Authority of New Zealand. 2010.

[60] NZG G. The assessment and management of cardiovascular risk. Wellington: New Zealand Guideline Group. 2003.

[61] NZG G. New Zealand cardiovascular guidelines handbook: a summary resource for primary care practitioners, 2nd ed. Wellington: New Zealand Guideline Group. 2009.

[62] Wirawan IM, Larsen PD, Aldington S, Griffiths RF, Ellis CJ. Cardiovascular risk score and cardiovascular events among airline pilots: a case-control study. Aviat Space Environ Med. 2012;83(5):465-471.

[63] Nicol ED, Rienks R, Gray G, Guettler NJ, Manen O, Syburra T, et al. An introduction to aviation cardiology. Heart (British Cardiac Society). 2019;105(Suppl 1):s3-s8.

[64] Kochar M, Min JK. Physiologic assessment of coronary artery disease by cardiac computed tomography. Korean Circ J. 2013;43(7):435-442.

[65] Smith D, Toff W, Joy M, Dowdall N, Johnston R, Clark L, et al. Fitness to fly for passengers with cardiovascular disease. Heart. 2010;96 Suppl 2:ii1-16.

[66] ICAO. Manual of Civil Aviation Medicine. 3rd Edition. 2012.

[67] Conlon DLaHA. Cardiovascular Risk Factors in Airline Pilots. Workplace Health & Safety.vol. 66 ■ no. 10.

[68] Pagan LU, Gomes MJ, Okoshi MP. Endothelial Function and Physical Exercise. Arq Bras Cardiol. 2018;111(4): 540-541.

[69] Rodríguez-Monforte M, Flores-Mateo G, Barrio F, Costa B, Sánchez E. Metabolic syndrome and dietary patterns: a systematic review and meta-analysis of observational studies-reply. Eur J Nutr. 2019;58(8):3383-3386.

[70] Ruiz-Ramie JJ, Barber JL, Sarzynski MA. Effects of exercise on HDL functionality. Curr Opin Lipidol. 2019;30(1):16-23.

[71] Eckel RH, Jakicic JM, Ard JD, de Jesus JM, Houston Miller N, Hubbard VS, et al. 2013 AHA/ACC guideline on lifestyle management to reduce cardiovascular risk: a report of the American College of Cardiology/ American Heart Association Task Force on Practice Guidelines. Circulation. 2014;129(25 Suppl 2):S76-S99.

[72] Ezzati M, Riboli E. Behavioral and dietary risk factors for noncommunicable diseases. N Engl J Med. 2013;369(10):954-964.

[73] Zhao CN, Meng X, Li Y, Li S, Liu Q, Tang GY, et al. Fruits for Prevention and Treatment of Cardiovascular Diseases. Nutrients. 2017;9(6).

[74] Staruschenko A. Beneficial Effects of High Potassium. Hypertension. 2018;71(6):1015-1022.

[75] Vidal J. Updated review on the benefits of weight loss. Int J Obes Relat Metab Disord. 2002;26 Suppl 4:S25-S28.

[76] Coughlin JW, Brantley PJ, Champagne CM, Vollmer WM, Stevens VJ, Funk K, et al. The impact of continued intervention on weight: Five-year results from the weight loss maintenance trial. Obesity (Silver Spring). 2016;24(5):1046-1053.

[77] Brown JD, Buscemi J, Milsom V, Malcolm R, O'Neil PM. Effects on cardiovascular risk factors of weight

losses limited to 5-10. Transl Behav Med. 2016;6(3):339-346.

[78] Ahern AL, Aveyard PN, Halford JCG, Mander A, Cresswell L, Cohn SR, et al. Weight loss referrals for adults in primary care (WRAP): protocol for a multi-centre randomised controlled trial comparing the clinical and cost-effectiveness of primary care referral to a commercial weight loss provider for 12 weeks, referral for 52 weeks, and a brief self-help intervention [ISRCTN82857232]. BMC Public Health. 2014;14(1):620.

[79] Cadegiani FA, Diniz GC, Alves G. Aggressive clinical approach to obesity improves metabolic and clinical outcomes and can prevent bariatric surgery: a single center experience. BMC Obesity. 2017;4(1):9.

[80] Marmot M, Brunner E. Alcohol and cardiovascular disease: the status of the U shaped curve. BMJ. 1991;303(6802): 565-568.

[81] Klatsky AL. Alcohol and cardiovascular diseases: where do we stand today? J Intern Med. 2015;278(3):238-250.

[82] Ronksley PE, Brien SE, Turner BJ, Mukamal KJ, Ghali WA. Association of alcohol consumption with selected cardiovascular disease outcomes: a systematic review and meta-analysis. BMJ. 2011;342:d671.

[83] Holmes J, Beard E, Brown J, Brennan A, Meier PS, Michie S, et al. Effects on alcohol consumption of announcing and implementing revised UK low-risk drinking guidelines: findings from an interrupted time series analysis. Journal of Epidemiology and Community Health. 2020;74(11): 942-949.

[84] Williams B, Mancia G, Spiering W, Agabiti Rosei E, Azizi M, Burnier M, et al. 2018 ESC/ESH Guidelines for the management of arterial hypertension. Eur Heart J. 2018;39(33):3021-3104.

[85] Bhatnagar A, Payne TJ, Robertson RM. Is There A Role for Electronic Cigarettes in Tobacco Cessation? Journal of the American Heart Association. 2019;8(12):e012742.

[86] Kaul S. Evidence for the Universal Blood Pressure Goal of <130/80 mm Hg Is Strong. Hypertension. 2020;76(5): 1391-1399.

[87] Mosenzon O, Pollack R, Raz I. Treatment of Type 2 Diabetes: From "Guidelines" to "Position Statements" and Back. Recommendations of the Israel National Diabetes Council. 2016;39(Supplement 2):S146-S53.

[88] Rosenson RS, Hegele RA, Koenig W. Cholesterol-Lowering Agents. Circulation Research. 2019;124(3): 364-385.

[89] Sumaili EK, Krzesinski JM, Zinga CV, Cohen EP, Delanaye P, Munyanga SM, et al. Prevalence of chronic kidney disease in Kinshasa: results of a pilot study from the Democratic Republic of Congo. Nephrol Dial Transplant. 2009;24(1):117-122.

Chapter 5

Cardiovascular Risk Factors in Children

Mirjam Močnik and Nataša Marčun Varda

Abstract

Cardiovascular morbidity and mortality are still increasing in developed countries with emphasis on the obesity epidemic. Children and young adults are no exception. With modern lifestyle, traditional cardiovascular risk factors, such as hypertension, obesity, dyslipidemia, insulin resistance, kidney damage, are increasingly present in children leading to premature cardiovascular events in adult life. Cardiovascular risk factor can accelerate naturally progressing atherosclerosis, which should be prevented to facilitate quality and longevity of life. Primary and primordial prevention in the pediatric population are of utmost importance. However, if a cardiovascular risk factor is already present, frequent monitoring of possible development of other cardiovascular risk factors and evaluation of end organ damage should be implemented to intervene in time.

Keywords: atherosclerosis, obesity, hypertension, dyslipidemia, insulin resistance, kidney damage, prevention

1. Introduction

Atherosclerosis, a common denominator for all cardiovascular diseases (CVD), is a complex process that starts in fetal life, and its natural course is a result of interplay between genetic and environmental factors [1]. Clinical manifestations of atherosclerosis, including coronary artery disease, cerebrovascular disease and peripheral arterial disease, will occur in two thirds of men and half of women after age 40 [2]. However, a positive association of coronary atherosclerosis and atherosclerosis in abdominal aorta with classic cardiovascular risk factors, such as hypertension, obesity, dyslipidemia and impaired glucose tolerance, has been shown already in adolescents and young adults [3]. Earlier incidence of CVD in at-risk groups of children has been suggested [4].

In recent decades, the cardiovascular risk burden has increased largely due to the obesity epidemic, contributing to the fact that now CVD are globally the leading cause of death. Since 1975, prevalence of obesity more than quadrupled among children and adolescents with an increased likelihood of becoming an adult with obesity [5, 6].

In this chapter, traditional cardiovascular risk factors in children are reviewed with proposed comprehensive management.

2. Obesity

The obesity epidemic in children is a well-known fact in recent decades and still a growing issue in some countries that needs to be tackled accordingly. Adipose tissue, an active endocrine organ, is closely involved in production of atherogenic adipokines, oxidative stress and chronic inflammation, that altogether promote atherosclerosis. Therefore, the presence of obesity alone is a risk factor for CVD [7]. Mostly, it is due to sedentary lifestyle, inappropriate food habits and genetic susceptibility, and rarely a consequence of endocrine (e.g. hypothyroidism, Cushing syndrome, hypothalamic obesity, persistent hyperinsulinism, etc), syndromic (Alström, Bardet-Biedl, Prader Willi, Beckwith-Wiedemann, Carpenter, Cohen, Albright hereditary osteodystrophy, etc.) or monogenic causes (defects in genes encoding melanocortin 4 receptor (MC4R), leptin (LEP), leptin receptor (LEPR), pro-opiomelanocortin (POMC), etc.) [8].

Obesity and overweight diagnosis are based on anthropometric measurements and body mass index (BMI) calculation. Due to the growth and development there is no single cut-off point to define obesity in children, but is dependent on age and sex. Several curves that give BMI distribution as a function of age and sex have been established [8]. Body fat can also be estimated with dual energy X-ray absorptiometry, bioelectrical impedance, computed tomography and magnetic resonance imaging of abdomen, measurement of skinfold thickness at multiple sites, air displacement plethysmography and stable isotope dilution techniques, which apply to newer methods and future perspectives in obesity assessment [9]. Waist circumference is another anthropometric measurement that correlates well with obesity and is useful in determination of central obesity, correlating even more strongly with several obesity complications, such as insulin resistance, dyslipidemia and non-alcoholic fatty liver disease [10].

Complications of obesity in children and adolescents are numerous and are in part responsible for further cardiovascular damage. They can be categorized by organ systems: cardiovascular (hypertension, left ventricular hypertrophy, atherosclerosis), metabolic (insulin resistance, dyslipidemia, metabolic syndrome, type 2 diabetes), pulmonary (asthma, obstructive sleep apnea), gastrointestinal (non-alcoholic fatty liver disease, gastroesophageal reflux), skeletal (tibia vara, slipped capital-femoral epiphysis), psychological, other (polycystic ovary syndrome, pseudotumor cerebri) [11].

Lifestyle changes are the cornerstone of obesity management and are partly age dependent. Young infants up to two years of age with high body weight should have age appropriate amounts of formula, preferably should be breastfed, and should not be given sweetened beverages, fast food and desserts, should not have any screen of any kind, should have at least 12 hours of sleep a day, and should be allowed to be as active as possible. A toddler, aged from two to four, should have a balanced diet, should not be offered sugar sweetened beverages and fast food, size of the portion should be age appropriate and they should have a routine sleep pattern. Screen time should be kept to a minimum. It is important to stress that parents are role models for children and should model the eating behavior they want their child to have. A good meal hygiene with family based meals is recommended. Children, aged 5–9, should have a balanced diet with the exclusion of sweetened beverages and fast food, they should start to be involved in organized sports along with active play. At least sixty minutes of moderate physical activity is recommended. Screen time should be limited to academic requirements. With further growth and puberty, management evolves. Mostly, recommendations are similar, however, in adolescents skipping meals with overindulgence at the next meal or eating mostly in afternoon or evening can become an inappropriate habit leading to excess calories intake. Regular exercise routine of sixty to ninety minutes per day is recommended. With modern technologies, which in this age group are unavoidable, progress can be tracked and comparison can sometimes be encouraged between peers [12].

As parents are strong role models for children, especially younger, a family oriented approach with lifestyle changes for the whole family is recommended [12].

Pharmacological treatment of obesity in children is discouraged, however, a few studies with metformin and orlistat showed some success with weight loss, but small or none for cardio-metabolic complications [13].

3. Hypertension

Historically, hypertension was believed to be a rare disease in children, mostly due to secondary causes, however, in the past two decades, its prevalence increased significantly, mostly due to obesity, and was estimated from 4.3% among children aged 6 years to 3.3% among those aged 19 years and peaked at 7.9% among those aged 14 years [14].

In children, physiologically, blood pressure increases with age and body size, making it impossible to define a single blood pressure level to establish hypertension, as in adults. Therefore, the definition is based on the normal distribution of blood pressure in healthy children. Hypertension is defined as systolic or diastolic blood pressure above 95th percentile for sex, age and height measured on at least three separate occasions. High-normal blood pressure is defined as above 90th, but less than 95th percentile. For boys and girls, aged 16 or above, the definition is as in adults. In addition, reference values for sex, age and height of ambulatory blood pressure measurement have been obtained from different European populations and provide useful information for diagnosis and management of hypertension. The blood pressure cuff must be appropriate to the size of the child [15, 16].

Secondary hypertension is more frequent in the pediatric population, however, the prevalence varies between studies and has yet to be confirmed. The causes of secondary hypertension are numerous and should be sought for systematically depending on history, examination and clinical results. In brief, they are presented in **Table 1** [16]. Some syndromes, such as Williams's, Turner's and Leigh's, have also been associated with hypertension [16].

After a thorough diagnostic work-up, secondary causes need to be treated appropriately. If none can be established, the diagnosis of essential hypertension is confirmed. Usually, essential hypertension is present among older children with a strong family history of hypertension [16].

First-line treatment, especially in obese, is lifestyle intervention with salt restriction and weight loss. Pharmacological treatment is indicated in hypertensive children unresponsive to lifestyle modifications, as well as in children with symptomatic hypertension, secondary hypertension, target organ damage, diabetes mellitus or chronic kidney disease [17, 18]. Antihypertensive treatment is started with the lowest dose of a single drug and titrated if needed until maximum recommended dose is reached. If blood pressure is still elevated, the second drug can be added and up-titrated. The choice of particular antihypertensive drug is partly dependent on underlying etiology, partly on other relevant factors, such as end organ damage, concurrent disorders, side effects and clinician's preference [17, 18].

Etiology subgroup	Possible underlying etiology
Immunological	Systemic lupus erythematosus Juvenile ankylosing spondylitis Antineutrophil cytoplasmic antibodies-associated vasculitis
Cardiovascular	Coarctation of aorta Atrioventricular malformation Renal artery stenosis
Endocrine	Hypo- and hyperthyroidism Adrenal neuroblastoma
Gastrointestinal	Gastroschisis
Hematological	Sickle cell disease
Medications related	Steroids Central stimulants Adrenocorticotropic hormone
Neurological	Severe intraventricular hemorrhage Hydrocephalus Brain tumor Neural tube defect Arnold Chiari malformation
Renal	Hydronephrosis Nephrotic syndrome Glomerulonephritis Renal dysplasia Cystic renal disease
Respiratory	Bronchopulmonary dysplasia Chronic lung disease Sleep disordered breathing related (e.g. obstructive sleep apnea)

Table 1.
Causes of secondary hypertension in children.

4. Dyslipidemia

Dyslipidemia is a known risk factor for atherosclerosis and should be identified in youth to intervene in time and to reduce not only future CVD disease [19], but also arterial ischemic stroke in children, where dyslipidemia and hypertriglyceridemia were found to be more prevalent [20].

Commonly, lipid screening includes measurement of total cholesterol, high-density lipoprotein cholesterol (HDL), low-density lipoprotein cholesterol (LDL) and triglycerides. Additionally, several other lipoproteins, such as apolipoprotein A1 and B can be evaluated and provide further information on cardiovascular risk.

The prevalence of dyslipidemia is increasing due to increasing obesity, where almost in a half of children with obesity, a type of dyslipidemia (hypertriglyceridemia, lowered HDL, elevated LDL) is present [21]. School children, who are overweight, are 2.4 to 7.1 more likely to have elevated total cholesterol, LDL and triglycerides in comparison to lean peers [22].

Dyslipidemia in children can be a consequence of inherited dyslipidemia syndrome. Familial hypercholesterolemia, a monogenic, autosomal dominant disorder, is caused by mutations of LDL receptor or other protein that affects LDL receptor activity. Homozygous forms are rare, but are associated with rapidly progressive atherosclerosis leading to CVD and mortality in the first two decades of life. More commonly, heterozygous form is present with accelerated atherosclerosis and cardiovascular events before age of 50 years. These patients mostly have isolated elevation of LDL [19].

Familial combined hyperlipidemia is characterized by mixed dyslipidemia (LDL and triglycerides may be high or normal, HDL normal or reduced) with significant production of very low-density lipoprotein (VLDL) cholesterol and increased risk for CVD. It is less likely to be diagnosed in children, since significant elevations in fats may not occur until late adolescence, however apolipoprotein B levels may rise earlier and may be a better marker for this condition. In adults it is associated with features of metabolic syndrome and insulin resistance [19].

Rarely, severe hypertriglyceridemia may also be of genetic origin. Patients are likely to have a defect in lipoprotein lipase [19].

Some forms of secondary dyslipidemia (**Table 2**) are more frequent in children than in adults, and should be evaluated for [19].

Correction of secondary causes should normalize lipid levels, if there is no underlying genetic factor. Otherwise, the core management of dyslipidemia is lifestyle change with regular exercise, reduced screen time and diet. Dietary change should include total fat in less than 30% of daily caloric intake, with 8–10% saturated fat, avoidance of trans-fats and cholesterol intake less than 300 mg/day. This may be advanced to restriction of saturated fat less than 7% and cholesterol intake less than 200 mg/day if dyslipidemia persists. This level of restriction was found to be safe for growth and development. Water-soluble fiber and plant sterols may complement the diet. Patients with hypertriglyceridemia should also limit their sugar intake with replacement of simple sugars with complex carbohydrates and increase of omega-3 fatty acid intake [19, 23].

If lifestyle change over 6–12 months is unsuccessful, pharmacological treatment may be added. Statins were shown to be efficacious in children with familial hypercholesterolemia with a good safety profile. In children above 10 years of age,

Etiology subgroup	Possible underlying etiology
Endocrine/Metabolic	Diabetes - type 1, type 2 Hypothyroidism Polycystic ovarian syndrome Lipodystrophy Klinefelter syndrome Glycogen storage disease Gaucher disease Niemann-Pick disease
Cardiac	Kawasaki disease Orthotopic heart transplant
Rheumatological	Juvenile inflammatory arthritis Systemic lupus erythematosus
Gastrointestinal	Obstructive liver disease/other cholestatic conditions Alagille syndrome Biliary cirrhosis Hepatitis
Renal	Nephrotic syndrome Chronic renal disease Renal transplant
Medications/Exogenous	Glucocorticoids Isotretinoin Oral contraceptive therapy ß blockers Antipsychotics Alcohol

Table 2.
Causes of secondary dyslipidemia in children.

cholesterol absorption inhibitors may be added as adjunctive therapy. Bile acid sequestrants (cholestyramine, colestipol) also lower cholesterol level, but may have adverse gastrointestinal effects, such as gas, bloating, constipation and cramps, that limit their use and decrease compliance. Fibrates, niacin and orlistat lower triglyceride levels. For some genetic causes, novel treatment options are emerging, such as PCSK9 monoclonal antibody therapy [19, 23, 24].

5. Diabetes mellitus and insulin resistance

Diabetes is an additional cardiovascular risk factor that needs to be addressed in children. Historically, diabetes mellitus type 1 was considered of main importance in children. With increasing obesity, diabetes mellitus type 2 is becoming more prevalent [25]. Other etiologies, causing diabetes mellitus in children, are presented in **Table 3** [26].

Etiology subgroup	Possible underlying etiology
Type 1	Immune mediated Idiopathic
Type 2	
Other specific types	Genetic defects of ß-cell function Maturity onset diabetes of the young (MODY) Mitochondrial diabetes Genetic defects in insulin action Type a insulin resistance Leprechaunism Rabson-Mendenhall syndrome Lipoatrophic diabetes
Diseases of the exocrine pancreas	Cystic fibrosis Hemochromatosis Pancreatectomy
Endocrinopathies	Cushing syndrome Pheochromocytoma Hyperthyroidism
Medications or chemical induced	Glucocorticoids Diazoxide ß adrenergic agonists Pentamidine Nicotinic acid Interferon α Tacrolimus
Infections	Congenital rubella Cytomegalovirus
Uncommon forms of immune-mediated diabetes	"stiff-man" syndrome Anti-insulin receptor antibodies
Other genetic syndromes sometimes associated with diabetes	Down syndrome Turner syndrome Klinefelter syndrome Wolfram syndrome Friedreich ataxia Prader-Willi syndrome Bardet-Biedl syndrome Myotonic dystrophy

Table 3.
Causes of diabetes mellitus in children.

Regardless of the type of diabetes mellitus, hyperglycemia leads to impaired cardiovascular function, which was demonstrated in type 1 diabetes mellitus with impaired carotid artery structure and function, and decreased elastic properties of the aorta, already in children [27]. Diabetes mellitus is associated with a two-fold increase in the risk of CVD with a premature cardiovascular mortality and further risk increment when other cardiovascular risk factors coexist [28]. Early onset of diabetes mellitus further worsens cardiovascular risk [28].

Studies in the last decades indicate that insulin resistance is the predecessor of type 2 diabetes mellitus and has been associated with obesity, metabolic syndrome, hypertension and heart disease. It is defined as decreased tissue response to insulin and its cellular actions, commonly associated with obesity, however, not always, and not all obese have insulin resistance. Clinically, methods for insulin resistance measurement are scarce and, in many cases, limited to the research environment, however, one of the consequences of insulin resistance is chronic compensatory hyperinsulinemia, which can be demonstrated [29].

The diagnosis of both, diabetes mellitus and insulin resistance, is based on clinical symptoms, blood glucose monitoring, oral glucose tolerance test, and additional optional investigations, such as autoantibodies associated with diabetes or insulin levels [30]. In diabetes mellitus type 1 insulin therapy should be initiated immediately with recommendation of eventual insulin pump application in all small children, in patients with dawn phenomenon, severe hypoglycemia events or severe blood glucose fluctuations, glycated hemoglobin (HbA1c) values outside target range despite intensified conventional therapy, incipient microvascular or macrovascular secondary disease, limitations of the quality of life, in children with great fear of needles, pregnant adolescents and competitive athletes [30]. Treatment of type 2 diabetes mellitus and preceding insulin resistance is similar to treatment in adults. Weight loss and lifestyle change is the cornerstone of initial management. Patients may also be treated with oral agents, most appropriately starting with metformin, the only registered oral agent in children with diabetes mellitus type 2, and some may require administration of insulin to achieve glycemic control [31, 32].

6. Cardiovascular risk and kidney disease

The relationship between cardiovascular risk factors and chronic kidney disease is reciprocal: chronic kidney disease is a risk factor for CVD and cardiovascular damage accelerates kidney damage. Therefore, when we talk about vascular damage, we are really also talking about kidney damage and vice versa.

CVD is responsible for the majority of deaths in children with chronic kidney disease because of a high prevalence of traditional and uremia-related cardiovascular risk factors, with the highest risk in patients on dialysis. The cardiovascular alterations begin early in pediatric chronic kidney disease. Early markers of cardiac involvement, such as left ventricular hypertrophy and dysfunction, and early markers of atherosclerosis, such as increased carotid artery intima media thickness and increased arterial stiffness, are frequently present in children with chronic kidney disease [33, 34]. In children with early chronic kidney disease, before needing dialysis, modifiable cardiovascular risk factors should be identified and appropriate interventions should take place to decrease or delay premature CVD. Slowing down the progression of chronic kidney disease with avoidance of dialysis might be the best strategy to decrease cardiovascular risk [35].

7. Selected novel cardio-vascular risk factors

Diagnostic work-up should also include other cardiovascular risk factors that do not belong to the traditional ones that were described above. For example, urate is believed to be an independent indicator of arterial hypertension in children associated also with renal dysfunction [36]. Lipoprotein (a) is not associated with obesity, such as other lipoproteins, but is regarded as an independent cardiovascular risk factor and was found to be high in children with a family history of premature cardiovascular events [37]. Elevated levels of homocysteine were found in children with abdominal obesity [38], however a genetic hyperhomocysteinemia with mutations in methylenetetrahydrofolate reductase (MTHFR gene) was associated with stroke in children and in affected children with hyperhomocysteinemia and recurrent risk of stroke might be prevented with folate supplementation [39]. Vitamin D is frequently deficient in obese potentially leading to osteomalacia, and was additionally associated with insulin resistance and elevated blood pressure [40, 41]. Some studies even showed a higher risk of CVD and mortality when vitamin D was deficient, emphasizing the need for its supplementation [42].

To assess end-organ damage, kidney function, heart anatomy, and ocular background examination are commonly implemented, however, blood vessels, directly damaged by atherosclerosis, can be evaluated with intima media thickness and vessel elasticity evaluation. Intima media thickness is regarded as a subclinical indicator of atherosclerosis but has a lesser predictive value in children than in adults. There were several studies indicating an association between intima media thickness and obesity, familial hypercholesterolemia and hypertension in children, but sometimes associations were not clear cut and intra- and interoperable comparability raised doubts in the method [43]. Arterial stiffness can be commonly assessed with pulse wave velocity measurement that can be performed by several different methods, such as applanation tonometry. The higher the velocity of the pulse wave, the less compliant artery is expected, suggesting subclinical atherosclerosis. In children, several cardiovascular risk factors were associated with higher pulse wave velocity, however, the method is not in routine use [44].

8. Diagnostic work-up of cardiovascular risk factors in children

Cardiovascular complications, such as myocardial infarction and stroke, are rare in children, however, cardiovascular risk factors are increasing in prevalence, mostly due to worldwide increment of obesity. Preventive measures are most important in children and young adults, where the atherosclerotic process can be slowed down and possibly clinical manifestations of cardiovascular disease delayed [45].

Preventive measures can be individualized or population-based. The individualized approach includes active search of at-risk children during health check, who are more likely to develop premature CVD due to an underlying disease, inappropriate lifestyle or genetic disposition. Population-based approach includes interventions that affect the entire population aiming to lower cardiovascular risk in the whole population [45].

In pediatrics, we are most commonly involved in an individualized approach. Established recommendations in cardiovascular risk management in children involve two different goals: the prevention of risk-factor development and prevention of future CVD by effective management of identified risk factors. Therefore, several risk factors should be evaluated for, namely family history, diet, physical inactivity, tobacco exposure, blood pressure, lipid levels, overweight or obesity, diabetes mellitus, metabolic syndrome and perinatal factors [45].

Investigations	
Laboratory work-up	• Blood tests: complete blood count, electrolytes, kidney function and liver damage markers, lipidogram, apolipoprotein A1 and B, lipoprotein (a), urate, homocysteine, cystatin C, TSH, blood sugar, HbA1c, vitamin D • Urine tests: urinalysis, 24-hour urine sampling for proteinuria, albumin/creatinine in morning void sample • Optional investigations to exclude secondary causes
Imaging	• Abdominal ultrasound • Intima media thickness • Heart ultrasound • Ocular background examination • Optional investigations to exclude secondary causes
Functional diagnostics	• ECG • Ambulatory blood pressure measurement • Oral glucose tolerance test with insulin levels • Pulse wave velocity • Optional investigations to exclude secondary causes

Table 4.
Common investigations in children with cardiovascular risk; TSH—thyroid stimulating hormone, HbA1c—glycosylated hemoglobin, ECG—electrocardiogram.

The management of children with cardiovascular risk factors should be tailored to identify other possible cardiovascular risks, to evaluate end organ damage and to advise proper therapy. It starts with a good history with focus on family history and lifestyle. Next, clinical examination with anthropometric measurements with respect to percentile curves and blood pressure measurement should be performed. If blood pressure is elevated on multiple occasions, an ambulatory blood pressure measurement is recommended. Further work-up depends on history and examination and involves several laboratory, imaging and functional diagnostics, presented in **Table 4**.

In addition to above diagnostics, selected novel cardiovascular factors can be determined. Quite a few new diagnostic options to better define cardiovascular risk are on horizon, investigated in prospective studies, shortly presented in the next section.

9. Psychosocial aspect

Along with the management of classic cardiovascular risk factors, psychosocial aspects should also be evaluated. They can be partly responsible for disease development or can be a consequence of a chronic disease.

Early-life psychosocial factors that may influence cardiovascular health in adulthood include self-regulation (the ability to manage behavior, emotion, attention and social interactions), cognitive ability and aspects of home environment. They influence life-long health by facilitating education, problem solving, memory, communication, sense of control and ability to cope with stressful situations. Higher levels of psychosocial features were associated with greater likelihood of favorable cardiovascular state in adulthood with healthy levels of blood pressure, cholesterol, body mass index, cardiovascular-related medication status, smoking and blood sugar [46].

On the other hand, a chronic disease present in a child can have an important impact in a child's life and his or her family. Psychosocial issues are under-recognized, persist into adulthood and may impede optimal outcome. Children with chronic illness are at increased risk for mental health and adjustment problems. Child's adjustment depends mostly on the way the family copes with the child's condition. In young people, especially adolescents, underlying psychosocial issues can be suggested when new medical symptoms arise that cannot be explained by organic disease, when poor compliance to therapy is evident, when school refusal is present and when risky behavior involving excessive use of substances or excessive sexual behavior arises. These signs should alert the pediatrician to refer the patient to psychological treatment in time. Interventions are family-based, educational and are building on strengthening relationships and positive support [47].

Childhood obesity, a major contributor to CVD risk in modern society, can profoundly affect a child's social and emotional well-being and self-esteem. Obesity is associated with increased anxiety, body dissatisfaction and lower self-esteem. In obese, higher prevalence of eating disorder is present. In addition, obesity affects children's and adolescent's social and emotional health. Obese children are often bullied for their weight, excluded from activities, particularly physical, and face numerous negative stereotypes, discrimination and social marginalization, leading to further lower self-esteem, self-confidence, negative body image and negative effect to academic performance. The latter is in part due to chronic health-related conditions responsible for missing school [48].

10. Future perspectives

Despite numerous investigations and several cardiovascular risk factors evaluation, we still do not have a marker or investigation with prognostic value that would predict future CVD and premature cardiovascular events in children at risk. Several new biomarkers and investigations are emerging in research environment to assess cardiovascular risk, such as kidney injury molecule 1, adropin, salusin-α and -ß, uromodulin, markers of oxidative stress, along with functional diagnostics such as body composition measurement and elastography. Kidney injury molecule 1, a known marker for kidney tubular necrosis, was found elevated in overweight children [49]. Salusin-α and -ß are involved directly in the process of atherosclerosis with salusin-α slowing down and salusin-ß promoting atherosclerosis. In children, salusin-α correlated negatively with diastolic pressure [50, 51]. Adropin was discovered recently as a regulator of endothelial function among its several other physiological roles, such as angiogenesis, metabolism of glucose, fatty acids and dyslipidemia. Its role is protective and in overweight children lowered levels were found [52]. Uromodulin has an immunomodulatory role. In urine, it serves as a marker of kidney damage, however, in blood serum in elderly it was found to be a marker in CVD prognosis [53]. Children with diabetes had lower levels of serum uromodulin that correlated negatively with albuminuria [54]. Atherosclerosis, nowadays considered a chronic inflammatory process, is also being extensively researched through inflammatory markers and markers of oxidative stress, and some association with overweight in children has already been shown [55]. Very recently, microRNA is emerging as another possible diagnostic or therapeutic target that is being increasingly studied. Its postranslational function involves role in lipid metabolism, however, additional research, especially in children, is warranted [56], as for all other above mentioned biomarkers.

Along with fat mass evaluation, discussed in the second section, ultrasound and magnetic elastography are emerging as novel techniques for organ elasticity determination. The use of ultrasound elastography opens up a new spectrum of ultrasound applications - its use has spread in liver and tumor stiffness evaluation, and several new indications are emerging in the research environment [57]. In the context of cardiovascular risk assessment, liver elasticity could be evaluated in obesity to assess the degree of steatosis or fibrosis without invasive liver biopsy [58]. Ultrasound elastography might also non-invasively assess elastic properties of the kidney aiming to quantify intrarenal fibrosis that could contribute to the overall assessment of renal function [59]. In children, liver elastography has been successfully performed, however, other areas remain a subject of research. The predictive value of elastography in the context of cardiovascular risk has yet to be determined.

Cardiovascular risk factors are strongly affected by environmental factors and unhealthy lifestyle choices. However, some susceptibility is inherited and related to the cumulative effect of many common genetic variants. With the progress of genetic diagnostics, made in recent years, there is also a place for the research of genetic susceptibility and the role of genetic markers and their possible implementation in clinical praxis. Genome-wide association studies have been successful in identifying some associations of single nucleotide polymorphisms for coronary artery disease. It has been shown that some of the manifestations of coronary heart disease, such as calcification, ectasia and main-stem stenosis, are more strongly inherited than others. The results of genome-wide association studies are believed to aid in individual risk prediction for cardiovascular risk and events development by molecular biological methods [60, 61].

11. Conclusions

Cardiovascular diseases are the main cause of morbidity and mortality in the world and several cardiovascular risk factors contribute to this fact already in childhood. With the obesity epidemic, risk is multiplying for next generations, with expectation of further increase in cardiovascular diseases. The prevention, or at least a delay, represents a challenge for pediatricians, because if treated early, cardiovascular complications may be potentially reversible. Interventions should be initiated as soon as possible to avoid the development of potentially untreatable disease.

Conflict of interest

The authors declare no conflict of interest.

Author details

Mirjam Močnik[1*] and Nataša Marčun Varda[2]

1 Department of Paediatrics, University Medical Centre Maribor, Maribor, Slovenia

2 Department of Paediatrics, University Medical Centre Maribor and Medical Faculty, University of Maribor, Maribor, Slovenia

*Address all correspondence to: mirjammocnik91@gmail.com

IntechOpen

© 2021 The Author(s). Licensee IntechOpen. This chapter is distributed under the terms of the Creative Commons Attribution License (http://creativecommons.org/licenses/by/3.0), which permits unrestricted use, distribution, and reproduction in any medium, provided the original work is properly cited.

References

[1] Kelishadi R. Inflammation-induced atherosclerosis as a target for prevention of cardiovascular diseases from early life. Open Cardiovasc Med J. 2010;4:24-29. DOI: 10.2174/187419401004020024

[2] Robinson JG, Fox KM, Bullano MF, Grandy S; SHIELD Study Group. Atherosclerosis profile and incidence of cardiovascular events: a population-based survey. BMC Cardiovasc Disord. 2009;9:46. DOI: 10.1186/1471-2261-9-46

[3] McGill HC Jr, McMahan CA, Herderick EE, Malcom GT, Tracy RE, Strong JP. Origin of atherosclerosis in childhood and adolescence. Am J Clin Nutr. 2000;72(5 Suppl):1307S-1315S. DOI: 10.1093/ajcn/72.5.1307s

[4] Raghuveer G. Lifetime cardiovascular risk of childhood obesity. Am J Clin Nutr. 2010;91:1514S-1519S. DOI: 10.3945/acjn.2010.28701D

[5] World Health Organization. Obesity and overweight [Internet]. Available from: https://www.who.int/health-topics/obesity#tab=tab_1 [Accessed: 2021-05-08]

[6] World Health Organization. Global health estimates: life expectancy and leading causes of death and disability [Internet]. Available from: https://www.who.int/data/gho/data/themes/mortality-and-global-health-estimates [Accessed: 2021-05-08]

[7] Meyers MR, Gocke N. Endothelial dysfunction in obesity: etiological role in atherosclerosis. Curr Opin Endocrinol Diabetes Obes. 2007;14:365-369. DOI: 10.1097/MED.0b013e3282be90a8

[8] Aggarwal B, Jain V. Obesity in children: definition, etiology and approach. Indian J Pediatr. 2018:85:463-471. DOI: 10.1007/s12098-017-2531-x

[9] Wells JC, Fewtrell MS. Measuring body composition. Arch Dis Child. 2006;91:612-617. DOI: 10.1136/adc.2005.085522

[10] Qiao Q, Nyamdorj R. The optimal cut-off values and their performance of waist circumference and waist-to-hip ratio for diagnosing type II diabetes. Eur J Clin Nutr. 2010;64:23-29. DOI: 10.1038/ecjn.2009.92

[11] Daniels SR. Complications of obesity in children and adolescents. Int J Obes (Lond). 2009;33 Suppl:SS60-SS65. DOI: 10.1038/ijo.2009.20

[12] Cuda SE, Censani M. Pediatric obesity algorithm: a practical approach to obesity diagnosis and management. Front Pediatr. 2019;6:431. DOI: 10.3389/fped.2018.00431

[13] O'Connor EA, Evans CV, Burda BU, Walsh ES, Eder M, Lozano P. Screening for obesity and intervention for weight management in children and adolescents: evidence report and systematic review for the US Preventive Services Task Force. JAMA. 2017;317:2427-2444. DOI: 10.1001/jama.2017.0332

[14] Song P, Zhang Y, Yu J, Zha M, Zhu Y, Rahimi K, et al. Global prevalence of hypertension in children: a systematic review and meta-analysis. JAMA Pediatr. 2019;173:1154-1163. DOI: 10.1001/jamapediatrics.2019.3310

[15] Lurbe E, Agabiti-Rosei E, Cruickshank JK, Dominiczak A, Erdine S, Hirth A, et al. 2016 European Society of Hypertension guidelines for the management of high blood pressure in children and adolescents. J Hypertens. 2016;34:1887-1920. DOI: 10.1097/HJH. 0000000000001039

[16] Gupta-Malhotra M, Benker A, Shete S, Hashmi SS, Tyson JE,

Barratt MS, et al. Essential hypertension vs. secondary hypertension among children. Am J Hypertens. 2015;28:73-80. DOI: 10.1093/ajh/hpu083

[17] Burrello J, Erhardt EM, Saint-Hilary G, Veglio F, Rabbia F, Mulatero P, et al. Treatment of arterial hypertension in children and adolescents: a network meta-analysis. Hypertension. 2018;72:306-313. DOI: 10.1161/HYPERTENSIONAHA.118.10862

[18] Flynn JT, Kaelber DC, Baker-Smith CM, Blowey D, Carroll AE, et al. Clinical practice guideline for screening and management of high blood pressure in children and adolescents 2017;140:e20171904. DOI: 10.1542/peds.2017-1904

[19] Bamba V. Update on screening, etiology and treatment of dyslipidemia in children. J Clin Endocrinol Metabol. 2014;99:3093-3102. DOI: 10.1210/jc.2013-3860

[20] Sultan S, Dowling M, Kirton A, DeVeber G, Linds A, Elkind MSV; IPSS investigators. Dyslipidemia in children with arterial ischemic stroke: prevalence and risk factors. Pediatr Neurol. 2018;78:46-54. DOI: 10.1016/j.pediatrneurol.2017.09.019

[21] Elmaoğulları S, Tepe D, Uçaktürk SA, Karaca Kara F, Demirel F. Prevalence of dyslipidemia and associated factors in obese children and adolescents. J Clin Res Pediatr Endocrinol. 2015;7:228-234. DOI: 10.4274/jcrpe.1867

[22] Freedman DS, Dietz WH, Srinivasan SR, Berenson GS. The relation of overweight to cardiovascular risk factors among children and adolescents: the Bogalusa Heart Study. Pediatrics. 1990;103:1175-1182. DOI: 10.1542/peds.103.6.1175

[23] Yoon JM. Dyslipidemia in children and adolescents: when and how to diagnose and treat? Pediatr Gastroenterol Hepatol Nutr. 2014;17:85-92. DOI: 10.5223/pghn.2014.17.2.85

[24] Wong ND, Rosenblit PD, Greenfield RS. Advances in dyslipidemia management for prevention of atherosclerosis: PCSK9 monoclonal antibody therapy and beyond. Cardiovasc Diagn Ther. 2017;7(Suppl 1): S11-S20. DOI: 10.21037/cdt.2017.03.02

[25] Bhupathiraju SN, Hu FB. Epidemiology of obesity and diabetes and their cardiovascular complications. Circ Res. 2016;118:1723-1735. DOI: 10.1161/CIRCRESAHA.115.306825

[26] Botero D, Wolfsdorf JI. Diabetes mellitus in children and adolescents. Arch Med Res. 2005;36:281-290. DOI: 10.1016/j.arcmed.2004.12.002

[27] Stakos DA, Schuster DP, Sparks EA, Wooley CF, Osei K, Boudoulas H. Cardiovascular effects of type 1 diabetes mellitus in children. Angiology. 2005;56:311-317. DOI: 10.1177/000331970505600311

[28] Pastore I, Bolla AM, Montefusco L, Lunati ME, Rossi A, Assi E, et al. The impact of diabetes mellitus on cardiovascular risk onset in children and adolescents. Int J Mol Sci. 2020;21:4928. DOI: 10.3390/ijms21144928

[29] Levy-Marchal C, Arslanian S, Cutfield W, Sinaiko A, Druet C, Marcovecchio ML, et al. ESPE-LWPES-ISPAD-APPES-APEG-SLEP-JSPE; insulin resistance in children Consensus Conference Group. Insulin resistance in children: consensus, perspective, and future directions. J Clin Endocrinol Metab. 2010;95:5189-5198. DOI: 10.1210/jc.2010-1047

[30] Neu A, Bürger-Büsing J, Danne T, Dost A, Holder M, Holl RW, et al.

Diagnosis, therapy and follow-up of diabetes mellitus in children and adolescents. Exp Clin Endocrinol Diabetes. 2019;127(S 01):S39-S72. DOI: 10.1055/a-1018-8963

[31] Steinberger J, Daniels SR; American Heart Association Atherosclerosis, Hypertension, and Obesity in the Young Committee (Council on Cardiovascular Disease in the Young); American Heart Association Diabetes Committee (Council on Nutrition, Physical Activity, and Metabolism). Obesity, insulin resistance, diabetes, and cardiovascular risk in children: an American Heart Association scientific statement from the Atherosclerosis Hypertension, and the Diabetes Committee (Council on Nutrition, Physical Activity, and Metabolism). Circulation. 2003;107:1448-1453. DOI: 10.1161/01.cir.0000060923.07573.f2

[32] Zeitler P, Arslanian S, Fu J, Pinhas-Hamiel O, Reinehr T, Tandon N, et al. ISPAD Clinical Practice Consensus Guidelines 2018: Type 2 diabetes mellitus in youth. Pediatr Diabetes. 2018; 19 Suppl 27:28-46. DOI: 10.1111/pedi.12719

[33] Weaver DJ, Mitsnefes M. Cardiovascular disease in children and adolescents with chronic kidney disease. Semin Nephrol. 2018;38:559-569. DOI: 10.1016/j.semnephrol.2018.08.002

[34] Schroff R, Dégi A, Kerti A, Kis E, Cseprekál O, Tory K, et al. Cardiovascular risk assessment in children with chronic kidney disease. Pediatr Nephrol. 2013;28:875-884. DOI: 10.1007/s00467-012-2325-3

[35] Mitsnefes MM. Cardiovascular disease in children with chronic kidney disease. J Am Soc Nephrol. 2012;23:578-585. DOI: 10.1681/ASN.2011111115

[36] Noone DG, Marks SD. Hyperuricemia is associated with hypertension, obesity, and albuminuria in children with chronic kidney disease. J Pediatr. 2013;162:128-132. DOI: 10.1016/j.jpeds.2012.06.008

[37] Glowinska B, Urban M, Koput A. Cardiovascular risk factors in children with obesity, hypertension and diabetes: lipoprotein(a) levels and body mass index correlate with family history of cardiovascular disease. Eur J Pediatr. 2002;161:511-518. DOI: 10.1007/s00431-002-1040-7

[38] Zhu W, Huang X, Li M, Neubauer H. Elevated plasma homocysteine in obese schoolchildren with early atherosclerosis. Eur J Pediatr. 2006;165:326-331. DOI: 10.1007/s00431-005-0033-8

[39] Cardo E, Monrós C, Artuch R, Campistol J, Pineda M, Vilaseca MA. Children with stroke: polymorphism of the MTHFR gene, mildy hyperhomocysteinemia and vitamin status. J Child Neurol. 2000;15:295-298. DOI: 10.1177/088307380001500505

[40] Gul A, Ozer S, Yilmaz R, Sonmezgoz E, Kasap T, Takcl S, et al. Association between vitamin D levels and cardiovascular risk factors in obese children and adolescents. Nutr Hosp. 2017;34:323-329. DOI: 10.20960/nh.412

[41] Liang X, Chen M, Qu P, Hao G, Huang Y, Chen J, et al. The association of vitamin A and vitamin D with hypertension in children: a case-control study. Int J Hypertens. 2018;9295147. DOI: 10.1155/2018/9295147

[42] Savastio S, Pozzi E, Tagliaferri F, Degrandi R, Cinquatti R, Rabbone I, et al. Vitamin D and cardiovascular risk: which implications in children? Int J Mol Sci. 2020;21:3536. DOI: 10.3390/ijms21103536

[43] Litwin M, Niemirska A. Intima-media thickness measurements in

children with cardiovascular risk factors. Pediatr Nephrol. 2009;24:707-719. DOI: 10.1007/s00467-008-0962-3

[44] Stoner L, Kucharska-Newton A, Meyer ML. Cardiometabolic health and carotid-femoral pulse wave velocity in children: a systematic review and meta-regression. J. Pediatr. 2020;218:98-105.e3. DOI: 10.1016/j.jpeds.2019.10.065

[45] Expert Panel on Integrated Guidelines for Cardiovascular Health and Risk Reduction in Children and Adolescents; National Heart, Lung, and Blood Institute. Expert panel on integrated guidelines for cardiovascular health and risk reduction in children and adolescents: summary report. Pediatrics. 2011;;128(Suppl 5): S213-S256. DOI: 10.1542/peds.2009-2107C

[46] Appleton AA, Buka SL, Loucks EB, Rimm EB, Martin LT, Kubzansky LD. A prospective study of positive early-life psychosocial factors and favorable cardiovascular risk in adulthood. Circulation. 2013;127:905-912. DOI: 10.1161/CIRCULATIONAHA.112.115782

[47] Geist R, Grdisa V, Otley A. Psychosocial issues in the child with chronic conditions. Best Pract Res Clin Gastroenterol. 2003;17:141-152. DOI: 10.1016/s1521-6918(02)00142-7

[48] Sahoo J, Sahoo B, Choudhury AK, Sofi NY, Kumar R, Bhadoria AS. Childhood obesity: causes and consequences. J Family Med Prim Care. 2015;4:187-192. DOI: 10.4103/2249-4863.154628

[49] Goknar N, Oktem F, Ozgen IT, Torun E, Kuçukkoc M, Demir AD, et al. Determination of early urinary renal injury markers in obese children. Pediatr Nephrol. 2015;30:139-144. DOI: 10.1007/s00467-014-2829-0

[50] Alpsoy S, Dogan B, Ozkaramanli Gur D, Akyüz A, Fidan Ç, Guzel S, et al. Assessment of salusin alpha and salusin beta levels in patients with newly diagnosed dipper and non-dipper hypertension. Clin Exp Hypertens. 2021;43:42-48. DOI: 10.1080/10641963.2020.1797086

[51] Dervişoğlu P, Elmas B, Kösecik M, Işgüven ŞP, Büyükavci M, Köroğlu M. Salusin-α levels are negatively correlated with diastolic blood pressure in children with obesity. Cardiol Young. 2019;29:1225-1229. DOI: 10.1017/S1047951119001173

[52] Altincik A, Sayin O. Evaluation of the relationship between serum adropin levels and blood pressure in obese children. J Pediatr Endocrinol Meba. 2015;28:1095-1100. DOI: 10.1515/jpem-2015-0051

[53] Leiherer A, Muendlein A, Saely CH, Ebner J, Brandtner EM, Fraunberger P, et al. Serum uromodulin is a predictive biomarker for cardiovascular events and overall mortality in coronary patients. Int J Cardiol. 2017;231:6-12. DOI: 10.1016/j.ijcard.2016.12.183

[54] Wiromat P, Bjornstad P, Roncal C, Pyle L, Johnson RJ, Cherney DZ, et al. Serum uromodulin is associated with urinary albumin excretion in adolescents with type 1 diabetes. J Diabetes Complications. 2019;33: 648-650. DOI: 10.1016/j.jdiacomp.2019.05.023

[55] Kilic E, Özer ÖF, Erek Toprak A, Erman H, Torun E, Kesgin Ayhan S, et al. Oxidative stress status in childhood obesity: a potential risk predictor. Med Sci Monit. 2016;22:3673-3679. DOI: 10.12659/msm.897965

[56] Barwari T, Joshi A, Mayr M. MicroRNAs in cardiovascular disease. J Am Coll Cardiol. 2016;68:2577-2584. DOI: 10.1016/j.jacc.2016.09.945

[57] Sigrist RMS, Liau J, Kaffas AE, Chammas MC, Willmann JK.

Ultrasound elastography: review of techniques and clinical applications. Theranostics. 2017;7:1303-1329. DOI: 10.7150/thno.18650

[58] Yoneda M, Suzuki K, Kato S, Fujita K, Nozaki Y, Hosono K, et al. Nonalcoholic fatty liver disease: US-based acoustic radiation force impulse elastography. Radiology. 2010;256:640-647. DOI: 10.1148/radiol.10091662

[59] Grenier N, Gennisson JL, Cornelis F, Le Bras Y, Couzi L. Renal ultrasound elastography. Diagn Interv Imaging. 2013;94:545-550. DOI: 10.1016/j.diii.2013.02.003

[60] Gullace G, Khalaf H. Preclinical diagnosis and risk assessment of atherosclerosis - at birth? At event? When is best? Eur Cardiol. 2011;7:164-166. DOI:10.15420/ecr.2011.7.3.164

[61] Khera AV, Chaffin M, Wade KH, Zahid S, Brancale J, Xia R, et al. Polygenic prediction of weight and obesity trajectories from birth to adulthood. Cell. 2019;177:587-596. DOI: 10.1016/j.cell.2019.03.028

Section 2

Miscellaneous

Chapter 6

Role of Arterial Pressure, Wall Stiffness, Pulse Pressure and Waveform in Arterial Wall Stress/Strain and Its Clinical Implications

Thomas K. Day

Abstract

Biomechanical stress applied to the intima of arteries has long been suspected as a factor in the initiation and localisation of atherosclerotic plaque, and it is implicated in the separation of plaque from the underlying arterial wall giving rise to the acute clinical consequences of thrombosis, dissection and embolism. The factors underlying transmural stress were investigated *in-vitro* using fresh porcine abdominal aortas on an experimental rig in which pulse pressure, pulse waveform, fluid viscosity, pulse rate, vessel wall compliance and systolic and diastolic blood pressure could be varied at will. Vessel wall compliance was progressively reduced by exposure of the artery to formaldehyde vapour for increased periods of time, a saline-treated artery being used as control. Centripetal transmural stress (CTS) and strain were studied by direct observation of the displacement of a compliant false intima (FI) using real-time B and M mode ultrasound, and by measuring the differential pressure between the space beneath the FI and the adjacent vessel lumen. CTS was found to be directly related to pulse pressure ($r = 0.907$, $p < 0.001$) and inversely related to vessel wall compliance. It was independently affected by ranked peak pressure waveform ($R = 0.93$, $p < 0.01$) being higher with sharp peak pressure and lower when the waveform was rounded, and it peaked in early diastole in untreated vessels, and both in diastole and peak systole in ones stiffened by formaldehyde vapour. Mean arterial pressure exerted a profound effect via its effect on vessel wall stiffness, which was found to rise 7-fold across the mean arterial pressure range 50-130 mmHg and continued to increase in a logarithmic fashion as the upper physiological range of mean arterial pressure was exceeded. There are two potential clinical implications: in mitigating the postulated biomechanical aspects atherogenesis and atherosclerotic plaque detachment, maintaining large vessel wall compliance is important, and the main factor determining this in a healthy artery is mean arterial pressure; if the arterial wall has already become stiffened as a result of disease, and in the absence of critical stenosis, the findings suggest that the appropriate therapeutic targets are modification of pulse pressure and pulse waveform profile. Simply reducing the diastolic pressure in elderly patients may be unwise if the result is a widened pulse pressure and increased transmural strain. The distribution of atheroma at points of focal mechanical strain in the vessel wall may be explicable if the stress induced by an excessive pulse pressure provokes the inflammatory changes seen in repetitive strain injury. Investigation of inflammatory signalling in the vessel wall provoked by repeated mechanical stress may represent a productive area for future research.

Keywords: atherosclerosis, hypertension, arterial wall elasticity, pulse waveform, mechano-sensitivity

1. Introduction

The central role of biomechanics in the pathogenesis of atheroma is supported by a body of circumstantial evidence [1]: atherosclerotic plaque is not laid down uniformly on the inner lining of arteries but at the junctions of branch vessels, at points where the external wall of the artery is fixed to surrounding structures and at kinks and bends where mechanical strain and flow turbulence occur. It is susceptible to the effects of blood pressure [2]. It is not seen in veins except when these are used as arterial grafts [3]. Blood pressure is a well-established risk factor for coronary artery disease [4]. Atherosclerosis occurs prematurely in situations where arterial wall stiffness is increased such as diabetes, pseudoxanthoma elasticum and progeria syndromes [5–7]. Blood viscosity, which contributes to the transmission of shear strain to the endothelium, is an independent risk factor for ischaemic heart disease [8]. Lastly, experimental and computer modelling studies have demonstrated an association between atherosclerosis-prone areas of the arterial tree and conditions of local blood flow characterised by high strain-low shear, and oscillatory reverse flow [9, 10].

There are two postulated mechanisms whereby such mechanical strain acting on the inner arterial wall might give rise to the development of atherosclerosis and explain its focal localisation within the arterial tree: firstly, the endothelium might be damaged directly by forces stripping it from the underlying intima or causing ultrastructural changes to the intercellular junctions thus exposing the underlying collagen network of the intima to blood components giving rise to collagen-platelet and collagen-fibrin interactions and the development of plaque according to the incrustation theory of atherogenesis. Such endothelial damage has been shown to give rise to atheroma-like lesions in experimental animals [11], and the attachment of the endothelium to underlying collagen is less strong in animals that are atheroma-prone compared to those that are resistant [12]. Direct mechanical damage to the endothelium would tend to occur at sites where there was maximum lifting and shear stress and this might explain its focal distribution. Secondly, endothelial cells are highly mechano-sensitive and certain conditions of shear stress and pulse waveform have been shown to provoke a stress response in endothelial cells favouring platelet and white cell adherence, translocation of white cells and expression of inflammatory mediators, processes that have been linked to the development of atherosclerosis [10, 13–16].

Experiments related to this latter mechanism have hitherto concentrated on the effect of shear stress, which may be likened to the aerodynamic equivalent of drag acting on the endothelial surface. Little work by contrast has been done on the inward "lift" effect in inducing stress acting at right angles to the endothelial surface, tending to lift the endothelium off the underlying substrate, and inducing conformational change on the inner wall of the artery. Conformational change in the inner arterial wall resulting from this lifting effect would tend to give rise to the boundary layer separation and local oscillatory flow reversal at low flow rate that appear to induce a pro-atherogenic endothelial cell phenotype in the tissue culture experiments [10, 15, 16].

The study of the factors affecting the inward stress/strain relationship to the arterial wall is consequently of interest both in relation to the initial development of atherosclerosis but also in relation to the stresses causing the developed atherosclerotic plaque to separate and thus cause clinical harm.

The aim of the present work was to examine directly the factors giving rise to transmural stress/strain and to their possible interactions. A bench-based test rig was employed similar to that described by Giussaniani et al. [17] modified to provide continuous pulsatile flow within fresh pig arteries.

2. Materials, methods

2.1 Arteries

Abdominal aortas from freshly slaughtered young white pigs were obtained from an abbattoir conforming to European animal welfare standards (EC Regulation 1099/2009) and were transported at 4°C Ringer's lactate solution. The average length of the test segment was 120 mm (SD 5 mm), the internal diameter of the proximal end 18.1 mm (SD+/− 0.54) and that of the distal end 13.8 mm (SD+/−2.7).

In each artery adherent loose areolar-lymphatic tissue was removed whist preserving the adventitia and all side branches were ligated at their origins with 2/0 silk whilst keeping the artery moist and cool in Ringers-lactate solution. The segments of artery used extended from the coeliac trunk to the aortic bifurcation.

For studies on the stress strain relationship across the intima in pulsatile flow conditions a fluid-filled 0.9 mm polythene saline-filled catheter was introduced through a side branch and secured by a ligature. The tip of the catheter was positioned near the midpoint of the test artery, this point being marked on the exterior wall of the artery using Gentian Violet to facilitate the subsequent positioning of the ultrasound probe. During each test run this catheter was perfused at 0.1 ml/hr. with saline using a syringe pump. Once the catheter was in position a thin deformable latex membrane (Préservatif classique, PHR Lab, Boulogne Billancourt, Fr) was introduced along the full length of the arterial lumen. The membrane overlapped the ends and was smoothed against the internal wall of the artery by filling the lumen with saline. This membrane was intended to take the role of a deformable FI. **Figure 1** shows the appearance of the lined artery and the movement of the FI in relation to the wall on B-mode ultrasound when the artery is subjected to pulsatile flow under test conditions. The presence of this lining membrane also had the advantage of preventing minor leaks. The specimen, consisting of the artery and the FI, was then mounted in the test bath illustrated in **Figure 2**, being secured over the tube at either end by sliding it over two O- rings positioned on the mounting tube and holding it between the rings with a double turn of a 4 mm Silastic sling.

The artery was rotated until the catheter tip lay inferiorly, directly opposite the ultrasound probe. The tubes upon which the artery was mounted were then slid far enough apart for the artery to be lie in a relaxed straight line, not under tension. The bath was filled with oxygenated Ringer's lactate at 37°C, up to but not over the top of the uppermost wall of the artery. Contact jelly was applied and the ultrasound probe set up over the tip of the catheter so as to give a view of the artery an the membrane in transverse section. The probe was held in a clamp in contact with the superior wall of the artery but not pressing sufficiently to deform it.

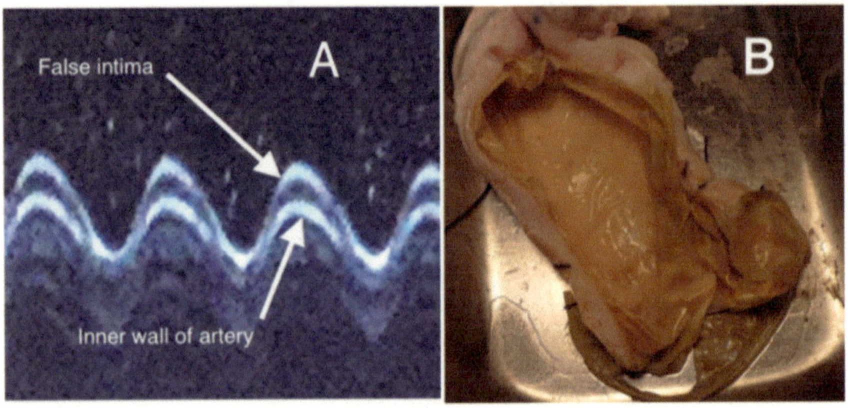

Figure 1.
A. The movement in B-mode ultrasound of the posterior wall of the artery and the false intima (FI) subjected to a pulse pressure of 60 mmHg and a peak pressure wave of an intermediate level of sharpness. B. The thin latex false intima lining the opened test artery; the perfused catheter is placed between the FI and the inner arterial wall to measure the differential pressure between this space and the adjacent arterial lumen.

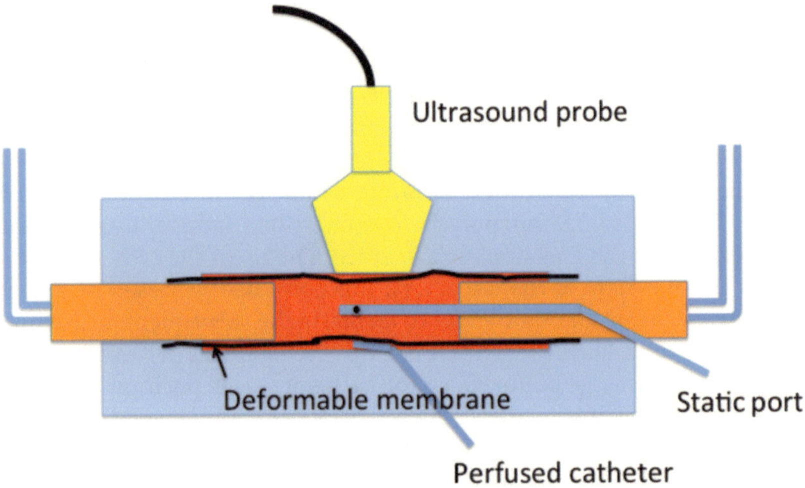

Figure 2.
The artery in its test bath. The stress imposed on the FI throughout the pressure cycle is observed by recording the differential pressure between the perfused catheter and the adjacent lumen, whilst the strain response of the FI to the passage of the pulse wave is observed using M-mode ultrasound.

2.2 Perfusion apparatus

The arteries were perfused with isotonic saline or sucrose/saline solutions with sucrose concentration adjusted to provide a range of viscosities using the apparatus shown in **Figure 3**. The perfusate was circulated from a 1 L reservoir by a centrifugal pump, forming a primary circuit by which an adjustable head of pressure could be obtained through adjustment of the return circuit valve. This circuit was tapped through a side branch to form a secondary circuit by means of which the test artery was perfused. This circuit circulated fluid at the established head of pressure through the test artery then back to the reservoir via a barostatic valve and flow meter. Pulsatile flow was imposed on the fluid by a 60 ml glass syringe pump which was operated by means of a series of cams of different profiles turned by a geared and governed slow speed electric motor. These cams were designed to reduplicate a variety of human aortic waveforms [18]. Eight cams were manufactured to deliver stroke volumes between 8 and 32mls.

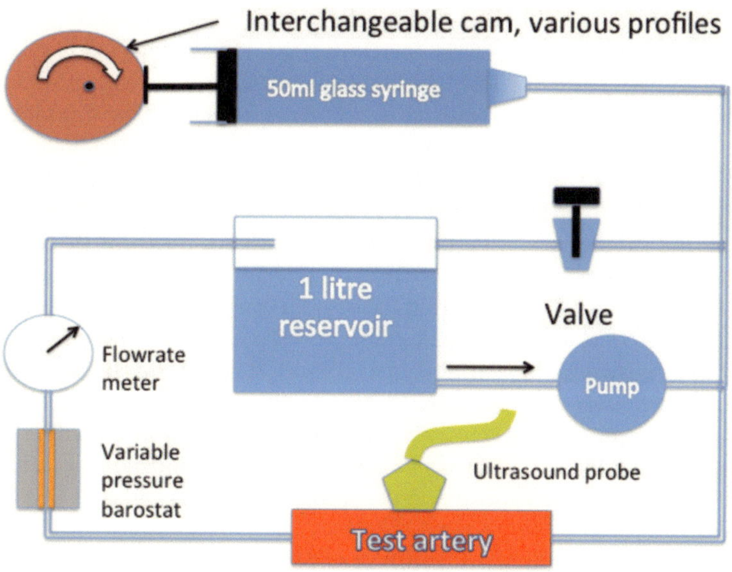

Figure 3.
Perfusion apparatus.

Arterial pressure and pulse pressure wave profile were recorded via side tap taken off the upstream side of the inflow tube enabling differential pressure to be measured between the arterial lumen and the water bath adjacent to the artery at the same level (the arterial pressure). CTS was measured by recording the differential pressure between the perfused catheter in the sub-membrane space and a static port in the adjacent arterial lumen. These two differential pressures were measured using Honeywell 24PCBPFAD transducers calibrated using a mercury manometer, and recorded simultaneously using a dual channel Thornton 464 (Waltham, Ma) chart recorder.

The deformation of the arterial wall in response to pressure change and the displacement of the FI during pulsatile flow was observed during different phases of the pressure cycle using a linear 7.5Mhz ultrasound probe, by means of which the transverse section artery, its wall and the FI could be visualised using split B and M-mode ultrasound, **Figure 1**. Care was taken to ensure that the artery itself and the catheters and tubes connected to the differential pressure transducers were free of bubbles.

2.3 Variables

2.3.1 Static observations, non-pulsatile flow

Observations on the effects of non-pulsatile arterial pressure on arterial wall diameter and thickness were made using the experimental apparatus described above omitting the perfused cannula beneath the FI. Pressure was raised in a stepwise fashion using the barostatic valve, having closed the primary return circuit valve, and measurements of the artery made in cross section using B mode ultrasound.

2.3.2 Direct and derived variables, pulsatile flow

The perfusion apparatus allowed one group of variables to be adjusted and controlled directly whilst the other parameters were held at set levels. These direct variables were: pulse rate, baseline ("diastolic") pressure, cam profile, outflow resistance and arterial wall stiffness. Outflow resistance was a directly set value achieved by adjusting the outflow barostat to a specific pressure in relation to flow. Fluid viscosity was adjusted by alternating saline as a perfusate with a viscosity of 1 mPa.s for sucrose/saline solutions at concentrations of 10, 20 and 30% providing a range of viscosities at 15 deg. C from 1.4 to 3.9 mPa.s [19]. Arterial wall stiffness was adjusted by exposing the test artery to formaldehyde vapour for periods up to 48 hours whilst another artery kept in Ringer's lactate for the same period acted as a control. The degree of increase in stiffness produced by formadelhyde exposure is similar in order of magnitude to that reported in post-mortem studies of athero-sclerotic human aortas [20] and to the effects of hypertension in the test vessels. The effect of altering a single variable on CTS and FI could thus be studied, and this was done so within series of individual arteries where the other parameters could be maintained at set levels. In this way, for example, the effect of changing the pulse rate on NS and false intima separation under different conditions of diastolic and systolic pressure and fluid viscosity could be explored in artery with an established elastic properties.

Changing the cams for ones of different stroke volume and profile created two derived variables, waveform and pulse pressure. Pulse pressure showed a direct physical link to CTS with some variation between cam profiles which was dependent on the shape of the pressure wave. In exploring this, different cams were used to alter the shape of the pressure wave and a schedule of machine settings worked through (**Table 1**) to harvest groups of identical pulse pressure for comparison of the effects of waveform and vice versa. In comparison of the effect of pulse pressure on CTS independent of waveform, peak waveform shape was ranked according to the area under each peak within 40 mmHg of peak pressure. The total number of pressure waves of equivalent peak sharpness thus harvested was 122 and the number of identical pulse pressures (tested at different pulse rates and baseline pressures) was 186. The schedule of machine settings permitted the independent effects of baseline pressure, pulse rate and viscosity to be studied whilst the other variables were kept constant (**Table 1**).

2.3.3 Measurement of hoop stress modulus

For the direct measurement of hoop stress elastic modulus, strips 10 mm in width were cut from the proximal end of each test aorta using a guillotine-guide which compressed and held the artery between two plates of Perspex provided with cutting slots, and measurement of stress/strain relationships was undertaken at stresses of between 0 and 100mN/mm^2 at 0.2 N intervals using the tensiometer device illustrated in **Figure 4**. Either end of each hoop was firmly held between two aluminium blocks lined with fine sandpaper that were screwed together and then

Pulse rate and test intervals bpm	Baseline pressure and test intervals mmHg	Cam no.	Viscosity mPa.s	Arterial wall stiffness Kpa	Derived Peak waveform sharpness	Derived upsweep velocity	Derived pulse pressure	CTS
40–180 (20)	40–160 (20)	1–8	1–3	400-7000	Ranked according to area below peak	Ranked according to gradient	Measured directly	Measured directly

Table 1.
Range of machine settings and direct and derived variables measured.

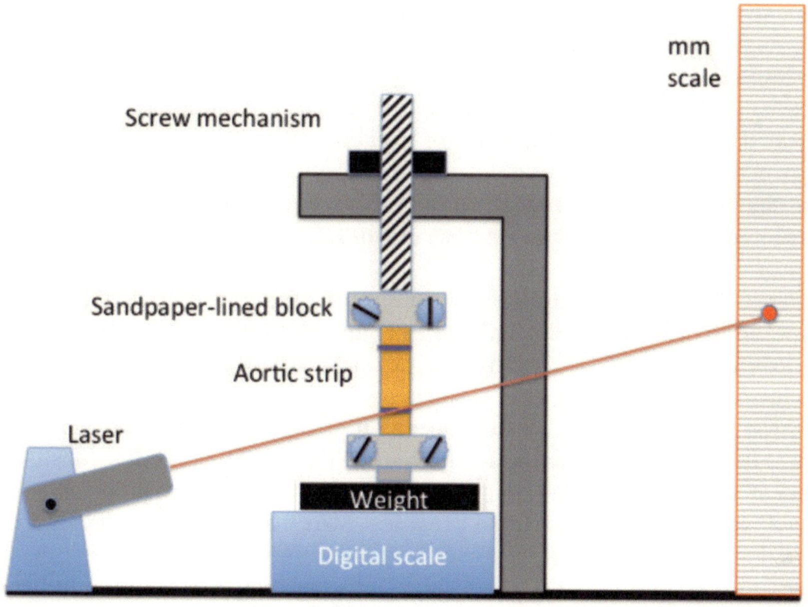

Figure 4.
Tensiometer apparatus for measurement of stress/strain relationship of aortic hoop strips.

attached with magnets to the tensiometer once the hoop strip was mounted. Two points about 4 cm apart were marked at the upper and lower extremity of each hoop with Gentian Violet and the laser was then used to project the relative position of these marks onto a scale as the progressive loads were applied. The average cross sectional area of each hoop was calculated by measuring the width and thickness of the arterial strip with a micrometer at three positions in the middle and at the junction of the central and upper and lower thirds at the beginning and end of each test, and taking the mean.

2.4 Statistics

Pearson's correlation was used for parametric variables and Spearman's ranking coefficient for the non-parametric relationship between sharpness of the peak pressure wave and DP. 95% confidence limits are shown in **Figure 4**. For the purpose of transposing hoop stress measurements into equivalent lumenal pressures the artery was treated as a thin walled cylinder and the relationship between the tension in the wall and the corresponding internal arterial pressure was derived mathematically from the formula: Pressure equivalent (mmHg) = 47 x Hoop stress (KPa) x t/d, where t/d is the thickness to diameter ratio.

3. Results

3.1 Elastic response of the arterial wall to changes in arterial pressure

In both pulsatile and non-pulsatile flow the arterial wall showed a 3-phase elastic response to rising arterial pressure (see figures below). In the first phase, corresponding to sub-physiological pressure, the artery is relatively flaccid and distends easily with no thinning. In the second phase, corresponding to the normal physiological range of pressure, the stress/strain relationship is almost linear and over this linear segment Young's modulus can be calculate at about 400–600 KPa and the wall begins to thin. As the pressure increases beyond the physiological range there is a marked loss of compliance with an 8 to 10 fold increase in Young's modulus. In this last phase the arterial wall thins to its minimum. **Figure 5** shows the proportional change in inner wall diameter and wall thickness of pig abdominal aortas (n = 5) subjected to stepwise changes in static (non-pulsatile) pressure over the range 0 – 250 mmHg.

The character of this 3-phase response to rises and fall in intralumenal pressure was explored using arterial hoop strips cut from the proximal end of the abdominal aortic segment.

Figure 6 illustrates how Young's modulus measured in this way rises steeply once the upper limit of the physiological range of pressure is exceeded. The implications of this loss of wall compliance with rising arterial pressure are seen once pulsatile flow is introduced (**Figure 7**).

In the studies using pulsatile flow over a range of arterial diastolic and systolic pressures induced by varying the stroke volume load and the baseline diastolic pressure at a constant outflow resistance, a similar negative correlation was observed between the mean arterial pressure (MAP) and arterial wall compliance expressed as the proportional increase in cross-section per mm Hg pressure change (Spearman's R = −0.74, $p < 0.001$). **Figure 7** is a semi-log plot of the compliance versus MAP using 11 runs at different pressure settings in a single fresh pig abdominal aorta. The fall in arterial wall compliance with increased MAP follows the same three-phase response as that shown in **Figures 5** and **6**. As MAP approaches the upper limit of the physiological range there is a logarithmic reduction in compliance as the artery enters the third phase of stress/strain relationship and this is associated with corresponding rise in the pulse pressure, CTS, FI separation and the sharpness of the pressure peak.

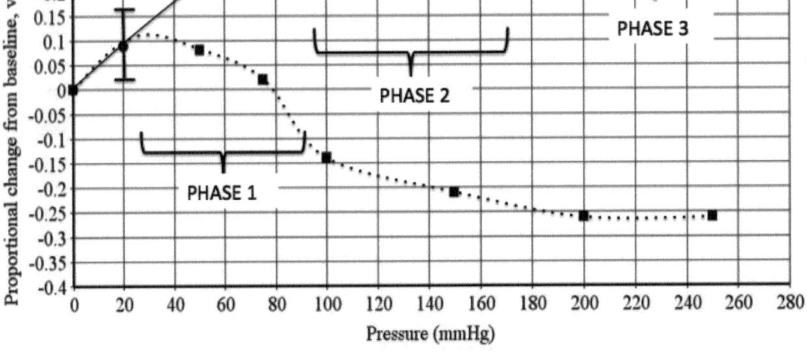

Figure 5.
*3-phase elastic response of the arterial wall to rising static pressure (non-pulsatile flow), n = 5 +/− SEM. Throughout the physiological range of pressure the arterial diameter increases in response to rising pressure and the wall thins; at the upper limit of pressure the arterial diameter reaches an elastic limit and the wall its minimum thickness. A similar 3-phase stiffening of the arterial wall in response to mean arterial pressure is seen under conditions of pulsatile flow (**Figure 7**) and as the wall stiffens pulse pressure increases and the strain across the inner arterial wall rises proportionately.*

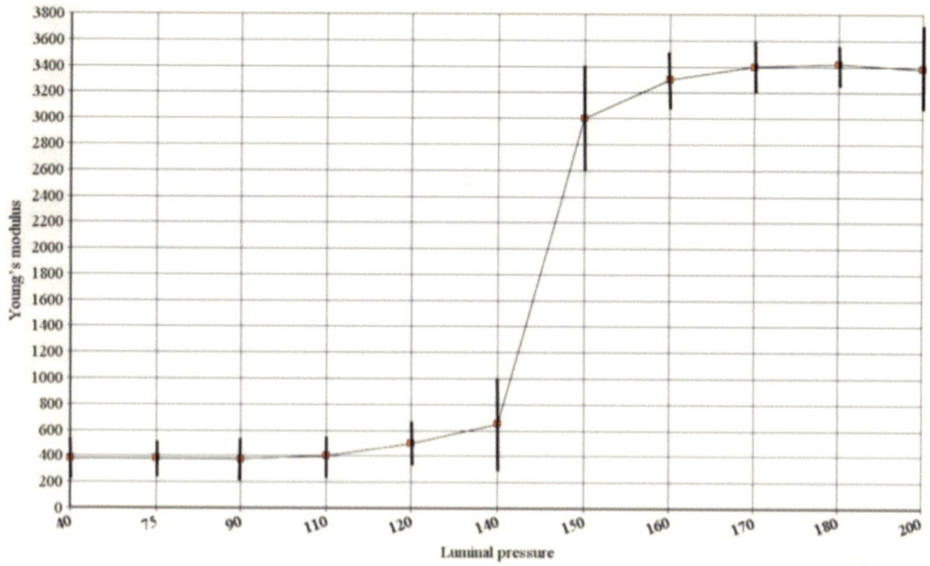

Figure 6.
Changes of Young's modulus (Kpa) in hoops trips of arterial wall subjected to increasing tension. Equivalent lumenal pressure derived from the Young-Laplace formula is shown on the X axis. N = 5, runs 20.

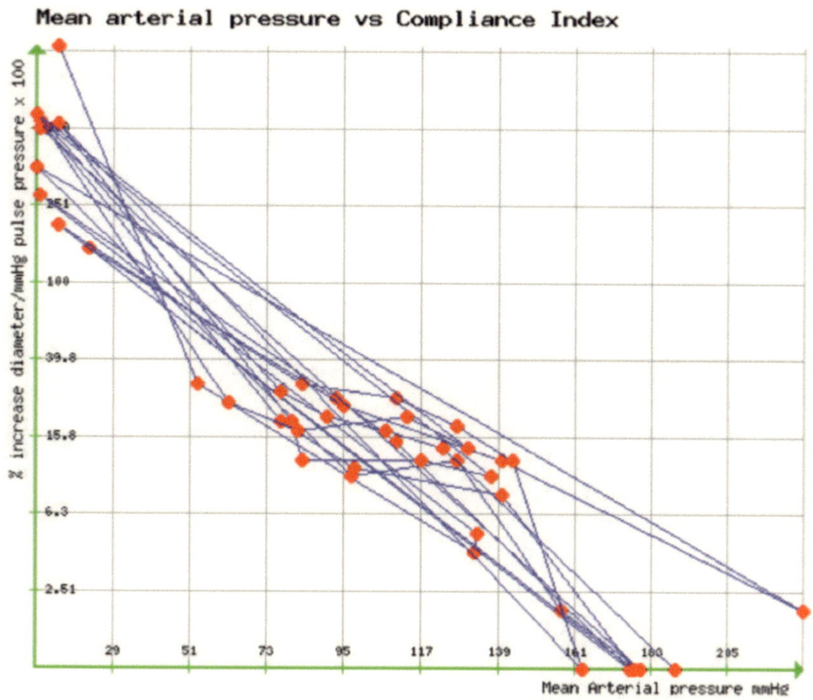

Figure 7.
Under pulsatile flow conditions a rise in mean arterial pressure just above the normal range for the pig [21] gives rise to an exponential loss of wall compliance which is correlated with a corresponding increase in transmural strain. 11 runs in a single artery.

3.2 Arterial wall compliance under pulsatile flow conditions

As arterial wall compliance drops, pulse pressure increases and the systolic peaks of the pressure wave sharpen. **Figure 8** compares the pressure traces where

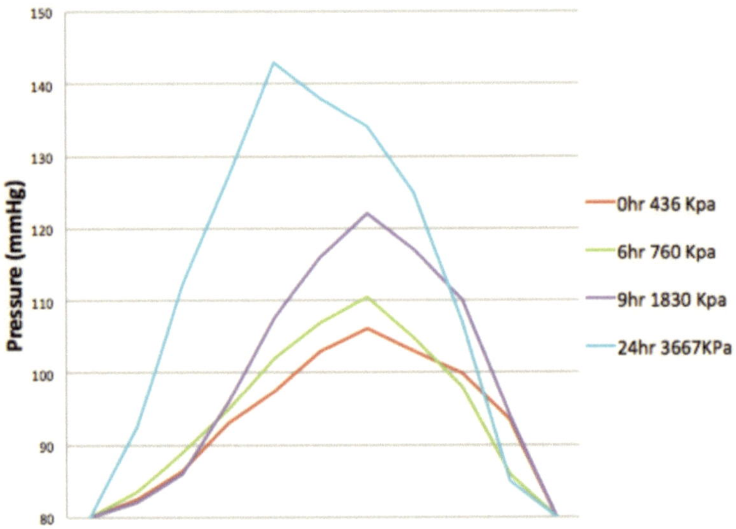

Figure 8.
Mean changes in pulse pressure and waveform profile with progressive loss of arterial wall compliance over a one-second pressure cycle. The key shows the period of exposure to formaldehyde vapour and resulting mean Young's modulus (Kpa) in relation to hoop strips cut from the proximal end of the test vessel after 6,9 and 24 hours of exposure. The volume load, cam profile and volume cycle and outflow resistance are held constant. n = 5, runs 20.

the arterial wall compliance alone has been changed by progressive formaldehyde exposure, the volume load, baseline pressure, pulse rate and outflow resistance being held constant. The corresponding Young's modulus for each period of formalin exposure measured at the equivalent of 100 mmHg pressure load using hoop strips cut from the proximal end of the test artery is shown in the key.

As arterial wall compliance decreases under pulsatile flow conditions the separation of the FI during passage of the pressure wave increases and reaches its maximum during the transition from systole to diastole and vice-versa. **Figure 9** shows the timing of the mean separation of the FI from the underlying vessel wall observed using B/M mode ultrasound throughout the phases of the pulse pressure wave cycle measured in five representative arteries as the wall is progressively stiffened. When the arterial wall is relatively compliant little separation of the FI occurs: as it stiffens increasing "lifting" separation of the FI is seen during passage of the pressure wave and occurs out of phase with the pressure wave itself, initially only in systolic/diastolic transitions but as the vessel stiffens further both in systolic and diastolic transitions.

3.3 Pulse pressure, centripetal strain and separation of the FI

The pulse pressure is very closely directly correlated to the CTS ($r = 0.907$, $p < 0.001$) and to the internal displacement of the FI when controlled for peak pressure waveform. **Figure 10** shows the relationship controlled for slightly blunted peaks characterised by an area under peak pressure 3.5 mm^2 (where each square represents 12 mmHg pressure over a period of 40 msec). Maximum proportional internal displacement of the FI is seen to occur as the peak pressure declines at the start of diastole (**Figure 9**) and is greatest when the pressure change is abrupt.

3.4 Waveform profile, viscosity, pulse rate, and diastolic pressure

No effect of pulse rate, or perfusate viscosity over the range 1 to 3.9 mPa.s on CTS or FI strain was observed independent of the effect of pulse pressure. This

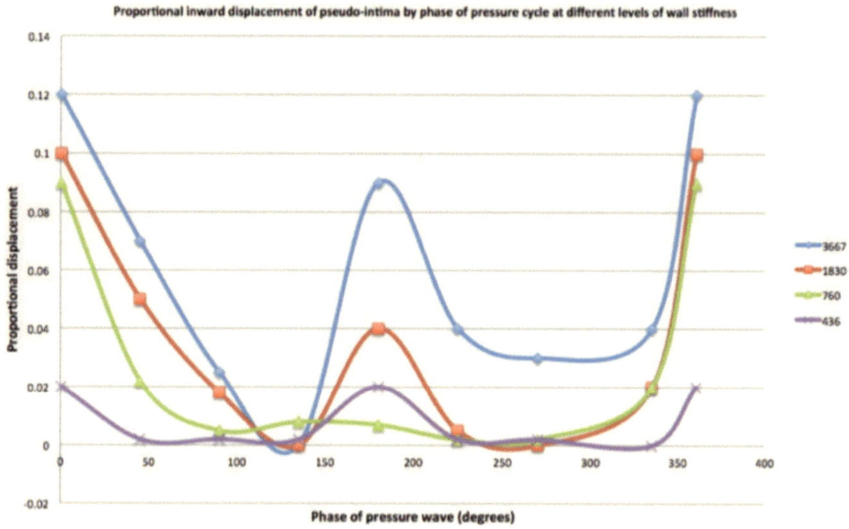

Figure 9.
Timing of strain response of the FI throughout the pressure cycle as the vessel wall is stiffened by progressive exposure to formaldehyde vapour. Figures in the key refer to corresponding mean Young's modulus derived from hoop strip tensiometry of the exposed formaldehyde vessels.

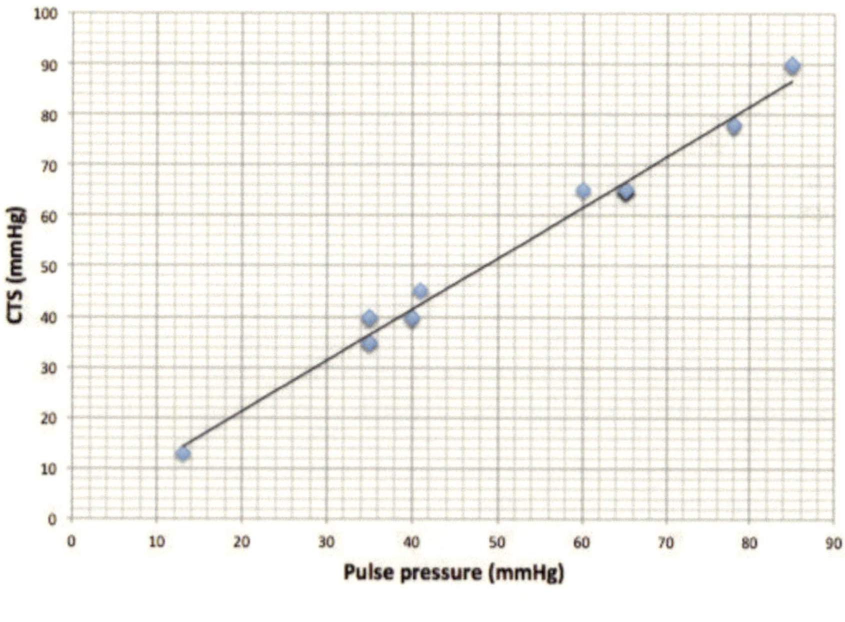

Figure 10.
Close relationship between pulse pressure and CTS controlled for the same waveform, area under peak (AUP) = 3.5 mm, n = 6 runs = 18.

does not exclude the possibility that viscosity may affect *shear strain* acting on the endothelium in pulsatile flow conditions which was not measured. Increased vessel wall stiffness is reflected in sharpening of the peak pressure wave and increased pulse pressure and both are associated with increased CTS. A close correlation was found between pulse pressure, CTS and FI separation irrespective of pulse rate, baseline ("diastolic") pressure, waveform or fluid viscosity. However this correlation depended on comparing like waveform profiles. When waveform profiles alone were altered by changing the cam profiles and selecting identical pulse pressures

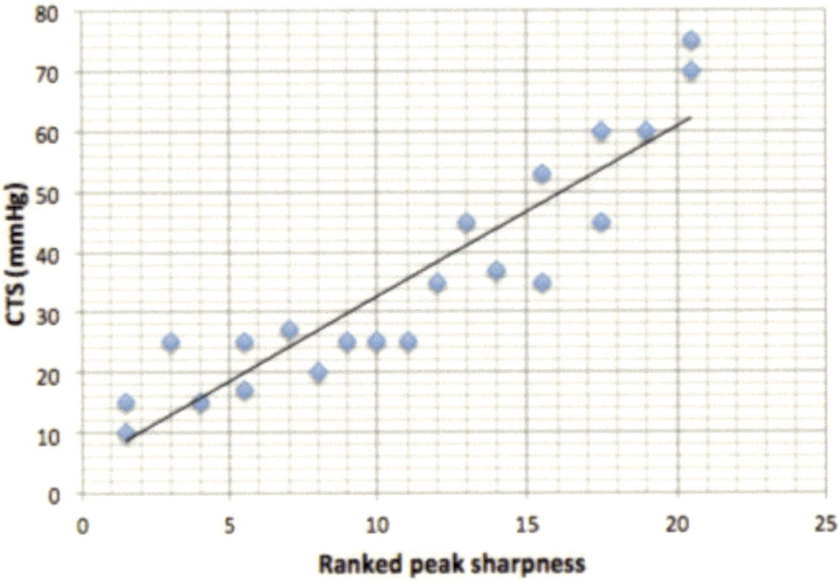

Figure 11.
Relationship between peak waveform profile and CTS when the pulse pressure remains the same, MAP in range 75-100 mmHg. Sharper peaks give rise to a greater CTS in pulsatile flow, whilst with blunted ones the CTS is reduced.

for analysis, the sharper the pressure transition the greater the CTS and false intima separation, (Spearman's R 0.93, $p < 0.001$), **Figure 11**).

4. Discussion

Blood pressure along with age, smoking habits and serum low-density lipoprotein cholesterol concentration (LDL-C) is a risk factor in the development of ischaemic heart disease and the risk of atherosclerotic large and middle-sized arterial disease throughout the body [22]. Much attention has been paid to the clinical management of blood pressure and LDL-C. By comparison relatively little attention has been given to the haemodynamic inter-relationships whereby blood pressure and other variables such as blood viscosity, vessel wall stiffness and pulse pressure waveform may interact to stress the arterial wall and influence the development of vascular disease. The presence of cholesterol in atherosclerotic plaques, the results of experimental animal studies and the clinical effectiveness of statins have tended to concentrate attention on the cholesterol accumulation theory of atherogenesis perhaps to the detriment of the study of these biomechanical factors. Although LDL-C undoubtedly plays a part in the atherogenic process in relation to atherogenic inflammatory changes in the vessel wall, the clinical relevance of targeting blood cholesterol in itself remains unclear especially in the elderly [23–25]. Recent studies suggest that non-statin lowering LDL-C in itself is not necessarily useful [26] and that statins exert their effect via an anti-inflammatory rather than cholesterol-lowering pathway, a pathway in which mechanical stress is also implicated [27–29]. It follows that pursuing blood cholesterol targets in a patient already on an appropriate does of statins may be less productive than pursuing blood pressure and lifestyle targets. Bearing in mind the focal distribution of atheroma in the vascular tree at points of mechanical strain alluded to in the introduction, and the established role of inflammatory signalling in atherogenesis, it may also be appropriate now to reappraise atherosclerosis in terms of a biomechanical-inflammatory disease akin to a repetition strain injury where similar inflammatory mediators and histological changes are involved [30, 31] rather than regarding it as a disease of principally metabolic origin.

In this context the study of haemodynamic variables in relation as to how they may interact to cause mechanical stress becomes relevant.

The weaknesses in the present model are that it is an in vitro study involving fresh specimens maintained as far as possible in physiological conditions. The haemodynamic parameters and dimensions of porcine vessels are similar but not identical to those of their human equivalents [21]. The model examines pulsatile flow in a moving column of fluid but the nature of the pulsatility and the flow may be different from that encountered in vivo. In terms of the broad principles the experimental set-up nevertheless provides a thought-provoking model of the stress/strain response of a major artery similar to the human equivalent. With this caveat in mind the principle mechanical findings, namely: (a) a rise in mean arterial pressure above the physiological range results in a precipitate increase in transmural strain consequent upon the vessel wall stiffening in response to pressure and (b) that this increased strain is proportional to pulse pressure and is affected by the shape of the pulse pressure peak and vessel wall compliance provide theoretical support for concentrating on blood pressure management and in particular on management of pulse pressure in the reduction of clinical risk both from atherogenesis and from plaque detachment. Artificially increasing vessel wall stiffness to the extent seen in hypertension also increases transmural strain and emphasises the central role of loss of large vessel compliance, whether caused by hypertension or disease, in the physical strain across the vessel wall under pulsatile flow conditions. Measures to preserve large vessel compliance such as regular exercise, blood pressure and diabetic control thus logically becomes a key element in the management of cardiovascular risk [32, 33] and in the reduction of the risk associated with onward transmission of damaging pressure waves to vulnerable distal vessels [34]. The possible role of heat therapy and garlic extracts in this respect requires further confirmation [35, 36]. In summary the parameters showing an effect in regard to CTS are: mean arterial pressure, pulse pressure, wall compliance and pressure waveform.

There is an interplay between these factors; this interplay with some postulated clinical correlations is illustrated in **Figure 12**.

With regard to further study it would be interesting to look into the effect of changing the characteristics of pulsatile flow in respect to pulse pressure and waveform on the expression of adhesion molecules, oxygen free radicals and nitric oxide by the endothelium, and to investigate further the possible repetitive strain nature of hypertensive atherogenesis. This experimental set-up may also prove useful in investigating the role of biomechanical variables in atheromatous plaque detachment and in helping to develop newer more compliant materials for arterial grafts and stents.

The postulated role of pulse pressure and pulse waveform in atherogenesis would be further supported if it could be shown in clinical studies that subjects with relatively low pulse pressure and rounded pulse pressure waveforms, such as those with untreated mild congenital aortic stenosis, had a lower burden of atheroma in distal vessels than in comparable controls. The role of blood pressure in the initiation of inflammatory changes in the vessel wall might be further explored by examining whether good blood pressure control reduces the expression of inflammatory mediators associated with cardiovascular risk such as CRP.

4.1 Clinical implications

The conclusion of the present study is a hypothesis based on observational evidence and *in-vitro* experimentation. Should the hypothesis be confirmed by

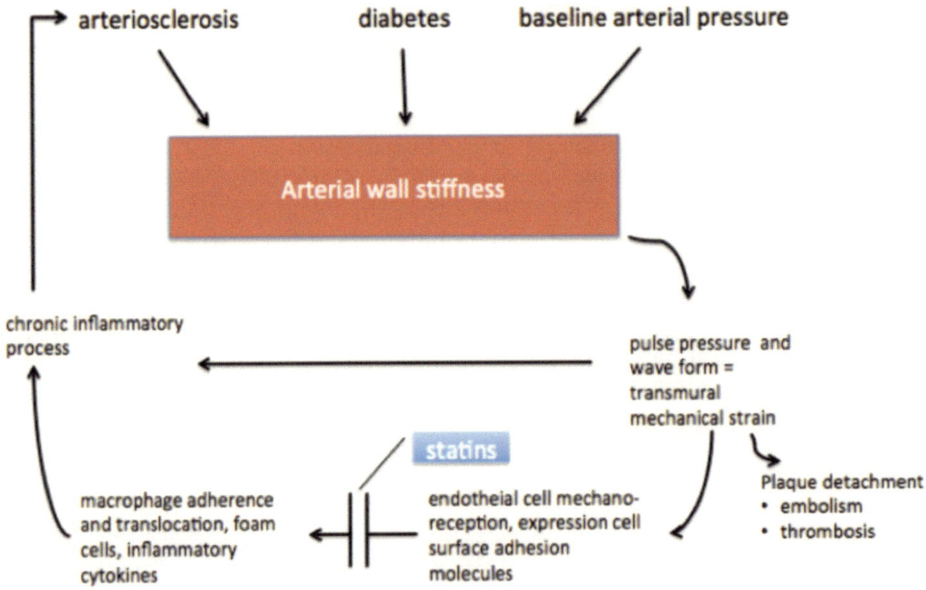

Figure 12.
Postulated relationship between vessel wall stiffness, blood pressure and mechanisms involved in the pathophysiology of atherosclerosis and cardiovascular risk.

clinical studies these findings provide theoretical support for the following clinical measures: control of mean arterial pressure and pulse pressure are particularly appropriate targets for prevention; large vessel wall compliance is important, and in a vessel already stiff, the transmural strain and hence the mechanical contribution to the risk of plaque separation is determined by pulse pressure and the sharpness of the systolic peak. The choice of treatment should be determined accordingly, and efforts to reduce the diastolic pressure in elderly hypertensive patients may be misplaced: the rational targets should be mean arterial pressure, pulse pressure and waveform. A key element is the role of arterial wall compliance in large vessels.

In brief it may be helpful to consider atherosclerosis as a disease of mechanical-inflammatory origin to which metabolic elements contribute a part rather than concentrating on the contribution of metabolic elements alone.

5. Conclusions

Pulse pressure, mean arterial pressure, pulse pressure waveform and arterial wall elasticity were found to affect transmural stress and strain in pig aortas subjected to a variety of haemodynamic stresses *in vitro*. Moderate rises in mean arterial pressure across and above the physiological range gave rise to exponential increases in wall stiffness and transmural stress. Transmural stress is implicated in both atherogenesis and plaque separation. It is proposed that atherosclerosis should be seen as a disease of mechanical-inflammatory origin whereby repeated excess mechanical stress gives rise to a state of sustained inflammatory healing in the vessel wall akin to a repetition strain injury. The way in which statins impair this inflammatory response is discussed. These studies suggest that preventative and therapeutic measures should target mean arterial pressure, pulse pressure, arterial pressure waveform and emphasises the importance of maintaining arterial wall elasticity in capacitance vessels. The possible link between mechanical transmural stress and inflammatory signalling in the vessel wall requires further evaluation. This study provides theoretical support for the central role of blood pressure management in the control of cardiovascular risk.

Author details

Thomas K. Day
Independent Researcher, London, UK

*Address all correspondence to: thomasday3@me.com

IntechOpen

© 2021 The Author(s). Licensee IntechOpen. This chapter is distributed under the terms of the Creative Commons Attribution License (http://creativecommons.org/licenses/by/3.0), which permits unrestricted use, distribution, and reproduction in any medium, provided the original work is properly cited.

References

[1] Texon M. The hemodynamic concept of atherosclerosis. Bul NY Acad Med. 1960;36(4):263-274.

[2] MacMahon S, Peto R, Cutler J, Collins R, Sorlie P, Neaton J, Abbott R, Godwin J, Dyer A, Stamier J. Blood pressure, stroke and coronary heart disease. Part 1, Prolonged differences in blood pressure: prospective observational studies corrected for the regeression dilutaion bias. *Lancet* 1990;335:765-774.

[3] Walton KW, Slaney G, Ashton F. Atherosclerosis in vascular grafts for peripheral vascular disease. Atherosclerosis 1985;54:49-64.

[4] Stokes J III, Kannel WB, Wpolf PA, D'Agostino RB, Cupples LA. Blood pressure as a risk factor for cardiovascular disease. The Framingham study – 30 years of follow-up. *Hypertesnion* 1989;13 (suppl I):I-13-I-18.

[5] Christensen T, Neubauer B. Arterial wall stiffness in insulin-dependant diabetes mellitus. Acta Radiol. 1988;29(3):299-302.

[6] Campens L, Vanakkar OM, Trachet B, Segers P, Leroy BP, De Zaeytijd J, Voet D, De Paepe A, De Backer T, De Bakkar J. Characterisation of cardiovascular involvement in pseudoxanthoma elasticum families. Arteriosclerosis, Thrombosis and Vasc Biol. 2013;33:2646-2652.

[7] Gerhard-Herman H, Smoot LB, Wake N. Mechanisms of premature vascular aging in children with Hutchinson-Gilford progeria syndrome. Hypertension. 2012;59(1):92-97.

[8] Low GD, Lee AJ, Rumey A, Price JF, Fowkes FG. Blood viscosity and the risk of cardiovascular events: the Edinburgh Artery Study. Brit J. Haematol. 1997;96(1):168-173.

[9] Dai G, Kaazempur-Morfrad MR, Natarajan S, Zhang Y, Vaughn S, Blackman BR, Kamm RD, Garcia-Cardeña G, Gimbrone MA. Distinct endothelial phenotypes evoked by arterial waveforms derived from atherosclerosis-susceptible and resistant regions of human vasculature. Proc Natl Acad Sci USA. 2004;101:14871-14876.

[10] Kwak BR, Bäck M, Bochaton-Piallat M-L, Caligiuri G, Daemen MJAP, Davies PF, Hoefer IE, Holvoet P, Jo H, Krams R, Lehoux S, Monaco C, Steffens S, Virmani R, Weber C, Wentzel JJ, Evans PC. Biomechanical factors in atherosclerosis: mechanisms and clinical implications. Eur Heart J. 2014:35;3013-3020.

[11] Moore S. Endothelial injury and atherosclerosis. Exp Mol Biol. 1979;31(1):182-190.

[12] Merrilees MJ, Scott L. Culture of rat and pig aortic endothelial cells. Difference in their growth rate and glycosaminoglycan synthesis. Atherosclerosis. 1981;38(1-2)19-26.

[13] Hansson G. Inflammation, atherosclerosis and coronary artery disease. N Engl J Med. 2005;16: 1685-1695.

[14] Fels B, Kuschen-Vihrag K. It takes more than two to tango: mechanosignaling of the endothelial surface. Pflugers Arch. 2020;472(4): 419-433.

[15] Davies PF. Flow-mediated mechanical transduction. Physiol Rev. 1995;75(3):519-560

[16] Nagel T, Resnick N, Atkinson WJ, Dewey CF, Gimbrone MA. Shear stress selectively upregulates adhesion

molecule-1 expression in cultured human vascular endothelial cells. J Clin Invest. 1994;94(2):885-891.

[17] Giussani DA, Moore PJ, Spencer JAD, Hanson MA. Changes in frequency and in complaince affect the pulsatility index of the Doppler flow velocity waveform at constant flow in an in vutre pulsatile flow model. J Matern Fetal Invest. 1995:5;78-82.

[18] Smulyan H, Safar ME. Systolic blood pressure revisited. J Amer Coll Cardiol. 1997;29:1407-1413.

[19] Telis VRN, Telis-Romero J, Mazzotti HB, Gabas AL. Viscosity of aqueous carbohydrate solutions at different temperatures and concentrations. J Food Prop. 2007:10(1);185-195.

[20] He C and Roach MR. The composition and mechanical properties of abdominal aortic aneurysms. *J Vasc Surg.* 1993:20 (1);6-13).

[21] Hannon JP, Bossone CA, Wade CE. *Normal Physiological Variables for Conscious Pigs used in Biomedical Research (1989)*. Letterman Army Institute of Research. Institute Report 379.

[22] Alexander WR. Hypertension and the pathogenesis of atherosclerosis. Hypertension 1995;25(2):155-161.

[23] Kannel WB, Castelli WP, Gordon T. Cholesterol in the prediction of atherosclerotic disease. New perspectives based on the Framingham study. Ann Intern Med. 1979;90:85-91.

[24] Ravnskov U, Diamond D, Hama R, Hamazaki T, Hammarskjöld B, Hynes N, Kendrick M, Langsjoen PH, Malhotra H, Mascitelli L, McCully KS, Ogushi Y, Okuyama H, Rosch PJ, Schersten T, Sultan S, Sunberg R. Lack of an association or an inverse association between low-density-lipoprotein cholesterol and mortality in the elderly: a systemic review. Brit Med J. 2016; 6:e010401.

[25] Wong AP, Mohamed AL, Niedzwiecki A. Atherosclerosis and Cholesterol Theory: a Reappraisal. World J Cardiovascular. Res. 2016; 6:391-409.

[26] Lincoff AM, Nicholls SJ, Riesmeyer JS for the ACCELERATE Investigators. Evacetrarib and cardiovascular outcomes in high-risk vascular disease. N Engl J Med. 2017;376:1933-1942.

[27] Teupser D, Bruegel M, Stein O, Stein Y, Thiery J. HMG-CoA reductase inhibitors reduce adhesion of human monocytes to endothelial cells. Biochem Biophys Res Commun. 2001; 289(4):838-844.

[28] Greenwood J Mason JC. Statins and the vascular endothelial inflammatory response. Trends Immunol. 2007; 28(2):88-98.

[29] Davignon J, Ganz P. Role of endothelial dysfunction in atherosclerosis. Circulation 2004; 109(23i):1227-1132.

[30] Exposure-dependent increases in IL-1beta, substance P, CTGF and tendinosis in flexor digitorum tendons with upper extremity repetitive strain injury. Fedorczyk JM, Barr AE, Rani S, Gao HG, Amin M Amin S, Litvin J, Barbe MF. *J Orth Res*. 2010:28(3)298-307.

[31] Landén NX, Dongqing L, Ståhle M. Transition from inflammation to proliferation: a critical step during wound healing. Cell Mol Life Sci. 2016:73(20);3861-3885.

[32] Lewington S, Clarke R, Qizilbash N, Peto R, Collins R; Prospective Studies Collaboration. Age-specific relevance of usual blood pressure to vascular mortality: a meta-analysis of individual data for one million adults in 61

prospective studies. Lancet. 2002;360:1903-1913.

[33] Steppan J, Barodka V, Berkowitz DE, Nyhan D. Vascular stiffness and increased pulse pressure in the aging cardiovascular system. Cardiol Res Pract. 2011; 2011:263-585. doi 10.4061/2011/263585.

[34] O'Rourke MF, Safar ME. Relationship between aortic stiffeniong and microvascular disease in the brain and kidney. Hypertesnion 2005;46:200-204.

[35] Breithaupt-Grögler K, Ling M, Boudoulas H, Belz GG. Protective effect of garlic intake on the elastic properties of the aorta in the elderly. Circulation 1997;96(8):2649-2655.

[36] Brunt VE, Howard MJ, Francisco MA, Ely BR, Minson CT. Passive heat therapy improves endothelial cell function, arterial stiffness and blood pressure in sedentary humans. J. Physiol. 2016:594(18);5329-5342.

Chapter 7

Importance of Resistance Training in the Management of Cardiovascular Disease Risk

Brandon S. Shaw, Gregory A. Brown and Ina Shaw

Abstract

Contrary to the longstanding taboo of resistance training (RT) as a therapeutic treatment, RT has been gaining importance as a safe therapeutic option in the management of numerous diseases. Although exercise has well-documented health benefits on cardiovascular disease (CVD), the benefit of RT on CVD risk factors is not yet as widely prescribed as other modes of exercise. Due to its efficacy in the management of CVD, RT should be regarded as a complementary therapeutic treatment rather than a substitute to other modes of exercise therapy. While it is clear that RT can result in an attenuation of CVD risk, the various RT design options related to intensity and volume and how they impact on CVD risk, especially in different populations (i.e. children, elderly, women) is not yet well documented. This chapter will discuss the physiological phenomenon and benefits of RT as a therapeutic intervention aiming to manage CVD risk.

Keywords: CVD Management, CVD Prevention, Resistance Exercise Prescription, Strength Training, Weight Training

1. Introduction

Cardiovascular disease (CVD) is the number one cause of death worldwide [1]. It includes diseases of the heart, blood vessels supplying the heart, brain, and other organs [2] and includes diseases such as angina, myocardial infarction (MI) (heart attack), cerebrovascular attacks (stroke), heart failure, cardiomyopathy, carditis, abnormal heart rhythms, congenital heart disease, rheumatic heart disease, valvular heart disease, hypertensive heart disease, aortic aneurysms, peripheral artery disease, thromboembolic disease and venous thrombosis [3].

The underlying cause of CVD varies depending on the disease and may be caused by a variety of factors [4]. These risk factors for developing CVD are traditionally divided into primary and secondary risk factors with primary risk factors being those risk factors that have conclusively shown to have a strong association with CVD. In this regard, smoking, hypertension, dyslipidemia and physical inactivity, are the four traditional primary risk factors [5]. On the other hand, secondary risk factors include diabetes mellitus, obesity, diet, psychological factors, age, hereditary/family history, gender, ethnicity/race, and personal (previous) history [5]. Thankfully, CVD risk factors can be classified into modifiable and non-modifiable risk factors. Of particular importance to healthcare practitioners

IntechOpen

are the modifiable CVD risk factors, since these factors can be impacted upon via various interventions [1, 4].

Although physical inactivity or a sedentary lifestyle is one of the major risk factors for developing CVD, physical activity has proved especially useful in the overall prevention and treatment of CVD [4]. Problematically, despite strong scientific evidence supporting the benefits of regular physical activity for the prevention and management of CVD, physical inactivity is highly prevalent worldwide.

In addition, while it is known that physical activity is a critical intervention in the prevention and management of CVD, numerous types of modalities of physical activity exist. This includes, amongst others, aerobic exercise including walking, jogging, swimming, skipping rope, muscular fitness training including, strength training, power training, hypertrophy training, muscle endurance training, flexibility exercises, balance exercises, martial arts, and other physical fitness systems, including Pilates, Yoga and CrossFit. This sheer diversity of physical activity and the various variables of exercise programme design, which are exercise selection, intensity, repetitions, tempo, rest interval, sets and frequency of exercise sessions further complicate our understanding of what physical activity actually works or is best for the prevention and management of CVD in general, or for a specific type of CVD [4].

1.1 Health benefits of physical activity

Regular physical activity has an ancient association with general health and today it is unquestionable by all those involved in healthcare that regular physical activity provides many physical and psychological benefits. In this regard, >100,000 studies demonstrate positive associations between exercise and health [6]. In fact, overwhelming evidence exists that regular physical activity is associated with delaying the onset of 40 chronic conditions/diseases [7]. As such, exercise has proven to be a critical medical intervention even in diseases with a non-locomotor component. Specifically, a significant amount of scientific evidence has established a causal relationship between non-communicable diseases (NCD) and physical activity. This is especially important in that NCDs, such as CVD, diabetes and cancer, cause 65% of all deaths worldwide and are projected to result in >75% of all deaths by 2030 [8].

The success of physical activity in preventing, delaying and rehabilitating a multitude of chronic conditions/diseases relates to physical activity's multisystem responses. While the benefits of physical activity have been attributed to several mechanisms, including improved blood hemodynamics [9], improved levels of circulating lipids [10], increased cardiorespiratory fitness (CRF) [11, 12] and a reduced adiposity and enhanced muscle mass [13], more recent research has shown that during physical activity, proteins, peptides, enzymes and metabolites are released from one organ (mainly contracting skeletal muscle) to affect the metabolism in another organ [14].

1.2 Physical activity and CVD

Regular physical activity has a long scientific association with a reduced risk of CVD [15]. Two of the most well-known such studies demonstrating the importance of physical activity in preventing CVD are the Framingham Heart Study and London Transport Workers Study.

Prior to the Framingham Heart Study began in 1948 in Framingham, Massachusetts, little was known about the epidemiology of CVD. However, that study demonstrated much of the now-common knowledge concerning CVD, such as the effects of physical activity on CVD. In fact, the Framingham Heart Study is the source of the term risk factor [16]. The London Transport Workers Study, published in 1953 by Jeremy N. Morris was the first rigorous epidemiological study investigating physical activity and CVD risk. In that study, drivers and conductors of the London Transport Executive were compared and CVD rates were found to be increased in physically inactive bus drivers versus active conductors [17, 18].

More recently, many leading international organisations have recognised the importance of physical activity as medicine in not only improving health, but also preventing and managing CVD and have issued calls to action to make physical activity a priority in this regard [19, 20].

In addition to its independent effects on traditional CVD risk factors, regular physical activity can also improve cardiovascular health and impact upon non-traditional or novel CVD risk factors, such as C-reactive protein and oxidative stress [21, 22]. Physical activities' effectiveness at preventing and managing CVD is due to its ability to target various pathways through which it influences different physiological systems, such as its ability to promote a healthy anti-inflammatory environment, largely through the release of muscle-derived myokines, its ability to stimulate myocardial regeneration and its ability to improve age-related loss of muscle mass and strength, a frequently overlooked non-traditional CVD risk factor [23–25].

What is particularly noteworthy about physical activity's role in CVD prevention and management are the findings that even a single session or brief periods of physical activity are known to be associated with improvements in cardiovascular health parameters [26], such as an immediate decrease in blood pressure, also called post-exercise hypotension (PEH) [27], improved blood levels of lipids [28], enhanced fat oxidation [29] and improved insulin sensitivity [30].

1.3 Health benefits of resistance training (RT)

While it is still argued that cardiorespiratory fitness (CRF) is the most important measure for health, numerous other primary health-related physical fitness parameters exist and include; musculoskeletal fitness, body composition and flexibility [31]. Not only does resistance training (RT) improve on these parameters, but RT has also shown to enhance several other important aspects of physical and mental health [32]. Further, RT has also been associated with reduced low back pain, decreased arthritic discomfort, increased functional independence, improved mobility, enhanced functional status, enhanced movement control, and increased walking speed [32, 33]. What is especially important to note is that RT is equally, and in some cases superior, to other modes of physical activity, such as aerobic training, in its health-promoting benefits. Examples of this are RT's superior ability to increase metabolic rate, lean body mass and bone mineral density [33]. It is for these reasons that RT is recommended by numerous health organisations (e.g., American College of Sports Medicine, American Heart Association, American Association of Cardiovascular and Cardiopulmonary Rehabilitation, Surgeon General's Office) for inclusion into a comprehensive fitness programme that includes aerobic and flexibility exercise [34].

1.4 Resistance training and prevention and management of cardiovascular disease (CVD)

It is explicit that RT has been recognised for its value in improving the health of athletes and the general public. However, only recently has scientific evidence emerged substantiating its benefits in the prevention and management of CVD [35]. This is especially true given RT's unique benefits over other modes of physical activity, especially improving the often overlooked non-traditional CVD risk factors of muscle mass and strength loss [23–25].

The evidence for a blood pressure-lowering effect of RT remains scarce [36]. However, when such evidence is forthcoming it provides confirmation for the potential of RT in the prevention and treatment of high blood pressure in normo- and even hypertensive patients [37, 38]. Additionally, some studies even demonstrate that RT is equally or more effective than aerobic training at doing so [39]. What is especially important to note is that little/no RT studies have reported serious adverse events in even hypertensive participants [36].

A reduction in cholesterol levels are considered the gold standard in preventative cardiovascular medicine [40]. This is why it is essential that much evidence supports the role that RT improves HDL-cholesterol whilst reducing total cholesterol, LDL-cholesterol and triglycerides in adults [41–43]. What is particularly interesting is that RT shows a stronger association than aerobic exercise when attempting to improve HDL-cholesterol [44, 45]. It appears that an increased volume (via increased numbers of sets or repetitions), rather than intensity or load, has a greater impact on lipid profiles [46].

While CRF improvements following RT are not as substantial as those following a period of aerobic training [47], the evidence that RT does indeed increase CRF [36] is critical, since an enhanced CRF is associated with a lower risk of all-cause mortality and cardiovascular events [48]. Interestingly, both low- and high-intensity RT have demonstrated to improve CRF, albeit via different proposed mechanisms, such as an increased Type IIa muscle activity, increases in leg strength (i.e. for pedal thrust and efficiency of movement), improvements in oxidative enzymes [49]. However, many of the CRF adaptations to RT appear to be dependent on a higher volume of training [50].

More than 39% (1.9 billion) of adults were found to be overweight and 13% (650 million) obese in 2016 [51]. This is in addition to over 340 million children and adolescents being found to be overweight or obese in 2016 [51]. This is problematic in that overweight and obesity are associated with an increased incidence of various CVDs, such as diabetes, hypertension, and metabolic syndrome [52]. It is this CVD risk factor in which the effect of RT on body composition is unique when compared to other modes of physical activity. Specifically, RT has the ability to increase muscle mass, while simultaneously reducing fat mass [33, 53]. Further, RT offers an alternative to other modes of physical activity that may not be tolerated as well by individuals who are already overweight or obese, due to the excess body weight increasing the intensity (and perceived exertion) of weight-bearing activity [54, 55]. Another reason or barrier limiting participation in aerobic-type activities may arise from an initially low CRF [54, 56].

The increasing prevalence of diabetes suggests a clear need for effective diabetes prevention and management approaches [57, 58]. As stated previously, RT is unique in its ability to prevent overweight and obesity and it is for this reason that RT is receiving increasing recognition as a cornerstone in the prevention and treatment of type 2 diabetes [59, 60]. In this regard, emerging research suggests that RT has the power to combat metabolic dysfunction in patients with type 2 diabetes. Some of the beneficial adaptations exerted by RT include increased GLUT4 translocation in skeletal muscle, increased insulin sensitivity and restored metabolic flexibility. Further, an increased energy expenditure and excess post-exercise oxygen consumption (EPOC) in response to RT may be other beneficial effects [60]. In fact, it appears that RT can improve glycemic control and insulin sensitivity likely even more than aerobic training [61, 62].

Epidemiological studies have demonstrated the role of diet as a secondary CVD risk factor, as it has an important role to play in other CVD risk factors, such as hypertension, dyslipidemia, diabetes and obesity [63]. The role of diet in CVD development is complex and involves many dietary factors, including *inter alia* an excessive dietary intake of fat (particularly saturated fat), excessive intake of cholesterol, high intakes of certain carbohydrates (i.e. fructose and sucrose), excessive salt intake, excessive alcohol consumption and an inadequate intake of fiber [64]. Although research on the effects of RT on dietary patterns and intake is limited, most studies demonstrate that RT is unable to alter self-selected food intake or food preference [64–67]. However, cross-sectional studies do exist that demonstrate athletes engaging in RT have a decreased dietary intake of fat, even when compared to aerobic athletes [68]. While it seems RT may have no effect on dietary preferences, RT may affect diet indirectly by offsetting the effects of a poor diet. In this regard, since RT increases nitrogen retention, enhances protein synthesis and improves the expression of insulin-like growth factor in skeletal muscle, the anabolic potential of RT is useful in counteracting the catabolism experienced during CVD, such as interleukin-mediated myopathy of chronic heart failure, myopathy secondary to corticosteroid use in cardiac transplantation and during energy restriction for obesity management [69].

Much evidence exists identifying the mechanisms by which psychological factors, such as stress, depression, and anxiety and impact CVD [70]. In addition to RT's numerous physical benefits, the effect of RT on psychological factors is well documented. In this regard, the demonstrated mental health benefits of RT include decreased symptoms of depression, increased self-esteem, increased self-efficacy, increased, physical self-concept, improved cognitive ability and enhanced social interaction [71–73]. Specifically relating to CVD, it appears that RT may provide unique psychological benefits when compared to other physical activity modalities. This is because psychological benefits may be more related to reductions in body fat than changes in strength or fitness [72, 73]. Therefore, RT could be an alternative to aerobic training for some individuals in the biological and psychological management of adolescent obesity [72, 73].

1.5 Safety of resistance training in the management of cardiovascular disease risk

Resistance training is an exercise modality that can potentially target many of the adverse effects of CVD. However, there have been concerns regarding the safety of strenuous RT and its application to existing and future clinical interventions.

In the past, RT has been regarded as hazardous due to inflated blood pressure responses, elevated double pressure products and an increase in ischemic events. However, more recent research has demonstrated that RT may be less risky than was once assumed. In this regard, previous research has established intra-arterial blood pressures during RT in cardiac patients to be within a clinically tolerable range at 40–60% of 1-RM [72, 73]. Further, research has also demonstrated that electrocardiographic (ECG) responses during RT at 20%, 40%, 60%, and 80% of 1-RM failed to induce clinically significant ST-segment depression, angina or ventricular arrhythmias [74]. In fact, RT has not been found elicit significant cardiovascular events even during 1-RM determination [75]. As such, light-to-moderate RT can be deemed safe for low- to moderate-risk CVD patients.

With regards to the use of RT in high-risk CVD patients, even though traditional RT participation guidelines have previously advised that surgical and post–myocardial infarction (MI) patients should avoid RT for at least four to six months [76], it has been demonstrated that these patients can safely complete static-dynamic activity corresponding to carrying up to 30 pounds or about 13 kilogrammes by three weeks after an acute MI [77]. As such, it is probable that RT could be introduced earlier in even these high-risk settings should low-load programmes be prescribed.

While moderate to good left ventricular function and cardiorespiratory fitness in the absence of anginal symptoms or ischemic ST-segment depression have been proposed as preconditions for participation in RT, contraindications to RT comprise unstable angina, uncontrolled hypertension (systolic blood pressure ≥ 160 mm/Hg and/or diastolic blood pressure ≥ 100 mm/Hg), uncontrolled dysrhythmias, recent history of congestive heart failure that has not been evaluated and effectively treated, severe stenotic or regurgitant valvular disease and hypertrophic cardiomyopathy [78].

1.6 Non-communicable disease intervention research unit (NCDIRU) resistance training guidelines for the prevention and management of CVD

Although RT is increasingly recommended as an integral component of an overall CVD prevention and management programme, many global guidelines impose specific RT programme design recommendations for each CVD risk, type of disease, even at each severity level, or fail to provide specific criteria for training progression [79]. Further, a significant barrier to increased implementation of RT as a clinical therapy is the complex, difficult-to-follow regimes compulsively focusing on design variables such as load, intensity and volume. As such, a more feasible and easier-to-adhere-to paradigm for RT should be explored and adopted as a prescription for public health [80, 81].

In this regard, for apparently healthy individuals or those at low-risk, the Non-Communicable Disease Intervention Research Unit (NCDIRU) recommends utilising 8–10 different RT exercises that train the major muscle groups, with multiple sets (i.e. 3–4 sets) of 8–12 repetitions, with minimal rest intervals (i.e. 30–60 seconds) for most days of a week.

In turn, the NCDIRU recommends that individuals with high-risk should utilise 8–10 different RT exercises that train the major muscle groups using multiple sets (i.e. 3 sets) of 10–12 repetitions, with moderate-long rest intervals (i.e. 60–90 seconds) for 3 days weekly. These high-risk individuals should also have increased patient monitoring and programme supervision when compared to low-risk patients.

Despite much overlap and impracticality, many international organisations have guidelines or position statements for each CVD. However, in an effort to develop a practical and easy-to-follow RT regime that will increase adherence and outcomes, the NCDIRU recommends the following for those patients with existing CVD to delay progression or assist in the management of CVDs: an RT prescription of 8–10 different exercises that train the major muscle groups using 1–2 sets of 10–15 repetitions, twice weekly. In this existing CVD group, exercise sessions should begin at a lower intensity level of 12–15 repetitions and progress more slowly than programmes designed for low-risk patients, allowing time for adaptation. These patients should also have the most patient monitoring and programme supervision. Further, variable resistance machines with selectorised weight stacks should be utilised. In this regard, variable resistance machines with selectorised weight stacks; (1) allow the initial weight applied to be at a low level and increased in small increments; (2) the equipment is usually designed to protect the lower back, thus reducing the risk of injury; (3) many machines are designed to avoid handgripping which reduces the risk of exercise-induced hypertension; (4) the machines are usually designed to allow the resistance to be applied evenly through the patients' full range of motion (ROM); (5) many types of equipment can be double pinned to allow the individual to exercise through their pain-free ROM and 6) many machines do not require the individual to balance or control the weight, as do dumbbells and barbells, which may reduce the likelihood of injury [82].

2. Conclusions

Despite the well-known benefits of exercise, most adults and many children lead relatively sedentary lifestyles and are not active enough to achieve the health benefits of exercise. Further, due to the stigma associated with RT (i.e. erroneous/unfounded issues related to safety and damage to growth plates), many children and adults fail to engage in RT as part of their overall health and prevention/management of CVD [83]. This is despite the accumulating and overwhelming evidence for health and CVD-protective effects of RT. Given its whole-body, health-promoting nature, the integrative responses to RT will continue to attract special interest as the notion of "exercise is medicine" continues its integration into clinical settings [6]. Given that RT has both direct and indirect effects on the mortality and morbidity of CVDs via its identified risk factors (e.g. hypertension, dyslipidemia, obesity and diabetes), health care professionals and health policy makers should incorporate RT advocacy in their daily clinical practice and public health policies.

Acknowledgements

The authors would like to acknowledge the contributions made by the Non-Communicable Disease Intervention Research Unit (NCDIRU).

Conflict of interest

The authors declare no conflict of interest.

Author details

Brandon S. Shaw[1]*, Gregory A. Brown[2] and Ina Shaw[1]

1 Department of Human Movement Science, University of Zululand, Kwadlangezwa, South Africa

2 Physical Activity and Wellness Laboratory, Department of Kinesiology and Sports Science, University of Nebraska Kearney, NE, United States of America

*Address all correspondence to: shawb@unizulu.ac.za

IntechOpen

© 2021 The Author(s). Licensee IntechOpen. This chapter is distributed under the terms of the Creative Commons Attribution License (http://creativecommons.org/licenses/by/3.0), which permits unrestricted use, distribution, and reproduction in any medium, provided the original work is properly cited.

References

[1] World Health Organization (WHO). Cardiovascular Diseases (CVDs). 2017. Available from: https://www.who.int/news-room/fact-sheets/detail/cardiovascular-diseases-(cvds)#:~:text=CVDs%20are%20the%20number%201%20cause%20of%20death,deaths%20take%20place%20in%20low-%20and%20middle-income%20countries [Accessed 04/06/2021].

[2] Gaziano T, Reddy KS, Paccaud F, Horton S, Chaturvedi V. Chapter 33: Cardiovascular Disease. In: Jamison DT, Breman JG, Measham AR, Alleyne G, Claeson M, Evans DB, Jha P, Mills A, Musgrove P, editors. Disease Control Priorities in Developing Countries. 2nd ed. Washington (DC): The International Bank for Reconstruction and Development/The World Bank; 2006. ISBN-10: 0-8213-6179-1.

[3] Shaw I, Shaw BS, Brown GA, Cilliers JF. Concurrent Resistance and Aerobic Training as Protection against Heart Disease. Cardiovascular Journal of Africa. 2010;21(4):224-227.

[4] Shaw, B.S. & Shaw, I. Resistance Training as a Countermeasure for Key Non-Communicable Diseases in Low-Resource Settings: A Review. Asian Journal of Sports Medicine. 2021;2(1):1-8, e106588. DOI: 10.5812/asjsm.106588.

[5] Lawrence, K.E., Shaw, I. & Shaw, B.S. Hemodynamic Changes in Normotensive Overweight and Obese Individuals Following Home-Based Calisthenics Training. African Journal for Physical, Health Education, Recreation and Dance. 2014;Supplement 2:82-90.

[6] Ruegsegger GN, Booth FW. Health Benefits of Exercise, In: Zierath JR, Joyner MJ, Hawley JA, editors. Additional Perspectives on the Biology of Exercise. Cold Spring Harbor Laboratory Press; 2018. DOI: 10.1101/cshperspect.a029694.

[7] Booth FW, Roberts CK, Laye MJ. 2012. Lack of Exercise is a Major Cause of Chronic Diseases. Comprehensive Physiology. 2012;2:1143-1211. DOI: 10.1002/cphy.c110025.

[8] Blair SN, Sallis RE, Hutber A, Archer E. Exercise Therapy – The Public Health Message. Scandinavian Journal of Medicine & Science in Sports. 2012;22(4):e24-e28. DOI: 10.1111/j.1600-0838.2012.01462.x.

[9] Pal S, Radavelli-Bagatini S, Ho S. Potential Benefits of Exercise on Blood Pressure and Vascular Function. Journal of the American Society of Hypertension. 2013;7(6):494-506. DOI: 10.1016/j.jash.2013.07.004

[10] Vella CA, Kravitz L, Janot JM. A Review of the Impact of Exercise on Cholesterol Levels. IDEA Health & Fitness Source. 2001;19(10):48.

[11] Kokkinos P, Myers J, Franklin B, Narayan P, Lavie CJ, Faselis C. Cardiorespiratory Fitness and Health Outcomes: A Call to Standardize Fitness Categories. Mayo Clinic Proceedings. 2018;93(3):333-336. DOI: 10.1016/j.mayocp.2017.10.011.

[12] Shaw BS, Shaw I. Chapter 3. Role of Aerobic Exercise. In Cardiopulmonary Health and Rehabilitation. In: Simmons JA, Brown AC, editors. Aerobic Exercise: Health Benefits, Types and Common Misconceptions. Nova Science Publishers, Hauppauge, NY. USA. 2013; p. 59-84. ISBN: 978-1-62618-578-4.

[13] Shaw, I. & Shaw, B.S. (2014). Resistance Training and the Prevention of Sports Injuries. In: Hopkins, G, editors. Sports Injuries: Prevention, Management and Risk Factors. Nova

Science Publishers, Hauppauge, NY. USA. 2014. p. 123-136. ISBN: 978-1-63463-305-5.

[14] Febbraio MA. Health Benefits of Exercise — More than Meets the Eye! Nature Reviews Endocrinology, 2017;13:72-74. DOI: 10.1038/nrendo.2016.218.

[15] Schroeder EC, Franke WD, Sharp RL, Lee D. Comparative Effectiveness of Aerobic, Resistance, and Combined Training on Cardiovascular Disease Risk Factors: A Randomized Controlled Trial. PloS one. 2019;14(1):e0210292. DOI: 10.1371/journal.pone.0210292.

[16] Levy M, Wang V. The Framingham Heart Study and the Epidemiology of Cardiovascular Disease: A Historical Perspective. Lancet. 2013;383 (9921):999-1008. DOI: 10.1016/S0140-6736(13)61752-3.

[17] Morris, J.N., Heady, J.A., Raffle, P.A.B., Roberts, C.G., and Parks, J.W., 1953. Coronary heart disease and physical activity of work. Lancet 265, 1111-1120. DOI: 10.1016/S0140-6736(53)91495-0.

[18] Morris, J.N., Heady, J.A., Raffle, P.A.B., Roberts, C.G., and Parks, J.W., 1953. Coronary heart disease and physical activity of work. Lancet 265, 1053-1057. DOI: 10.1016/S0140-6736 (53)90665-5.

[19] Beaglehole R, Bonita R, Alleyne G, Horton R, Li L, Lincoln P, Mbanya JC, McKee M, Moodie R, Nishtar S, Piot P, Reddy KS, Stuckler D. UN High-Level Meeting on Non-Communicable Diseases: Addressing Four Questions. Lancet. 2011;378: 449-455. DOI: 10.1016/S0140-6736(11)60879-9.

[20] World Health Organization (WHO). 2020. WHO Guidelines on Physical Activity and Sedentary Behaviour. Geneva: World Health Organization. https://www.who.int/publications/i/item/9789240015128. ISBN 978-92-4-001512-8. [Accessed 23/05/2021].

[21] Afzalpour ME, Bashafaat H, Shariat A, Sadeghi H, Shaw I, Dashtiyan AA, Shaw BS. Plasma protein carbonyl responses to anaerobic exercise in female cyclists. International Journal of Applied Exercise Physiology. 2016;5(1): March.

[22] Oliveira e Silva VR, Stringuetta Belik F, Hueb JC, de Souza Gonçalves R, Costa Teixeira Caramori J, Perez Vogt B, Barretti P, Zanati Bazan SG, De Stefano GMM, Martin LC, da Silva Franco RJ. Aerobic Exercise Training and Nontraditional Cardiovascular Risk Factors in Hemodialysis Patients: Results from a Prospective Randomized Trial. 2019;9(6):391-399. DOI: 10.1159/000501589.

[23] Fiuza-Luces C, Santos-Lozano A, Joyner M, Carrera-Bastos P, Picazo O, Zugaza JL, Izquierdo M, Ruilope LM, Lucia A. Exercise Benefits in Cardiovascular Disease: Beyond Attenuation of Traditional Risk Factors. Nature Reviews Cardiology. 2018;15:731-743. DOI: 10.1038/s41569-018-0065-1.

[24] Shaw BS, Shaw I, Brown GA. Resistance Training and its Effect on Total, Central and Abdominal Adiposity. South African Journal for Research in Sport, Physical Education and Recreation. 2009;31(2):97-108. DOI: 10.4314/sajrs.v31i2.46331.

[25] Shaw BS, Shaw I, Mamen A. Contrasting Effects in Body Composition Following Endurance, Resistance and Concurrent Endurance and Resistance Training. Journal of Sports Medicine and Physical Fitness. 2010;50(2):207-213.

[26] Shaw BS, Dullabh M, Forbes G, Brandkamp J, Shaw I. Analysis of Physiological Determinants during a

Single Bout of Crossfit. International Journal of Performance Analysis in Sport. 2015;15:809-815. DOI: 10.1080/24748668.2015.11868832.

[27] Kleinnibbelink G, Stens NA, Fornasiero A, Speretta GF, Van Dijk APJ, Low DA, Oxborough DL, Thijssen DHJ. The Acute and Chronic Effects of High-Intensity Exercise in Hypoxia on Blood Pressure and Post-Exercise Hypotension: A Randomized Cross-Over Trial. Medicine. 2020;25;99 (39):e22411. DOI: 10.1097/MD.0000 000000022411.

[28] Lira FS, Zanchi NE, Lima-Silva AE, Pires FO, Bertuzzi RC, Santos RV, Caperuto EC, Kiss MA, Seelaender M. Acute High-Intensity Exercise with Low Energy Expenditure Reduced LDL-C and Total Cholesterol in Men. European Journal of Applied Physiology. 2009;107:203-210. DOI: 10.1007/ s00421-009-1115-5.

[29] Pearson RC, Olenick AA, Green ES, Jenkins NT. Acute Exercise Effects on Postprandial Fat Oxidation: Meta-Analysis and Systematic Review. Applied Physiology, Nutrition, and Metabolism. 2020;45(10):1081-1091. DOI: 10.1139/apnm-2019-0917.

[30] Henriksen EJ. Insulin resistance Effects of Acute exercise and exercise training on insulin resistance. Journal of Applied Physiology. 2002;93(2):788-796. DOI: 10.1152/japplphysiol. 01219.2001.

[31] Sener U, Ucok K, Ulasli AM, Genc A, Karabacak H, Coban NF, Simsek H, Cevik H. Evaluation of Health-Related Physical Fitness Parameters and Association Analysis with Depression, Anxiety, and Quality of Life in Patients with Fibromyalgia. International Journal of Rheumatic Diseases. 2016;19(8):763-772. DOI: 10.1111/1756-185X.12237.

[32] Westcott WL, Resistance Training is Medicine - Effects of Strength Training on Health. Current Sports Medicine Reports. 2012;11(4):209-216. DOI: 10.1249/JSR.0b013e31825dabb8

[33] Shaw BS, Shaw I, Brown GA. Resistance exercise is medicine: Strength training in health promotion and rehabilitation. International Journal of Therapy and Rehabilitation. 2015;22(8):385-389. DOI: 10.12968/ ijtr.2015.22.8.385.

[34] Kraemer WJ, Ratamess NA, French DN. Resistance Training for Health and Performance. Current Sports Medicine Reports. 2002;1:165-171 (). DOI: 10.1007/s11932-002-0017-7

[35] Graves JE, Franklin BA. Resistance Training for Health and Rehabilitation. Champaign, Ill: Human Kinetics; 2001. ISBN: 0736001786.

[36] Cornelissen VA, Fagard RF, Coeckelberghs E, Vanhees L. Impact of Resistance Training on Blood Pressure and Other Cardiovascular Risk Factors: A Meta-Analysis of Randomized, Controlled Trials. Hypertension. 2011;58:950-958. DOI: 10.1161/ HYPERTENSIONAHA.111.177071.

[37] Cornelissen VA, Smart NA. Exercise Training for Blood Pressure: A Systematic Review and Meta-analysis. Journal of the American Heart Association. 2013;2(1):e004473. DOI: 10.1161/JAHA.112.004473.

[38] Fagard RH. Exercise is Good for your Blood Pressure: Effects of Endurance Training and Resistance Training. Clinical and Experimental Pharmacology and Physiology. 2006;33:853-856. DOI: 10.1111/j. 1440-1681.2006.04453.x.

[39] Shaw I, Shaw BS. Effects of Aerobic, Resistance and Combination Exercise Training on Resting Blood Pressure: A Comparative Study. African Journal for Physical, Health Education, Recreation

and Dance. 2006;12(4):384-393. DOI: 10.4314/ajpherd.v12i4.24762.

[40] Mann S, Beedie C, Jimenez A. Differential Effects of Aerobic Exercise, Resistance Training and Combined Exercise Modalities on Cholesterol and the Lipid Profile: Review, Synthesis and Recommendations. Sports Medicine. 2014;44:211-221. DOI: 10.1007/s40279-013-0110-5.

[41] Kelley GA, Kelley KS. Impact of Progressive RT on Lipids and Lipoproteins in Adults: A Meta-Analysis of Randomized Controlled Trials. Preventative Medicine. 2009;48:9-19. DOI: 10.1016/j.ypmed.2008.10.010.

[42] Shaw BS, Shaw I, Goon DT. Resistance Training and Blood Lipid Regulation: A Review of the Evidence. Medicina Dello Sport. 2011;64(4): 511-521.

[43] Shaw I, Shaw BS. Relationship between Resistance Training and Lipoprotein Profiles in Sedentary Male Smokers. Cardiovascular Journal of Africa. 2008;19(4):194-197.

[44] Hsu C, Chang S, Nfor ON, Lee K, Lee S, Liaw Y. Effects of Regular Aerobic Exercise and Resistance Training on High-Density Lipoprotein Cholesterol Levels in Taiwanese Adults. International Journal of Environmental Research and Public Health. 2019; 16:2003. DOI: 10.3390/ijerph16112003.

[45] Shaw BS, Shaw I. Physical Activity and High-Density Lipoprotein Cholesterol in Sedentary Male Smokers. African Journal for Physical, Health Education, Recreation and Dance. 2007;13(4):441-452.

[46] Lira F, Yamashita A, Uchida M, Zanchi NE, Gualano B, Martins Jr E, Caperuto EC, Seelaender M. Low and moderate, rather than high intensity strength exercise induces benefit regarding plasma lipid profile. Diabetology & Metabolic Syndrome. 2010;2:31. doi:10.1186/1758-5996-2-31.

[47] Shaw BS, Shaw I. Effect of Resistance Training on Cardiorespiratory Endurance and Coronary Artery Disease Risk. Cardiovascular Journal of South Africa. 2005;16(5):200-204.

[48] Kodama S, Saito K, Tanaka S, Maki M, Yachi Y, Asumi M, Sugawara A, Totsuka K, Shimano H, Ohashi Y, Yamada N, Sone H. Cardiorespiratory Fitness as a Quantitative Predictor of All-Cause Mortality and Cardiovascular Events in Healthy Men and Women. JAMA. 2009;301:2024. DOI: 10.1001/jama.2009.681.

[49] Staron RS, Leonardi MJ, Karapondo DL, Malicky ES, Falkel JE, Hagerman FC, Hikida RS. Skeletal Muscle Adaptations during Early Phase of Resistance Training in Men and Women. Journal of Applied Physiology. 199;76:1247-1255. DOI: 10.1152/jappl.1994.76.3.1247.

[50] Bishop D, Jenkins DG, Mackinnon LT, Mceniery M, Carey MF. The Effects of Strength Training on Endurance Performance and Muscle Characteristics. Medicine & Science in Sports & Exercise. 1999;31(6):886-891. DOI: 10.1097/00005768-199906000-00018.

[51] World Health Organization (WHO). Obesity and Overweight. 2020. Available from: https://www.who.int/news-room/fact-sheets/detail/obesity-and-overweight. [Accessed 12/05/2021].

[52] Mandviwala T, Khalid U, Deswal A. Obesity and Cardiovascular Disease: A Risk Factor or a Risk Marker? Current Atherosclerosis Reports. 2016;18(5):21. DOI: 10.1007/s11883-016-0575-4.

[53] Shaw I, Shaw BS. Consequence of Resistance Training on Body Composition and Coronary Artery

Disease Risk. Cardiovascular Journal of South Africa. 2006;17(3):19-24.

[54] Dietz P, Hoffmann S, Lachtermann E, Simon P. Influence of Exclusive Resistance Training on Body Composition and Cardiovascular Risk Factors in Overweight or Obese Children: A Systematic Review. Obesity Facts. 2012;5:546-560. DOI: 10.1159/000341560

[55] McGuigan M, Tatasciore M, Newton R, Pettigrew S. Eight Weeks of Resistance Training Can Significantly Alter Body Composition in Children Who Are Overweight or Obese. Journal of Strength and Conditioning Research. 2009;23(1):80-85. DOI: 10.1519/JSC.0b013e3181876a56.

[56] Shaw BS, Shaw I. Determinants of Physical Activity in Children and Adolescents: Implications for the Increasing Prevalence of Childhood Obesity. African Journal for Physical, Health Education, Recreation and Dance. 2014;2:91-101.

[57] Flack KD, Davy KP, Hulver MW, Winett RA, Frisard MI, Davy BM. Aging, Resistance Training, and Diabetes Prevention. Journal of Aging Research. 2011:1-2. DOI: 10.4061/2011/127315

[58] Amati F, Dubé JJ, Coen PM, Stefanovic-Racic M, Toledo FGS, Goodpaster BH. Physical Inactivity and Obesity Underlie the Insulin Resistance of Aging. Diabetes Care. 2009;32(8):1547-1549. DOI: 10.2337/dc09-0267.

[59] Shaw BS, Shaw I. Exercise Therapy and its Role in Glucose Maintenance. African Journal for Physical, Health Education, Recreation and Dance. 2008;14(4):417-427. DOI: 10.4314/ajpherd.v14i4.24817.

[60] Strasser B, Pesta D. Resistance Training for Diabetes Prevention and Therapy: Experimental Findings and Molecular Mechanisms. BioMed Research International. 2013. DOI: 10.1155/2013/805217.

[61] Bacchi C, Negri ME, Zanolin, Milanese C, Faccioli N, Trombetta M, Zoppini G, Cevese A, Bonadonna RC, Schena F, Bonora E, Lanza M, Moghetti P. Metabolic Effects of Aerobic Training and Resistance Training in Type 2 Diabetic Subjects. A Randomized Controlled Trial (the READ2 Study). Diabetes Care. 2012;35:676-682. DOI: 10.2337/dc11-1655.

[62] Cauza U, Hanusch-Enserer B, Strasser B, Ludvik B, Metz-Schimmerl S, Pacini G, Wagner O, Georg P, Prager R, Kostner K, Dunky A, Haber P. The Relative Benefits of Endurance and Strength Training on the Metabolic Factors and Muscle Function of People with type 2 Diabetes Mellitus. Archives of Physical Medicine and Rehabilitation. 2005;86(8):1527-1533. DOI: 10.1016/j.apmr.2005.01.007.

[63] Brubaker PH, Kaminsky LA, Whaley MH. Coronary Artery Disease: Essentials of Prevention and Rehabilitation Programs. Champaign, IL: Human Kinetics; 2002

[64] Shaw BS, Shaw I, Brown GA. Relationship between Resistance Training and Self-Reported Habitual Nutrient Intake. South African Journal for Research in Sport, Physical Education and Recreation, 2010;32(2): 109-116. DOI: 10.4314/sajrs.v32i2.59300.

[65] Hurley BF, Hagberg JM, Goldberg AP, Seals DR, Ehsani AA, Brennan RE, Holloszy JO. Resistive Training can Reduce Coronary Risk Factors Without Altering VO2max or Percent Body Fat. Medicine and Science in Sport and Exercise. 1988;20(2):150-154. DOI: 10.1249/00005768-198820020-00008.

[66] Keim NL, Canty DJ, Barbieri TF, Wu MM. Effect of Exercise and Dietary Restraint on Energy Intake of Reduced-Obese Women. Appetite. 1996;26(1):55-70. DOI: 10.1006/appe.1996.0005.

[67] Shaw BS, Shaw I, Brown GA. Self-Reported Dietary Intake Following Endurance, Resistance and Concurrent Endurance and Resistance Training. Journal of Sports Science and Medicine. 2008;7(2):255-259.

[68] Morgan DW, Cruise RJ, Giradin BW, Lutz-Schneider V, Morgan DH, Qi WM. HDL-C Concentrations in Weight-Trained, Endurance-Trained and Sedentary Females. Physician and SportsMedicine. 1986;14(3):166-172, 177, 180-181. DOI: 10.1080/00913847.1986.11709017.

[69] Castaneda C, Gordon PL, Uhlin KL, Levey AS, Kehayias JJ, Dwyer JT, Fielding RA, Roubenoff R, Fiatarone Singh M. Resistance Training to Counteract the Catabolism of a Low-Protein Diet in Patients with Chronic Renal Insufficiency: A Randomized, Controlled Trial. Ann Intern Med. 2001;135:965-976. DOI: 10.7326/0003-4819-135-11-200112040-00008.

[70] Menezes AR, Lavie CJ, Milani RV, O'Keefe J, Lavie TJ. Psychological Risk Factors and Cardiovascular Disease: Is it All in Your Head? Postgraduate Medicine. 2011;123(5):165-176. DOI: 10.3810/pgm.2011.09.2472.

[71] Dionigi R. Resistance Training and Older Adults' Beliefs About Psychological Benefits: The Importance of Self-Efficacy and Social Interaction. Journal of Sport & Exercise Psychology. 2007;29:723-746. DOI: 10.1123/jsep.29.6.723.

[72] Goldfield GS, Kenny GP, Alberga AS, Prud'homme D, Hadjiyannakis S, Stasia GR, Phillip P, Tulloch H, Malcolm J, Doucette S, Wells GA, Ma J, Cameron JD, Sigal RJ. Effects of Aerobic Training, Resistance Training, or Both on Psychological Health in Adolescents with Obesity: The HEARTY Randomized Controlled Trial. Journal of Consulting and Clinical Psychology. 2015;83(6):1123-1135. DOI: 10.1037/ccp0000038.

[73] Haslam DR, McCartney SN, McKelvie RS, MacDougall JD. Direct Measurements of Arterial Blood Pressure During Formal Weightlifting in Cardiac Patients. Journal of Cardiopulmonary Rehabilitation. 1988;8:213-225; DOI: 10.1097/00008483-198806000-00002.

[74] Sagiv M. Safety of Resistance Training in the Elderly. European Review of Aging and Physical Activity. 2009;6:1. DOI: 10.1007/s11556-009-0047-8.

[75] Gordon NF, Kohl HW III, Pollock ML, Vaandrager H, Gibbons LW, Blair SN. Cardiovascular Safety of Maximal Strength Testing in Healthy Adults. American Journal of Cardiology. 1995;76:851-853. DOI: 10.1016/S0002-9149(99)80245-8.

[76] Sparling PB, Cantwell JD, Dolan CM, Niederman RK. Strength Training in a Cardiac Rehabilitation Program: A Six-month Follow-up. Archives of Physical Medicine and Rehabilitation. 1990;71:148-152.

[77] Wilke NA, Sheldahl LM, Tristani FE, Hughes CV, Kalbfleisch JH. The Safety of Static-Dynamic Effort Soon after Myocardial Infarction. American Heart Journal. 1985;110:542-545. DOI: 10.1016/0002-8703(85)90072-9.

[78] American College of Sports Medicine. ACSM's Guidelines for Exercise Testing and Prescription. 6th edition. Baltimore, Md: Lippincott Williams & Wilkins; 2000. ISBN: 0-683-30355-4.

[79] Fidalgo ASF, Parinatti P, Borges JP, de Paula T, Monteiro W. Institutional Guidelines for Resistance Exercise Training in Cardiovascular Disease: A Systematic Review. Sports Medicine. 2019;49(3):463-475. DOI: 10.1007/s40279-019-01059-z.

[80] Shaw BS, Turner S, Shaw I. Comparison of Muscle Endurance and Hypertrophy Resistance Training on Cardiovascular Disease Risk in Smokers. Asian Journal of Sports Medicine. 2021;12(1):1-6,e106589. DOI: 10.5812/asjsm.106589.

[81] Shaw BS, Shaw I. Resistance Training as a Countermeasure for Key Non-Communicable Diseases in Low-Resource Settings: A Review. Asian Journal of Sports Medicine. 2021;12(1):1-8,e106588. DOI: 10.5812/asjsm.106588.

[82] Kraemer WJ, Ratamess NA. Fundamentals of Resistance Training: Progression and Exercise Prescription. Medicine and Science in Sports and Exercise. 2004;36(4):674-88. DOI: 10.1249/01.mss.0000121945.36635.61.

[83] Shaw I, Boshoff VE, Coetzee S, Shaw BS. Efficacy of Home-Based Callisthenic Resistance Training on Cardiovascular Disease Risk in Overweight Compared to Normal Weight Preadolescents. Asian Journal of Sports Medicine. 2021;12(1)1-5,e106591. DOI: 10.5812/asjsm.106591.

Chapter 8

The Effects of Linoleic Acid Consumption on Lipid Risk Markers for Cardiovascular Disease

Erik Froyen

Abstract

Cardiovascular disease (CVD) is the number one contributor to death in the United States and worldwide. Lipid risk markers for CVD include high serum concentrations of total cholesterol, low-density lipoprotein cholesterol (LDL-C), very-low-density lipoprotein cholesterol (VLDL-C), lipoprotein (a), and triglycerides, as well as low serum concentrations of high-density lipoprotein cholesterol (HDL-C). Additional factors to assess CVD risk include apolipoprotein A (associated with HDL) and apolipoprotein B (associated with LDL). A suggested dietary strategy to decrease these risk factors is to replace a portion of saturated fatty acids with unsaturated fatty acids – especially polyunsaturated fatty acids (PUFAs). One PUFA, in particular, is the essential omega-6 PUFA linoleic acid, which has been demonstrated to affect these CVD risk markers. Therefore, this chapter will discuss the effects of linoleic acid consumption on lipid risk markers for CVD in healthy individuals, the associated mechanisms, and dietary recommendations to decrease CVD risk.

Keywords: linoleic acid, fatty acids, lipid risk markers, cardiovascular disease, humans

1. Introduction

Cardiovascular disease (CVD) (includes heart disease and stroke) is the leading cause of death in the United States [1] and worldwide [2]. In the United States, heart disease is the number one contributor to death, causing 647,457 deaths (23% of total deaths), while stroke is the fifth leading cause of death, contributing to 146,383 deaths (5.2% of total deaths) in 2017 [1]. Worldwide, heart disease is the leading cause of death, leading to 8.9 million deaths, or 16% of the total deaths globally in 2019. Stroke is the second leading contributor to deaths worldwide, causing more than 6 million deaths, or 11% of the deaths, worldwide [2].

A suggested dietary strategy to decrease the risk factors for CVD is to replace a portion of saturated fatty acids (SFAs) with monounsaturated fatty acids (MUFAs) and polyunsaturated fatty acids (PUFAs) [3–10]. For example, the Nurses' Health Study [11] demonstrated that replacing 5% of energy from SFAs with equivalent

IntechOpen

energy from MUFAs, PUFAs, or carbohydrates from whole grains, decreased the risk for coronary heart disease (CHD). A meta-analysis of randomized controlled trials reported that replacing saturated fat with polyunsaturated fat reduced CHD events [12].

However, certain authors and publications are not in agreement with these recommendations to decrease the risk factors for CVD, cardiovascular events, and/or mortality [13–22]. The PURE prospective cohort study concluded that intakes of total, saturated, and unsaturated fats were not significantly associated with the risk of myocardial infarction or CVD mortality [23]. Meta-analyses of prospective cohort studies demonstrated that consumption of saturated fat was not associated with an increased risk of CVD [24]. Interestingly, there was an inverse association between saturated fat intake and the risk of stroke [25]. Additionally, a meta-analysis of randomized controlled trials reported that replacing saturated fat with primarily polyunsaturated fat is "unlikely" to reduce CVD events or mortality [26]. Hooper et al. [27], in a review of randomized controlled trials, stated that there is "little or no effect of reducing saturated fat on all-cause mortality or cardiovascular mortality."

As noted, there is controversy regarding the effects of the consumption of fatty acids on CVD risk. One such controversy is the recommendation of linoleic acid, which is the essential omega-6 (or n-6) PUFA [28–30]. For example, it has been found that replacing saturated fat with linoleic acid lowers serum cholesterol, but does not lower the risk of death from CHD [21, 22]. Furthermore, there is concern regarding whether linoleic acid increases the risk for inflammation [31].

An analysis of prospective observational studies demonstrated that higher tissue and serum concentrations of linoleic acid decreased the risk for cardiovascular events [32]. The Cardiovascular Health Study, a prospective cohort study, discovered that higher circulating linoleic acid concentrations reduced total and CHD mortality [33]. A meta-analysis of prospective cohort studies found that decreased consumption of omega-6 PUFAs and increased intakes of saturated and trans-fatty acids increased CHD mortality [34]. Linoleic acid consumption reduced the risk of CHD events and death, according to another meta-analysis of prospective cohort studies [35]. A systematic review of randomized controlled trials, in which there was a replacement of dietary saturated and monounsaturated fatty acids with omega-6 fatty acids, concluded that omega-6 fatty acids lowered the risk of myocardial infarction. Additionally, the intake of omega-6 fatty acids reduced total serum cholesterol, but not "other blood fat fractions". It was also highlighted that "the benefits of omega-6 fats remain to be proven" [36].

According to the diet-heart hypothesis, a high consumption of saturated fat and cholesterol – and a low intake of polyunsaturated fat – increase the build-up of cholesterol and plaques in artery walls; these developments, therefore, increase the risks for atherosclerosis, cardiovascular disease, and myocardial infarction [18, 21, 37]. However, the diet-heart hypothesis has been evolving, and thus, some individuals recommend focusing more on overall dietary patterns, rather than individual fatty acids [37]. Moreover, there are a variety of factors that contribute to increasing the risk for CVD, such as high blood pressure, arrhythmia, inflammation, thrombosis, insulin resistance, endothelial dysfunction, obesity, cigarette smoke, genetics, the microbiome, a lack of exercise, a high alcohol consumption, and overall dietary patterns [14, 18, 37–42].

Lipid levels have also been proposed to be "strong" risk factors for CVD and mortality. These lipid risk factors include the following: high serum concentrations of total cholesterol, triglycerides, low-density lipoprotein cholesterol (LDL-C), lipoprotein(a), and very-low-density lipoprotein cholesterol (VLDL-C), as well as low serum concentrations of high-density lipoprotein cholesterol (HDL-C). In addition, apolipoprotein A1 (associated with HDL) and apolipoprotein B (associated with LDL) have been used as CVD risk markers [18, 43]. Interestingly, LDL particle size has also been utilized as a risk marker for CVD. The small, dense LDL subclass, compared to large, buoyant LDL particles, has been reported to be more atherogenic [44–50].

Therefore, this chapter will focus on the consumption of linoleic acid on lipid risk markers for CVD in healthy individuals, such as total cholesterol, triglycerides, LDL-C, LDL particle size, lipoprotein(a), VLDL-C, HDL-C, apolipoprotein A1, and apolipoprotein B. The associated mechanisms of action will also be covered. The chapter will conclude with recommendations to decrease the risk factors for CVD. Significant dietary sources of linoleic acid are presented in **Tables 1** and **2**. The chemical structure of linoleic acid is illustrated in **Figure 1**.

Oils	Linoleic acid (grams)
Corn oil	53.5
Cottonseed oil	51.9
Grapeseed oil	69.6
Peanut oil	32.0
Safflower oil	12.7
Sesame oil	41.3
Soybean oil	51.0
Sunflower oil	65.7
Walnut oil	52.9

Table 1.
Oil sources of linoleic acid (per 100 grams) [51, 52].

Nuts and seeds	Linoleic acid (grams)
Almonds	3.49
Brazil nuts	6.82
Pecans	5.85
Pine nuts	9.4
Pistachios	4.0
Pumpkin seeds	5.55
Sesame seeds	5.78
Sunflower seeds	9.29
Walnuts	10.8

Table 2.
Linoleic acid content in nuts and seeds (per 1 ounce or 28.3495 grams) [51, 52].

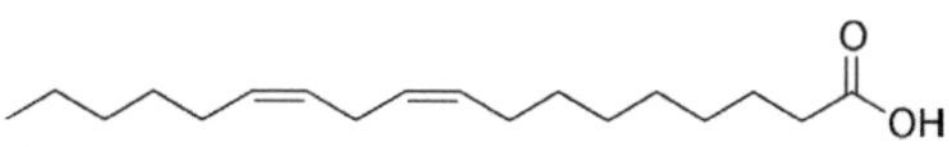

Figure 1.
The chemical structure of linoleic acid [53].

2. The effects of linoleic acid consumption on lipid risk markers for cardiovascular disease in healthy individuals

The consumption of linoleic acid has been demonstrated to affect lipid risk markers for cardiovascular disease. The discussed studies include intervention trials that investigated the effects of linoleic acid consumption, in grams or percentage of energy, on CVD lipid risk markers in healthy individuals. Therefore, epidemiological, postprandial, and animal studies are not covered. The results are organized by the respective CVD lipid risk marker.

2.1 Total cholesterol

The consumption of linoleic acid decreased total cholesterol compared to a usual U.S. diet (high in saturated fat and cholesterol) [54], and diets high in SFAs [55] (including stearic acid [56] and palmitic acid [57]), MUFAs [58], or medium-chain fatty acids [59]. A high intake of alpha-linolenic acid, the essential omega-3 fatty acid, decreased cholesterol concentrations compared to the control diet with the same percentage of linoleic acid [60]. In contrast, no significant differences in total cholesterol were observed after linoleic acid consumption compared to diets containing eicosapentaenoic acid (EPA) and docosahexaenoic acid (DHA) (omega-3 fatty acids) [61, 62], alpha-linolenic acid [63], high and low amounts of linoleic acid [64], oleic acid (a MUFA) [65, 66], or stearic acid [66]. Interestingly, intakes of SFA- or linoleic acid-rich diets – both supplemented with EPA and DHA – produced no significant differences in cholesterol concentrations [67].

2.2 Triglycerides

The consumption of linoleic acid decreased triglycerides compared to diets with significant amounts of oleic acid [58], stearic acid [56], or medium-chain fatty acids [59]. Intakes of linoleic acid, supplemented with EPA and DHA, reduced triglyceride concentrations versus a linoleic acid diet rich in oleic acid [62]. A SFA-rich diet and a diet high in linoleic acid, both with added EPA and DHA, lowered triglyceride concentrations, with no significant differences between diets [67]. In contrast, diets supplemented with EPA and DHA decreased triglycerides compared to linoleic acid intakes [55, 61]. No significant differences were observed regarding triglyceride concentrations between lower and higher linoleic acid intakes [54, 60, 64], and diets rich in linoleic acid versus diets high in alpha-linolenic acid [63], oleic acid [65], or stearic acid [66].

2.3 Low-density lipoprotein cholesterol (LDL-C)

Intakes of linoleic acid decreased LDL-C versus diets rich in oleic acid [58], SFAs [55], palmitic acid [57], stearic acid [56, 68], trans-fatty acids [68], or medium-chain fatty acids [59]. Furthermore, higher amounts of linoleic acid more significantly lowered LDL-C concentrations [54, 57]. There were mixed results or no significant differences in comparison to oleic acid [62, 65, 66, 68]. Additionally, there were no significant differences when comparing linoleic acid consumption to alpha-linolenic acid [63] or stearic acid [66]. Consuming low and high amounts of linoleic acid – along with significant amounts of alpha-linolenic acid [64] or EPA and DHA [62] – also did not differ. Moreover, no significant differences were observed with respect to LDL-C after following a SFA-rich diet or a diet high in linoleic acid – both supplemented with EPA and DHA [67].

2.4 LDL particle size

There were no significant differences in LDL particle size after consumption of low and high amounts of linoleic acid [60, 69], and intakes of linoleic acid compared to oleic acid or stearic acid [66]. Interestingly, there were decreases in large and small LDL particle concentrations after 10 days of a linoleic acid-rich diet compared to a diet high in SFAs, with both diets supplemented with EPA and DHA [70]. In contrast, no significant differences were observed in LDL particle size after 6 weeks of a linoleic acid-rich diet comparted to a SFA-rich diet (both supplemented with EPA and DHA) [67].

2.5 Very-low-density lipoprotein cholesterol (VLDL-C)

Following consumption of diets rich in linoleic acid, there were decreases in VLDL-C concentrations compared to diets containing significant amounts of oleic acid [58] or medium-chain fatty acids [59]. In contrast, intakes of a SFA- or linoleic acid-rich diet (both containing significant amounts of EPA and DHA) resulted in no significant differences between diets; however, both diets decreased VLDL-C concentrations [67].

2.6 High-density lipoprotein cholesterol (HDL-C)

HDL-C increased following consumption of linoleic acid compared to stearic acid [56]. In contrast, intakes of linoleic acid decreased HDL-C compared to EPA and DHA [61] or palmitic acid [57]. However, most studies noticed no significant differences regarding HDL-C concentrations after consuming low and high amounts of linoleic acid [54, 60, 62, 64], and linoleic acid compared to oleic acid [58, 65, 66], alpha-linolenic acid [60, 63], or stearic acid [66]. Interestingly, intakes of SFAs or linoleic acid (both diets supplemented with EPA and DHA) displayed no significant differences in HDL-C concentrations [67].

2.7 Lipoprotein(a)

Linoleic acid consumption reduced lipoprotein(a) concentrations compared with a diet high in trans-fatty acids [68]. However, linoleic acid intake increased lipoprotein(a) compared to a diet rich in SFAs [55]. In contrast, no significant differences were found after consuming linoleic acid compared to SFAs, oleic acid, or stearic acid [68].

2.8 Apolipoproteins A1, A2, and B

The consumption of linoleic acid increased apolipoprotein A1 compared to a typical U.S. diet [54]. Additionally, linoleic acid increased apolipoprotein A2 compared to EPA and DHA [55]. In contrast, apolipoproteins A1 and A2 decreased after following a diet rich in linoleic acid compared to a diet high in oleic acid [65]. Apolipoprotein A1 concentrations did not differ when comparing low and high linoleic acid intakes [60], and consumption of linoleic acid compared to diets containing high amounts of stearic acid or oleic acid [66]. There were decreases in apolipoprotein B concentrations after linoleic consumption compared to a typical U.S. diet [54], stearic acid, elaidic acid (a trans-fatty acid) [56], or SFAs [55]. There were no significant differences with respect to apolipoprotein B after intakes of linoleic acid compared with oleic acid [65, 66] or stearic acid [66].

3. The mechanisms by which linoleic acid affects lipid risk markers for cardiovascular disease

Linoleic acid (or PUFAs) has been demonstrated to affect CVD lipid risk markers. The mechanisms involved in altering these risk markers will be discussed in this section.

3.1 Total cholesterol

PUFAs have been shown to increase liver X receptor alpha (LXRα) gene expression [71, 72] via peroxisome proliferator activated receptors (PPARs) [71]. LXRα stimulates the expression of cholesterol 7 α-hydroxylase (CYP7), thereby converting cholesterol to bile acids. Therefore, by increasing CYP7 activity, PUFAs participate in cholesterol catabolism [73].

3.2 Triglycerides

PUFAs interact more strongly with PPARα compared to SFAs [74]. PPARα binds to peroxisome proliferator response elements (PPREs) located in the promotor regions of genes, such as apoC-III and lipoprotein lipase (LPL) [75]. It has been proposed that LPL may demonstrate increased activity towards VLDL triglycerides containing polyunsaturated fatty acids, thereby leading to increased breakdown of triglyceride-rich lipoproteins (chylomicrons and VLDL particles) [73, 76, 77]. LPL activity is inhibited by apoC-III, and thus, increases triglyceride concentrations [78]. It has been reported that PUFAs decrease apoC-III, thereby increasing LPL activity and, indeed, VLDL catabolism [73]. Moreover, omega-3 PUFAs have been shown to reduce triglycerides by lowering diacylglycerol acyltransferase, fatty acid synthase, and acetyl coenzyme A (CoA) carboxylase [79–84].

3.3 LDL-C

Intakes of linoleic acid [85] or PUFAs [73] have been demonstrated to increase LDL receptor activity, protein, and mRNA compared to SFAs. Furthermore, PUFAs increase membrane fluidity [73, 85, 86], which increases LDL receptor activity, and thus, increases LDL catabolism [87–89].

3.4 LDL particle size

It has been reported that consumption of SFAs increases large, buoyant LDL particles compared to lower SFA-containing diets [69, 90], whereas consumption of diets rich in PUFAs decreases large, buoyant LDL particles versus diets high in SFAs [70, 91]. It has been suggested that SFAs increase LPL and hepatic lipase activities [92, 93]. As such, LPL increases large, buoyant LDL particles, whereas hepatic lipase may stimulate the catabolism of triglyceride-rich lipoprotein remnants [92]. However, additional research is needed in this area regarding the mechanisms by which individual fatty acids affect LDL particle size.

3.5 VLDL-C

The sterol regulatory element-binding protein-1 (SREBP-1) is associated with lipogenesis and cholesterol synthesis in the liver [94, 95]. PUFAs have been shown to inhibit SREBP-1 gene transcription and/or protein [96], thereby lowering VLDL secretion from the liver [73, 96]. In addition, intakes of PUFAs increase VLDL catabolism and uptake [59, 81].

3.6 HDL-C

Replacing SFAs with MUFAs and/or PUFAs generates lower total cholesterol and LDL-C concentrations, with modest HDL-C reductions; however, a lower total cholesterol: HDL-C ratio results [4, 97]. It is thought that dietary fat increases the "transport rate" and decreases the "fractional catabolic rate" of HDL cholesterol ester and apolipoprotein A1 [98]. However, more research is needed to describe the mechanisms by which individual fatty acids impact HDL-C.

3.7 Lipoprotein(a)

Lipoprotein(a) is synthesized in the liver and contains apolipoprotein A, which is bound to apolipoprotein B-100 [99–101]. The biological activity of lipoprotein(a) is unknown [102]; however, high concentrations have been associated with CVD [101, 103, 104]. Genetics seem to be the primary determinant of lipoprotein(a) [105]. Hence, diet and exercise do not appear to be significant contributors to lipoprotein(a) concentrations. There have also been inconsistent findings of fatty acid consumption (including PUFAs) on lipoprotein(a) concentrations [106]. However, it has been suggested that fatty acids may affect liver apolipoprotein(a) synthesis, thereby impacting lipoprotein(a) [106–108]. As such, more research is needed to determine the effects of dietary composition on lipoprotein(a) concentrations.

3.8 Apolipoprotein A1

HDL particles contain apolipoprotein A1, which interacts with the ATP-binding cassette transporter on the surface of cells. Furthermore, apolipoprotein A1 is a cofactor for lecithin cholesterol acyl transferase, which generates mature HDL particles [43, 109]. Plasma apolipoprotein A1 concentration typically coincide with HDL-C concentrations [43]. The significance of apolipoprotein A2 is less clear [110]. Interestingly, PPARα also interacts with PPREs in the promoter region of the apolipoprotein A1 gene in the liver [75]. Hence, PUFAs may exert their effects on apolipoprotein A1 via PPARα [73].

3.9 Apolipoprotein B

Apolipoprotein B also occurs in two forms: apolipoprotein B-48 and apolipoprotein B-100. The intestine synthesizes apolipoprotein B-48, which is a component of chylomicrons. The liver produces apolipoprotein B-100, which is associated with VLDL and LDL particles. Apolipoprotein B is necessary for the binding of lipoproteins to the LDL receptor. Apolipoprotein B plasma concentrations are significantly associated with LDL-C concentrations [43, 111]. It has been reported that high apolipoprotein B concentrations increase the risk for CVD, whereas apolipoprotein A1 concentrations decrease CVD risk [43, 112]. As mentioned previously, PUFAs increase LDL catabolism, thereby reducing apolipoprotein B [87].

4. Linoleic acid recommendations

The adequate intake (AI) values for linoleic acid for males and females (19-50 years) are 17 grams/day and 12 grams/day, respectively. Regarding males and females ages 51-70 years, the AI values for linoleic acid are 14 grams/day and 11 grams/day, respectively. The American Heart Association recommends consuming 5 to 10% of energy as linoleic acid to decrease CVD risk [29, 31]. Additionally, the World Health Organization recommends consuming 2.5 to 9% of energy from linoleic acid to decrease LDL and total cholesterol concentrations, and thus, lower the risk for CVD [113]. It is not recommended to consume more than 10% of energy as linoleic acid due to limited research.

5. Fat recommendations

In addition to linoleic acid recommendations, there are fat recommendations to reduce CVD risk, cardiovascular events, and/or mortality. For example, it has been suggested to replace approximately 5% of energy from SFAs with MUFAs and/or PUFAs [4, 8–12, 38, 113], and to consume less than 10% of energy as SFAs [113, 114]. On the other hand, certain studies do not coincide with these recommendations [14–17, 21–27, 115]. In addition, low-fat, and in-turn, high-carbohydrate diets, decrease LDL-C; however, there is also a reduction in HDL-C and increased concentrations of VLDLs or triglycerides [37, 97, 116–118], which may produce higher amounts of small, dense LDL particles [41, 119, 120]. It has been reported that higher-fat versus lower-fat diets increase large, buoyant LDL and/or decrease small, dense LDL particles [69, 92, 121–123]. Interestingly, higher SFA intakes also increase large LDL and/or decrease small LDL particles [69, 90, 124–126]. These small, dense LDL particles may increase the risk for CVD in the following ways: 1) increased transport into arterial walls [127]; 2) increased attachment to proteoglycans [128]; 3) increased oxidation [129, 130]; and 4) reduced binding to the LDL receptor [127, 131, 132].

Various organizations have published dietary recommendations to decrease the risk factors for CVD. The American College of Cardiology/American Heart Association Task Force suggests consuming a diet rich in fruits, vegetables, whole grains, nuts, legumes, lean animal or plant protein sources, and fish. Additionally, it is recommended to decrease the consumption of red and processed meats, refined carbohydrates, trans-fatty acids, sodium, cholesterol, and sugar-sweetened drinks [38]. The Dietary Guidelines for Americans suggest consuming vegetable oils to replace sources rich in SFAs, such as butter, shortening, lard, palm oil, palm kernel oil, coconut oil, full-fat dairy products, and high-fat meats [114]. The World Health Organization also recommends replacing SFAs with unsaturated fatty acids, such as sunflower, safflower, corn, soybean, canola, and olive oils, as well as nuts, avocado, and fish [113].

It has been recently proposed, however, that guidelines to lower the risk for CVD should focus on overall dietary patterns, rather than individual fatty acids [14, 133]. The consumption of low-fat diets, for example, did not reduce CVD risk [134, 135]. Furthermore, certain individuals with higher intakes of saturated fat and cholesterol do not possess high CVD mortality rates, as they have an increased consumption of plant foods – in addition to MUFAs and PUFAs [15]. Furthermore, some foods that are higher in SFAs have not been demonstrated to increase the risk for CVD. A proposed explanation for these outcomes is the food matrix of these items, such as macro- and micronutrients, phytochemicals, and probiotics [14, 37].

6. Conclusions

This chapter focused on the effects of linoleic acid consumption on lipid risk markers for CVD in healthy individuals. Interestingly, linoleic acid reduced total cholesterol and LDL-C compared to diets that were lower in PUFAs and/or higher in

SFAs. In contrast, linoleic acid generated inconsistent outcomes regarding triglycerides, whereas EPA and DHA more significantly reduced triglyceride concentrations. In limited studies, linoleic acid decreased VLDL-C compared to diets containing oleic acid or medium-chain fatty acids, and decreased HDL-C compared to palmitic acid or EPA and DHA; however, linoleic acid increased HDL-C compared with stearic acid. Additionally, linoleic acid reduced apolipoprotein B in comparison to a typical U.S. diet, SFAs, or trans-fatty acids. Interestingly, there were inconsistent

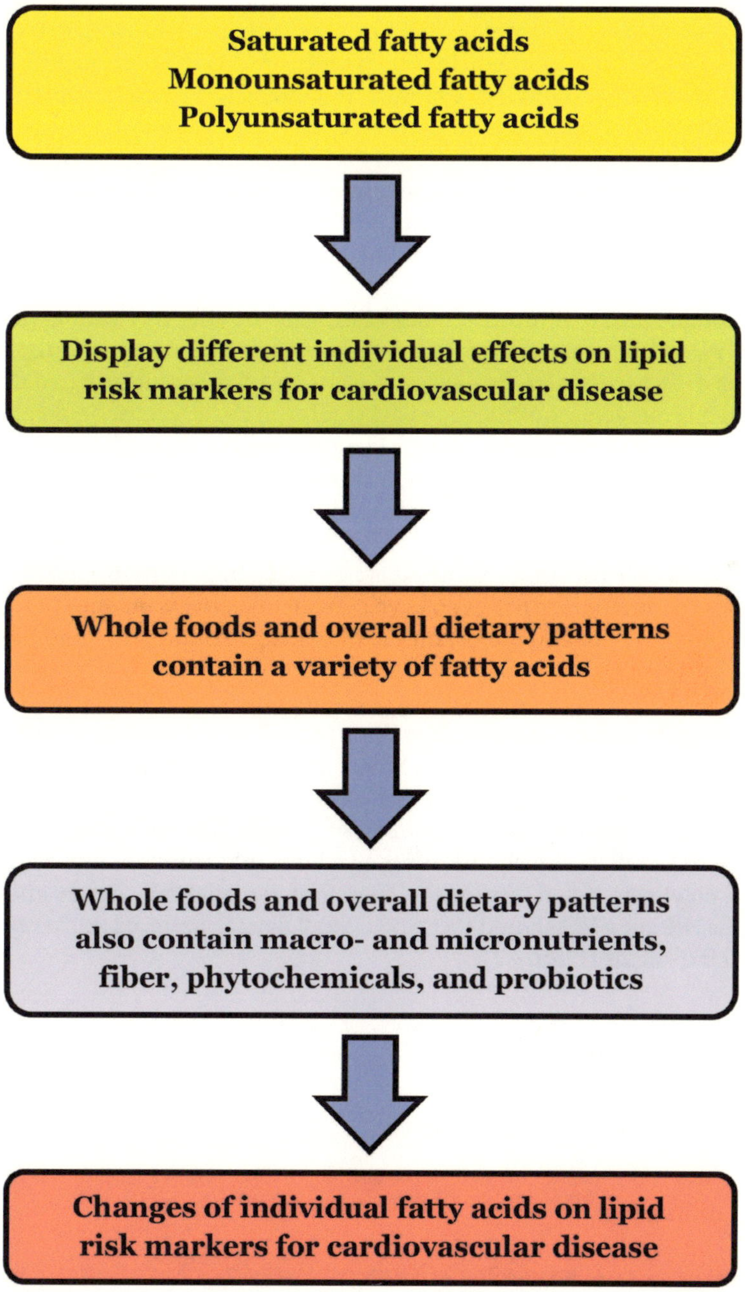

Figure 2.
The progression from individual fatty acids to whole foods and overall dietary patterns on lipid risk markers for cardiovascular disease.

results or no significant differences for selected CVD lipid risk markers – particularly when comparing linoleic acid to oleic acid. Therefore, additional research is needed regarding the effects of fatty acids on markers that increase the risk for CVD – in addition to the associated mechanisms.

The development of CVD is a complex process which involves many factors that influence the discussed lipid risk markers, such as exercise patterns, overweight/obesity, cigarette smoke, hypertension, high alcohol consumption, and genetics. To add to this complexity is our dietary patterns. As discussed, there are mixed results regarding the consumption of linoleic acid on CVD lipid risk markers. One such dietary explanation is the complex food matrices of these items, which may, therefore, influence CVD risk markers. In other words, we do not consume individual fatty acids; we consume food. For example, individual saturated and unsaturated fatty acids have differing effects on CVD risk markers; however, these individual effects may be diminished when these fatty acids are components of whole food items. This attribute may explain, in part, for the differing outcomes of saturated and unsaturated fat on CVD risk, events, and/or mortality. Perhaps, therefore, we should focus on whole foods and overall dietary patterns when providing guidelines to reduce the risk for CVD.

It is recommended that future studies investigate the effects of various dietary patterns on CVD risk markers, such as lower-carbohydrate versus higher-carbohydrate diets, lower-fat versus higher-fat diets, and plant-based versus meat-based diets. Based on the heterogeneity of the reviewed studies on the effects of linoleic acid consumption on lipid risk markers for CVD, future studies should be longer in duration – with more participants. Moreover, it should be clarified, in future publications, whether the discussed CVD lipid risk markers exist as strong and independent risk factors for CVD.

It is clear that the consumption of fat is a critical component to a healthy diet; consuming too much or too little can have detrimental effects on one's health. Therefore, moderation is an important factor to keep in mind regarding fat consumption. It seems, however, that certain dietary recommendations focus on decreasing the intakes of saturated fatty acids, and increasing the consumption of monounsaturated and polyunsaturated fatty acids. These recommendations may not be optimal in the following ways: 1) foods consist of individual fatty acids, which have different effects on CVD lipid risk markers; 2) overall dietary patterns and food components may offset the effects of specific fatty acids; and 3) individuals may not be familiar with significant food sources of saturated, monounsaturated, and polyunsaturated fatty acids. Therefore, it seems that dietary guidelines to lower the risk for CVD should focus on overall dietary patterns, rather than individual fatty acids (**Figure 2**).

Acknowledgements

No funding was used for this project.

Conflict of interest

The author declares no conflict of interest.

Author details

Erik Froyen
California State Polytechnic University, Pomona, USA

*Address all correspondence to: ebfroyen@cpp.edu

IntechOpen

© 2021 The Author(s). Licensee IntechOpen. This chapter is distributed under the terms of the Creative Commons Attribution License (http://creativecommons.org/licenses/by/3.0), which permits unrestricted use, distribution, and reproduction in any medium, provided the original work is properly cited.

References

[1] Deaths: Leading Causes for 2017 [Internet]. Available from: https://www.cdc.gov/nchs/nvss/leading-causes-of-death.htm [Accessed: 2021-05-16].

[2] World Health Organization. The top 10 causes of death [Internet]. Available from: https://www.who.int/news-room/fact-sheets/detail/the-top-10-causes-of-death [Accessed: 2021-05-16].

[3] Anton SD, Heekin K, Simkins C, Acosta A. Differential effects of adulterated versus unadulterated forms of linoleic acid on cardiovascular health. J Integr Med. 2013 Jan;11(1):2-10.

[4] Wang DD, Hu FB. Dietary Fat and Risk of Cardiovascular Disease: Recent Controversies and Advances. Annu Rev Nutr. 2017 Aug 21;37:423-46.

[5] Hu FB, Willett WC. Optimal diets for prevention of coronary heart disease. Jama. 2002 Nov 27;288(20):2569-78.

[6] Zock PL, Blom WA, Nettleton JA, Hornstra G. Progressing Insights into the Role of Dietary Fats in the Prevention of Cardiovascular Disease. Curr Cardiol Rep. 2016 Nov;18(11):111.

[7] Millen BE, Wolongevicz DM, de Jesus JM, Nonas CA, Lichtenstein AH. 2013 American Heart Association/American College of Cardiology Guideline on Lifestyle Management to Reduce Cardiovascular Risk: practice opportunities for registered dietitian nutritionists. J Acad Nutr Diet. 2014 Nov;114(11):1723-9.

[8] Sacks FM, Lichtenstein AH, Wu JHY, Appel LJ, Creager MA, Kris-Etherton PM, et al. Dietary Fats and Cardiovascular Disease: A Presidential Advisory From the American Heart Association. Circulation. 2017 Jul 18;136(3):e1-e23.

[9] Clifton PM, Keogh JB. A systematic review of the effect of dietary saturated and polyunsaturated fat on heart disease. Nutr Metab Cardiovasc Dis. 2017 Dec;27(12):1060-80.

[10] Wang DD, Li Y, Chiuve SE, Stampfer MJ, Manson JE, Rimm EB, et al. Association of Specific Dietary Fats With Total and Cause-Specific Mortality. JAMA Intern Med. 2016 Aug 1;176(8):1134-45.

[11] Li Y, Hruby A, Bernstein AM, Ley SH, Wang DD, Chiuve SE, et al. Saturated Fats Compared With Unsaturated Fats and Sources of Carbohydrates in Relation to Risk of Coronary Heart Disease: A Prospective Cohort Study. J Am Coll Cardiol. 2015 Oct 6;66(14):1538-48.

[12] Mozaffarian D, Micha R, Wallace S. Effects on coronary heart disease of increasing polyunsaturated fat in place of saturated fat: a systematic review and meta-analysis of randomized controlled trials. PLoS Med. 2010 Mar 23;7(3): e1000252.

[13] Harcombe Z, Baker JS, Cooper SM, Davies B, Sculthorpe N, DiNicolantonio JJ, et al. Evidence from randomised controlled trials did not support the introduction of dietary fat guidelines in 1977 and 1983: a systematic review and meta-analysis. Open Heart. 2015;2(1):e000196.

[14] Astrup A, Magkos F, Bier DM, Brenna JT, de Oliveira Otto MC, Hill JO, et al. Saturated Fats and Health: A Reassessment and Proposal for Food-Based Recommendations: JACC State-of-the-Art Review. J Am Coll Cardiol. 2020 Aug 18;76(7):844-57.

[15] Artaud-Wild SM, Connor SL, Sexton G, Connor WE. Differences in coronary mortality can be explained by differences in cholesterol and saturated fat intakes in 40 countries but not in France and Finland. A paradox. Circulation. 1993 Dec;88(6):2771-9.

[16] de Oliveira Otto MC, Mozaffarian D, Kromhout D, Bertoni AG, Sibley CT, Jacobs DR, Jr., et al. Dietary intake of saturated fat by food source and incident cardiovascular disease: the Multi-Ethnic Study of Atherosclerosis. Am J Clin Nutr. 2012 Aug;96(2):397-404.

[17] de Souza RJ, Mente A, Maroleanu A, Cozma AI, Ha V, Kishibe T, et al. Intake of saturated and trans unsaturated fatty acids and risk of all cause mortality, cardiovascular disease, and type 2 diabetes: systematic review and meta-analysis of observational studies. Bmj. 2015 Aug 11;351:h3978.

[18] Willett WC. Dietary fats and coronary heart disease. J Intern Med. 2012 Jul;272(1):13-24.

[19] Whelan J. The health implications of changing linoleic acid intakes. Prostaglandins Leukot Essent Fatty Acids. 2008 Sep-Nov;79(3-5):165-7.

[20] Kris-Etherton PM, Krauss RM. Public health guidelines should recommend reducing saturated fat consumption as much as possible: YES. Am J Clin Nutr. 2020 Jun 3;112(1):13-8.

[21] Ramsden CE, Zamora D, Majchrzak-Hong S, Faurot KR, Broste SK, Frantz RP, et al. Re-evaluation of the traditional diet-heart hypothesis: analysis of recovered data from Minnesota Coronary Experiment (1968-73). Bmj. 2016 Apr 12;353:i1246.

[22] Ramsden CE, Zamora D, Leelarthaepin B, Majchrzak-Hong SF, Faurot KR, Suchindran CM, et al. Use of dietary linoleic acid for secondary prevention of coronary heart disease and death: evaluation of recovered data from the Sydney Diet Heart Study and updated meta-analysis. Bmj. 2013 Feb 4;346:e8707.

[23] Dehghan M, Mente A, Zhang X, Swaminathan S, Li W, Mohan V, et al. Associations of fats and carbohydrate intake with cardiovascular disease and mortality in 18 countries from five continents (PURE): a prospective cohort study. Lancet. 2017 Nov 4;390(10107): 2050-62.

[24] Siri-Tarino PW, Sun Q, Hu FB, Krauss RM. Meta-analysis of prospective cohort studies evaluating the association of saturated fat with cardiovascular disease. Am J Clin Nutr. 2010 Mar;91(3):535-46.

[25] Kang ZQ, Yang Y, Xiao B. Dietary saturated fat intake and risk of stroke: Systematic review and dose-response meta-analysis of prospective cohort studies. Nutr Metab Cardiovasc Dis. 2020 Feb 10;30(2):179-89.

[26] Hamley S. The effect of replacing saturated fat with mostly n-6 polyunsaturated fat on coronary heart disease: a meta-analysis of randomised controlled trials. Nutr J. 2017 May 19;16(1):30.

[27] Hooper L, Martin N, Jimoh OF, Kirk C, Foster E, Abdelhamid AS. Reduction in saturated fat intake for cardiovascular disease. Cochrane Database Syst Rev. 2020 Aug 21;8:CD011737.

[28] Jandacek RJ. Linoleic Acid: A Nutritional Quandary. Healthcare (Basel). 2017 May 20;5(2):25.

[29] Harris WS, Mozaffarian D, Rimm E, Kris-Etherton P, Rudel LL, Appel LJ, et al. Omega-6 fatty acids and risk for cardiovascular disease: a science advisory from the American Heart Association Nutrition Subcommittee of the Council on Nutrition, Physical Activity, and Metabolism; Council on Cardiovascular Nursing; and Council on Epidemiology and Prevention. Circulation. 2009 Feb 17;119(6):902-7.

[30] Vannice G, Rasmussen H. Position of the academy of nutrition and dietetics: dietary fatty acids for healthy

adults. J Acad Nutr Diet. 2014 Jan; 114(1):136-53.

[31] Whelan J, Fritsche K. Linoleic acid. Adv Nutr. 2013 May 1;4(3):311-2.

[32] Marklund M, Wu JHY, Imamura F, Del Gobbo LC, Fretts A, de Goede J, et al. Biomarkers of Dietary Omega-6 Fatty Acids and Incident Cardiovascular Disease and Mortality. Circulation. 2019 May 21;139(21):2422-36.

[33] Wu JH, Lemaitre RN, King IB, Song X, Psaty BM, Siscovick DS, et al. Circulating omega-6 polyunsaturated fatty acids and total and cause-specific mortality: the Cardiovascular Health Study. Circulation. 2014 Oct 7;130(15):1245-53.

[34] Wang Q, Afshin A, Yakoob MY, Singh GM, Rehm CD, Khatibzadeh S, et al. Impact of Nonoptimal Intakes of Saturated, Polyunsaturated, and Trans Fat on Global Burdens of Coronary Heart Disease. J Am Heart Assoc. 2016 Jan 20;5(1):e002891.

[35] Farvid MS, Ding M, Pan A, Sun Q, Chiuve SE, Steffen LM, et al. Dietary linoleic acid and risk of coronary heart disease: a systematic review and meta-analysis of prospective cohort studies. Circulation. 2014 Oct 28;130(18): 1568-78.

[36] Hooper L, Al-Khudairy L, Abdelhamid AS, Rees K, Brainard JS, Brown TJ, et al. Omega-6 fats for the primary and secondary prevention of cardiovascular disease. Cochrane Database Syst Rev. 2018 Nov 29;11:CD011094.

[37] Forouhi NG, Krauss RM, Taubes G, Willett W. Dietary fat and cardiometabolic health: evidence, controversies, and consensus for guidance. Bmj. 2018 Jun 13;361:k2139.

[38] Arnett DK, Blumenthal RS, Albert MA, Buroker AB, Goldberger ZD, Hahn EJ, et al. 2019 ACC/AHA Guideline on the Primary Prevention of Cardiovascular Disease: A Report of the American College of Cardiology/American Heart Association Task Force on Clinical Practice Guidelines. J Am Coll Cardiol. 2019 Sep 10;74(10):e177-e232.

[39] Xu LB, Zhou YF, Yao JL, Sun SJ, Rui Q, Yang XJ, et al. Apolipoprotein A1 polymorphisms and risk of coronary artery disease: a meta-analysis. Arch Med Sci. 2017 Jun;13(4):813-9.

[40] Austin MA. Triglyceride, small, dense low-density lipoprotein, and the atherogenic lipoprotein phenotype. Curr Atheroscler Rep. 2000 May;2(3): 200-7.

[41] Kwiterovich PO, Jr. Clinical relevance of the biochemical, metabolic, and genetic factors that influence low-density lipoprotein heterogeneity. Am J Cardiol. 2002 Oct 17;90(8A):30i-47i.

[42] Krauss RM. Dietary and genetic effects on low-density lipoprotein heterogeneity. Annu Rev Nutr. 2001;21: 283-95.

[43] Florvall G, Basu S, Larsson A. Apolipoprotein A1 is a stronger prognostic marker than are HDL and LDL cholesterol for cardiovascular disease and mortality in elderly men. J Gerontol A Biol Sci Med Sci. 2006 Dec;61(12):1262-6.

[44] Carr MC, Ayyobi AF, Murdoch SJ, Deeb SS, Brunzell JD. Contribution of hepatic lipase, lipoprotein lipase, and cholesteryl ester transfer protein to LDL and HDL heterogeneity in healthy women. Arterioscler Thromb Vasc Biol. 2002 Apr 1;22(4):667-73.

[45] Krauss RM, Burke DJ. Identification of multiple subclasses of plasma low density lipoproteins in normal humans. J Lipid Res. 1982 Jan;23(1):97-104.

[46] Blake GJ, Otvos JD, Rifai N, Ridker PM. Low-density lipoprotein particle concentration and size as determined by nuclear magnetic resonance spectroscopy as predictors of cardiovascular disease in women. Circulation. 2002 Oct 8;106(15):1930-7.

[47] Duran EK, Aday AW, Cook NR, Buring JE, Ridker PM, Pradhan AD. Triglyceride-Rich Lipoprotein Cholesterol, Small Dense LDL Cholesterol, and Incident Cardiovascular Disease. J Am Coll Cardiol. 2020 May 5;75(17):2122-35.

[48] Williams PT, Superko HR, Haskell WL, Alderman EL, Blanche PJ, Holl LG, et al. Smallest LDL particles are most strongly related to coronary disease progression in men. Arterioscler Thromb Vasc Biol. 2003 Feb 1;23(2):314-21.

[49] Coresh J, Kwiterovich PO, Jr., Smith HH, Bachorik PS. Association of plasma triglyceride concentration and LDL particle diameter, density, and chemical composition with premature coronary artery disease in men and women. J Lipid Res. 1993 Oct;34(10):1687-97.

[50] DiNicolantonio JJ, O'Keefe JH. Effects of dietary fats on blood lipids: a review of direct comparison trials. Open Heart. 2018;5(2):e000871.

[51] U.S. Department of Agriculture (USDA). Food Data Central [Internet]. Available from: https://fdc.nal.usda.gov/ [Accessed: 2021-05-26].

[52] Froyen E, Burns-Whitmore B. The Effects of Linoleic Acid Consumption on Lipid Risk Markers for Cardiovascular Disease in Healthy Individuals: A Review of Human Intervention Trials. Nutrients. 2020 Aug 4;12(8).

[53] Chemical structure of linoleic acid [Internet]. Available from: https://commons.wikimedia.org/wiki/File:Linoleic_acid.png [Accessed: 2021-05-26].

[54] Iacono JM, Dougherty RM. Lack of effect of linoleic acid on the high-density-lipoprotein-cholesterol fraction of plasma lipoproteins. Am J Clin Nutr. 1991 Mar;53(3):660-4.

[55] Sanders TA, Oakley FR, Miller GJ, Mitropoulos KA, Crook D, Oliver MF. Influence of n-6 versus n-3 polyunsaturated fatty acids in diets low in saturated fatty acids on plasma lipoproteins and hemostatic factors. Arterioscler Thromb Vasc Biol. 1997 Dec;17(12):3449-60.

[56] Zock PL, Katan MB. Hydrogenation alternatives: effects of trans fatty acids and stearic acid versus linoleic acid on serum lipids and lipoproteins in humans. J Lipid Res. 1992 Mar;33(3):399-410.

[57] French MA, Sundram K, Clandinin MT. Cholesterolaemic effect of palmitic acid in relation to other dietary fatty acids. Asia Pac J Clin Nutr. 2002;11 Suppl 7:S401-7.

[58] Wagner KH, Tomasch R, Elmadfa I. Impact of diets containing corn oil or olive/sunflower oil mixture on the human plasma and lipoprotein lipid metabolism. Eur J Nutr. 2001 Aug;40(4):161-7.

[59] van Schalkwijk DB, Pasman WJ, Hendriks HF, Verheij ER, Rubingh CM, van Bochove K, et al. Dietary medium chain fatty acid supplementation leads to reduced VLDL lipolysis and uptake rates in comparison to linoleic acid supplementation. PLoS One. 2014;9(7): e100376.

[60] Goyens PL, Mensink RP. The dietary alpha-linolenic acid to linoleic acid ratio does not affect the serum lipoprotein profile in humans. J Nutr. 2005 Dec;135(12):2799-804.

[61] Sanders TA, Hochland MC. A comparison of the influence on plasma lipids and platelet function of supplements of omega 3 and omega 6 polyunsaturated fatty acids. Br J Nutr. 1983 Nov;50(3):521-9.

[62] Damsgaard CT, Frokiaer H, Andersen AD, Lauritzen L. Fish oil in combination with high or low intakes of linoleic acid lowers plasma triacylglycerols but does not affect other cardiovascular risk markers in healthy men. J Nutr. 2008 Jun;138(6):1061-6.

[63] Pang D, Allman-Farinelli MA, Wong T, Barnes R, Kingham KM. Replacement of linoleic acid with alpha-linolenic acid does not alter blood lipids in normolipidaemic men. Br J Nutr. 1998 Aug;80(2):163-7.

[64] Liou YA, King DJ, Zibrik D, Innis SM. Decreasing linoleic acid with constant alpha-linolenic acid in dietary fats increases (n-3) eicosapentaenoic acid in plasma phospholipids in healthy men. J Nutr. 2007 Apr;137(4):945-52.

[65] Sola R, La Ville AE, Richard JL, Motta C, Bargallo MT, Girona J, et al. Oleic acid rich diet protects against the oxidative modification of high density lipoprotein. Free Radic Biol Med. 1997;22(6):1037-45.

[66] Thijssen MA, Mensink RP. Small differences in the effects of stearic acid, oleic acid, and linoleic acid on the serum lipoprotein profile of humans. Am J Clin Nutr. 2005 Sep;82(3):510-6.

[67] Dias CB, Amigo N, Wood LG, Correig X, Garg ML. Effect of diets rich in either saturated fat or n-6 polyunsaturated fatty acids and supplemented with long-chain n-3 polyunsaturated fatty acids on plasma lipoprotein profiles. Eur J Clin Nutr. 2017 Nov;71(11):1297-302.

[68] Mensink RP, Zock PL, Katan MB, Hornstra G. Effect of dietary cis and trans fatty acids on serum lipoprotein[a] levels in humans. J Lipid Res. 1992 Oct;33(10):1493-501.

[69] Dreon DM, Fernstrom HA, Campos H, Blanche P, Williams PT, Krauss RM. Change in dietary saturated fat intake is correlated with change in mass of large low-density-lipoprotein particles in men. Am J Clin Nutr. 1998 May;67(5):828-36.

[70] Dias CB, Amigo N, Wood LG, Mallol R, Correig X, Garg ML. Improvement of the omega 3 index of healthy subjects does not alter the effects of dietary saturated fats or n-6PUFA on LDL profiles. Metabolism. 2017 Mar;68:11-9.

[71] Tobin KA, Steineger HH, Alberti S, Spydevold O, Auwerx J, Gustafsson JA, et al. Cross-talk between fatty acid and cholesterol metabolism mediated by liver X receptor-alpha. Mol Endocrinol. 2000 May;14(5):741-52.

[72] Ide T, Shimano H, Yoshikawa T, Yahagi N, Amemiya-Kudo M, Matsuzaka T, et al. Cross-talk between peroxisome proliferator-activated receptor (PPAR) alpha and liver X receptor (LXR) in nutritional regulation of fatty acid metabolism. II. LXRs suppress lipid degradation gene promoters through inhibition of PPAR signaling. Mol Endocrinol. 2003 Jul;17(7):1255-67.

[73] Fernandez ML, West KL. Mechanisms by which dietary fatty acids modulate plasma lipids. J Nutr. 2005 Sep;135(9):2075-8.

[74] Ferre P. The biology of peroxisome proliferator-activated receptors: relationship with lipid metabolism and insulin sensitivity. Diabetes. 2004 Feb;53 Suppl 1:S43-50.

[75] Schoonjans K, Staels B, Auwerx J. Role of the peroxisome proliferator-activated receptor (PPAR) in mediating

the effects of fibrates and fatty acids on gene expression. J Lipid Res. 1996 May;37(5):907-25.

[76] Schoonjans K, Peinado-Onsurbe J, Lefebvre AM, Heyman RA, Briggs M, Deeb S, et al. PPARalpha and PPARgamma activators direct a distinct tissue-specific transcriptional response via a PPRE in the lipoprotein lipase gene. Embo J. 1996 Oct 1;15(19):5336-48.

[77] Vasandani C, Kafrouni AI, Caronna A, Bashmakov Y, Gotthardt M, Horton JD, et al. Upregulation of hepatic LDL transport by n-3 fatty acids in LDL receptor knockout mice. J Lipid Res. 2002 May;43(5):772-84.

[78] Shachter NS. Apolipoproteins C-I and C-III as important modulators of lipoprotein metabolism. Curr Opin Lipidol. 2001 Jun;12(3):297-304.

[79] Cottin SC, Sanders TA, Hall WL. The differential effects of EPA and DHA on cardiovascular risk factors. Proc Nutr Soc. 2011 May;70(2):215-31.

[80] Mozaffarian D, Wu JH. (n-3) fatty acids and cardiovascular health: are effects of EPA and DHA shared or complementary? J Nutr. 2012 Mar;142(3):614S-25S.

[81] Ooi EM, Watts GF, Ng TW, Barrett PH. Effect of dietary Fatty acids on human lipoprotein metabolism: a comprehensive update. Nutrients. 2015 Jun 2;7(6):4416-25.

[82] Mozaffarian D, Wu JH. Omega-3 fatty acids and cardiovascular disease: effects on risk factors, molecular pathways, and clinical events. J Am Coll Cardiol. 2011 Nov 8;58(20):2047-67.

[83] Grimsgaard S, Bonaa KH, Hansen JB, Nordoy A. Highly purified eicosapentaenoic acid and docosahexaenoic acid in humans have similar triacylglycerol-lowering effects but divergent effects on serum fatty acids. Am J Clin Nutr. 1997 Sep;66(3): 649-59.

[84] Allaire J, Couture P, Leclerc M, Charest A, Marin J, Lepine MC, et al. A randomized, crossover, head-to-head comparison of eicosapentaenoic acid and docosahexaenoic acid supplementation to reduce inflammation markers in men and women: the Comparing EPA to DHA (ComparED) Study. Am J Clin Nutr. 2016 Aug;104(2):280-7.

[85] Mustad VA, Ellsworth JL, Cooper AD, Kris-Etherton PM, Etherton TD. Dietary linoleic acid increases and palmitic acid decreases hepatic LDL receptor protein and mRNA abundance in young pigs. J Lipid Res. 1996 Nov;37(11):2310-23.

[86] Tripodi A, Loria P, Dilengite MA, Carulli N. Effect of fish oil and coconut oil diet on the LDL receptor activity of rat liver plasma membranes. Biochim Biophys Acta. 1991 Jun 3;1083(3): 298-304.

[87] Fernandez ML, Lin EC, McNamara DJ. Differential effects of saturated fatty acids on low density lipoprotein metabolism in the guinea pig. J Lipid Res. 1992 Dec;33(12): 1833-42.

[88] Caviglia JM, Gayet C, Ota T, Hernandez-Ono A, Conlon DM, Jiang H, et al. Different fatty acids inhibit apoB100 secretion by different pathways: unique roles for ER stress, ceramide, and autophagy. J Lipid Res. 2011 Sep;52(9):1636-51.

[89] Shepherd J, Packard CJ, Grundy SM, Yeshurun D, Gotto AM, Jr., Taunton OD. Effects of saturated and polyunsaturated fat diets on the chemical composition and metabolism of low density lipoproteins in man. J Lipid Res. 1980 Jan;21(1):91-9.

[90] Bergeron N, Chiu S, Williams PT, S MK, Krauss RM. Effects of red meat, white meat, and nonmeat protein sources on atherogenic lipoprotein measures in the context of low compared with high saturated fat intake: a randomized controlled trial. Am J Clin Nutr. 2019 Jul 1;110(1):24-33.

[91] Ulven SM, Christensen JJ, Nygard O, Svardal A, Leder L, Ottestad I, et al. Using metabolic profiling and gene expression analyses to explore molecular effects of replacing saturated fat with polyunsaturated fat-a randomized controlled dietary intervention study. Am J Clin Nutr. 2019 May 1;109(5): 1239-50.

[92] Campos H, Dreon DM, Krauss RM. Associations of hepatic and lipoprotein lipase activities with changes in dietary composition and low density lipoprotein subclasses. J Lipid Res. 1995 Mar;36(3):462-72.

[93] Wang CS, Weingand KW, Anthony MS. Effect of atherogenic diet on lipoprotein lipase activity in cynomolgus monkeys. Atherosclerosis. 1987 Oct;67(2-3):173-80.

[94] Xu J, Nakamura MT, Cho HP, Clarke SD. Sterol regulatory element binding protein-1 expression is suppressed by dietary polyunsaturated fatty acids. A mechanism for the coordinate suppression of lipogenic genes by polyunsaturated fats. J Biol Chem. 1999 Aug 13;274(33):23577-83.

[95] Shimomura I, Bashmakov Y, Ikemoto S, Horton JD, Brown MS, Goldstein JL. Insulin selectively increases SREBP-1c mRNA in the livers of rats with streptozotocin-induced diabetes. Proc Natl Acad Sci U S A. 1999 Nov 23;96(24):13656-61.

[96] Field FJ, Born E, Mathur SN. Fatty acid flux suppresses fatty acid synthesis in hamster intestine independently of SREBP-1 expression. J Lipid Res. 2003 Jun;44(6):1199-208.

[97] Mensink RP, Zock PL, Kester AD, Katan MB. Effects of dietary fatty acids and carbohydrates on the ratio of serum total to HDL cholesterol and on serum lipids and apolipoproteins: a meta-analysis of 60 controlled trials. Am J Clin Nutr. 2003 May;77(5):1146-55.

[98] Hayek T, Ito Y, Azrolan N, Verdery RB, Aalto-Setala K, Walsh A, et al. Dietary fat increases high density lipoprotein (HDL) levels both by increasing the transport rates and decreasing the fractional catabolic rates of HDL cholesterol ester and apolipoprotein (Apo) A-I. Presentation of a new animal model and mechanistic studies in human Apo A-I transgenic and control mice. J Clin Invest. 1993 Apr;91(4):1665-71.

[99] Tsimikas S. A Test in Context: Lipoprotein(a): Diagnosis, Prognosis, Controversies, and Emerging Therapies. J Am Coll Cardiol. 2017 Feb 14;69(6): 692-711.

[100] Schmidt K, Noureen A, Kronenberg F, Utermann G. Structure, function, and genetics of lipoprotein (a). J Lipid Res. 2016 Aug;57(8): 1339-59.

[101] Malaguarnera M, Vacante M, Russo C, Malaguarnera G, Antic T, Malaguarnera L, et al. Lipoprotein(a) in cardiovascular diseases. Biomed Res Int. 2013;2013:650989.

[102] Tholstrup T, Marckmann P, Vessby B, Sandstrom B. Effect of fats high in individual saturated fatty acids on plasma lipoprotein[a] levels in young healthy men. J Lipid Res. 1995 Jul;36(7):1447-52.

[103] Gudbjartsson DF, Thorgeirsson G, Sulem P, Helgadottir A, Gylfason A, Saemundsdottir J, et al. Lipoprotein(a) Concentration and Risks of Cardiovascular Disease and Diabetes. J Am Coll Cardiol. 2019 Dec 17;74(24): 2982-94.

[104] Ljungberg J, Holmgren A, Bergdahl IA, Hultdin J, Norberg M, Naslund U, et al. Lipoprotein(a) and the Apolipoprotein B/A1 Ratio Independently Associate With Surgery for Aortic Stenosis Only in Patients With Concomitant Coronary Artery Disease. J Am Heart Assoc. 2017 Dec 15;6(12):e007160.

[105] Boerwinkle E, Leffert CC, Lin J, Lackner C, Chiesa G, Hobbs HH. Apolipoprotein(a) gene accounts for greater than 90% of the variation in plasma lipoprotein(a) concentrations. J Clin Invest. 1992 Jul;90(1):52-60.

[106] Enkhmaa B, Petersen KS, Kris-Etherton PM, Berglund L. Diet and Lp(a): Does Dietary Change Modify Residual Cardiovascular Risk Conferred by Lp(a)? Nutrients. 2020 Jul 7;12(7).

[107] Brousseau ME, Ordovas JM, Nicolosi RJ, Schaefer EJ. Effects of dietary fat saturation on plasma lipoprotein(a) and hepatic apolipoprotein(a) mRNA concentrations in cynomolgus monkeys. Atherosclerosis. 1994 Mar;106(1): 109-18.

[108] Azrolan N, Gavish D, Breslow JL. Plasma lipoprotein(a) concentration is controlled by apolipoprotein(a) (apo(a)) protein size and the abundance of hepatic apo(a) mRNA in a cynomolgus monkey model. J Biol Chem. 1991 Jul 25;266(21):13866-72.

[109] Fielding CJ, Shore VG, Fielding PE. A protein cofactor of lecithin:cholesterol acyltransferase. Biochem Biophys Res Commun. 1972 Feb 25;46(4):1493-8.

[110] Gao X, Yuan S, Jayaraman S, Gursky O. Role of apolipoprotein A-II in the structure and remodeling of human high-density lipoprotein (HDL): protein conformational ensemble on HDL. Biochemistry. 2012 Jun 12;51(23): 4633-41.

[111] Kuyl JM, Mendelsohn D. Observed relationship between ratios HDL-cholesterol/total cholesterol and apolipoprotein A1/apolipoprotein B. Clin Biochem. 1992 Oct;25(5):313-6.

[112] Walldius G, Jungner I, Holme I, Aastveit AH, Kolar W, Steiner E. High apolipoprotein B, low apolipoprotein A-I, and improvement in the prediction of fatal myocardial infarction (AMORIS study): a prospective study. Lancet. 2001 Dec 15;358(9298):2026-33.

[113] World Health Organization. Interim Summary of Conclusions and Dietary Recommendations on Total Fat & Fatty Acids [Internet]. Available from: https://www.who.int/nutrition/topics/FFA_summary_rec_conclusion.pdf?ua=1 [Accessed: 2021-06-05].

[114] Dietary Guidelines for Americans 2020-2025 [Internet]. Available from: https://www.dietaryguidelines.gov/ [Accessed: 2021-07-02].

[115] Schwingshackl L, Hoffmann G. Dietary fatty acids in the secondary prevention of coronary heart disease: a systematic review, meta-analysis and meta-regression. BMJ Open. 2014 Apr 19;4(4):e004487.

[116] Krauss RM. Dietary and genetic probes of atherogenic dyslipidemia. Arterioscler Thromb Vasc Biol. 2005 Nov;25(11):2265-72.

[117] Siri-Tarino PW, Sun Q, Hu FB, Krauss RM. Saturated fat, carbohydrate, and cardiovascular disease. Am J Clin Nutr. 2010 Mar;91(3):502-9.

[118] Parks EJ, Krauss RM, Christiansen MP, Neese RA, Hellerstein MK. Effects of a low-fat, high-carbohydrate diet on VLDL-triglyceride assembly, production, and clearance. J Clin Invest. 1999 Oct;104(8):1087-96.

[119] Berneis KK, Krauss RM. Metabolic origins and clinical significance of LDL

heterogeneity. J Lipid Res. 2002 Sep;43(9):1363-79.

[120] Krauss RM. Lipids and lipoproteins in patients with type 2 diabetes. Diabetes Care. 2004 Jun;27(6):1496-504.

[121] Krauss RM, Dreon DM. Low-density-lipoprotein subclasses and response to a low-fat diet in healthy men. Am J Clin Nutr. 1995 Aug;62(2):478S-87S.

[122] Faghihnia N, Tsimikas S, Miller ER, Witztum JL, Krauss RM. Changes in lipoprotein(a), oxidized phospholipids, and LDL subclasses with a low-fat high-carbohydrate diet. J Lipid Res. 2010 Nov;51(11):3324-30.

[123] Guay V, Lamarche B, Charest A, Tremblay AJ, Couture P. Effect of short-term low- and high-fat diets on low-density lipoprotein particle size in normolipidemic subjects. Metabolism. 2012 Jan;61(1):76-83.

[124] Egert S, Kratz M, Kannenberg F, Fobker M, Wahrburg U. Effects of high-fat and low-fat diets rich in monounsaturated fatty acids on serum lipids, LDL size and indices of lipid peroxidation in healthy non-obese men and women when consumed under controlled conditions. Eur J Nutr. 2011 Feb;50(1):71-9.

[125] Wang L, Bordi PL, Fleming JA, Hill AM, Kris-Etherton PM. Effect of a moderate fat diet with and without avocados on lipoprotein particle number, size and subclasses in overweight and obese adults: a randomized, controlled trial. J Am Heart Assoc. 2015 Jan 7;4(1):e001355.

[126] Kratz M, Gulbahce E, von Eckardstein A, Cullen P, Cignarella A, Assmann G, et al. Dietary mono- and polyunsaturated fatty acids similarly affect LDL size in healthy men and women. J Nutr. 2002 Apr;132(4): 715-8.

[127] Griffin BA. Lipoprotein atherogenicity: an overview of current mechanisms. Proc Nutr Soc. 1999 Feb;58(1):163-9.

[128] Anber V, Millar JS, McConnell M, Shepherd J, Packard CJ. Interaction of very-low-density, intermediate-density, and low-density lipoproteins with human arterial wall proteoglycans. Arterioscler Thromb Vasc Biol. 1997 Nov;17(11):2507-14.

[129] Taskinen MR. LDL-cholesterol, HDL-cholesterol or triglycerides--which is the culprit? Diabetes Res Clin Pract. 2003 Jul;61 Suppl 1:S19-26.

[130] Dejager S, Bruckert E, Chapman MJ. Dense low density lipoprotein subspecies with diminished oxidative resistance predominate in combined hyperlipidemia. J Lipid Res. 1993 Feb;34(2):295-308.

[131] Nigon F, Lesnik P, Rouis M, Chapman MJ. Discrete subspecies of human low density lipoproteins are heterogeneous in their interaction with the cellular LDL receptor. J Lipid Res. 1991 Nov;32(11):1741-53.

[132] Galeano NF, Milne R, Marcel YL, Walsh MT, Levy E, Ngu'yen TD, et al. Apoprotein B structure and receptor recognition of triglyceride-rich low density lipoprotein (LDL) is modified in small LDL but not in triglyceride-rich LDL of normal size. J Biol Chem. 1994 Jan 7;269(1):511-9.

[133] Liu AG, Ford NA, Hu FB, Zelman KM, Mozaffarian D, Kris-Etherton PM. A healthy approach to dietary fats: understanding the science and taking action to reduce consumer confusion. Nutr J. 2017 Aug 30;16(1):53.

[134] Estruch R, Ros E, Salas-Salvado J, Covas MI, Corella D, Aros F, et al. Primary Prevention of Cardiovascular Disease with a Mediterranean Diet

Supplemented with Extra-Virgin Olive Oil or Nuts. N Engl J Med. 2018 Jun 21;378(25):e34.

[135] Howard BV, Van Horn L, Hsia J, Manson JE, Stefanick ML, Wassertheil-Smoller S, et al. Low-fat dietary pattern and risk of cardiovascular disease: the Women's Health Initiative Randomized Controlled Dietary Modification Trial. Jama. 2006 Feb 8;295(6):655-66.

Chapter 9

Residual Cardiovascular Risk Factors in Dyslipidemia

Van Si Nguyen, Xuan Truong Tran, Thanh Duy Vo and Quang Truong Le

Abstract

Cardiovascular disease poses a major challenge for the 21st century. Although good control of blood pressure and type 2 diabetes and reducing low-density lipoprotein-cholesterol levels can improve cardiovascular outcomes, a substantial residual risk remains existed after treatment in most patient populations. Recently, many efforts have been directed at finding the important role of low high-density-lipoprotein cholesterol, high triglycerides, especially triglyceride-rich lipoproteins and lipoprotein (a) in the metabolism of atherosclerotic plaque formation Therefore, based on the recent evidence, identification and treatment of these risk factors may play a role in optimizing therapeutic strategy, particularly in high risk subjects along with conventional treatment. In clinical practice, adequate attention should be paid when screening and managing residual cardiovascular risk factors in dyslipidemia in term of individualized approach. The ongoing trials will give more answers to elucidate this important area.

Keywords: cardiovascular disease, dyslipidemia, residual risk factors, hypertriglyceridemia, low HDL-C, lipoprotein (a)

1. Introduction

Risk factors for cardiovascular disease (CVD) are specific lifestyles, behaviors and a set of conditions that increase likelihood of CVD. An individual may have more than one cardiovascular (CV) risk factors. In fact, CV risk factors often appear coherently. The more risk factors, the greater the risk of CVD. However, the individual with increased risk does not necessarily develop cardiovascular diseases.

A number of factors have been linked to an increased risk of cardiovascular disease which can be classified as (1) Unmodifiable risk factors: age (men over 45 years old, women over 55 years old), gender and family history of early CVD (men under 55 years old, women under 65 years old) and (2) Modifiable risk factors: unhealthy diets, high blood pressure, dyslipidemia, smoking, overweight, obesity, pre-diabetes or diabetes, sedentary lifestyle [1–3].

In addition, extended CV risk factors were proposed, including: metabolic syndrome (insulin resistance syndrome, syndrome X) including triglyceridemia, chronic kidney disease (CKD) with reduced glomerular filtration rate [15–59 ml/min/1.73 m^2], chronic inflammatory conditions (rheumatic disease, HIV), early menopause (< 40 years), history of eclampsia, high-risk ethnicity (South Asian), elevated lipoprotein (a) [Lp(a)] ≥ 50 mg/dL (≥ 125 nmol/L) or elevated apolipoprotein B

(ApoB) ≥ 130 mg/dL, C-reactive protein (CRP) ≥ 2 mg/L and ankle-brachial index <0.9 [4].

Residual CV risk factor is defined as the risk of CV events that persists despite achieving treatment goals for low-density lipoprotein cholesterol (LDL-C), blood pressure and blood glucose as recommended by current evidence-based guidelines [5, 6]. Residual CV risk factors include LDL-C > 100 mg/dL, high-sensitive C-reactive protein (hsCRP) > 2 mg/l, triglyceride (TG) > 200 mg/dL, high-density lipoprotein cholesterol (HDL-C) < 40 mg/dL, Lp(a) > 50 mg/dL [7]. The origin of residual CV risk factors in dyslipidemia is based on atherogenic dyslipidemia characterized by elevated TG and triglyceride-rich lipoproteins (TRLs), decreased HDL-C, and qualitative changes of lipoprotein particles [8–10].

2. Epidemiology

Most large studies extending over the last 25 years suggested that the leading cause of atheroslerotic cardiovascular disease (ASCVD) is high LDL-C levels and this has been widely recognized and accepted [9, 11]. Furthermore, there is also growing evidence that increased levels of LDL-C and other ApoB containers, including very low density lipoprotein cholesterol (VLDL-C), intermediate density lipoprotein cholesterol (IDL-C) and Lp(a), are directly related to the progression of ASCVD [12, 13]. In 2010, a multicenter study analyzing data from 26 randomized clinical trials in 2009 demonstrated that statins are effective in lowering LDL-C blood levels and controlling blood glucose levels. LDL-C at the recommended level is beneficial in reducing atherosclerotic CV events and CV mortality [14].

However, studies in recent years have revealed that control of plasma LDL-C concentrations is not the only goal of reducing the risk of CVD [15]. Based on the results of their study, Cannon et al. demonstrated an ongoing risk of major CV events after treatment with high doses of atorvastatin or pravastatin. The data signified that up to 26.3% in the atorvastatin-treated group and 22.4% in the pravastatin-treated group experienced a major CV event or death [16]. This evidence suggests that the goal of reducing the risk of CVD requires control not only of blood LDL-C levels but also of residual CV risk factors in other dyslipidemia, including TG and TRLs, HDL-C and Lp(a) [9].

3. Residual risk factors in dyslipidemia

3.1 Pathogenesis of atherosclerosis

Atherosclerosis is a complex phenomenon that is involved by a number of factors. Firstly, when the vascular endothelial cell layer is injured, the synthesis of nitrite oxide (NO), a chemical that protects blood vessels, is reduced, while the production of oxidants rises [17, 18]. Infiltration of ApoBs including remnants of chylomicron, VLDL-C, IDL-C, LDL-C and Lp(a) into the endothelial layer. The ApoBs that are retained in the vessel wall oxidize, triggering a cascade of biological events that result in an inflammatory response [19, 20]. Furthermore, platelets are stimulated to cause chronic vascular inflammation which leads to leukocyte recruitment [21, 22]. Monocytes and neutrophils penetrate the endothelial layer into the arterial wall. Macrophages that have been differentiated from monocytes amplify lipid absorption and produce foam cells, which play a key role in the formation and instability of atherosclerotic plaques. T lymphocytes, mastocytes, and other inflammatory cells penetrate the lesion and help to continue the noxious inflammatory response [20–24]. This process is also maintained and enhanced through signaling pathways such as MCP-1, M-CFS, GM-CFS [25–27]. As a result, the plaque ruptures and leads to clinical manifestations for example, myocardial infarction or stroke.

3.2 Hypertriglyceridemia and related markers

The function of TG in the etiology of atherosclerosis has garnered limited attention in recent years, with most studies focusing on the benefits of raising HDL-C. Contemporary clinical and genetic evidence, on the other hand, suggests that TG, especially TRLs, and apoprotein C3, play essential roles in the etiology of atherosclerosis. Therefore, TG and TRLs are getting increasing attention and are becoming one of the therapeutic targets for lowering the risk of ASCVD [28].

TG is the main component in the structure of the TRL group including VLDL-C and chylomicrons which are synthesized in the liver and small intestine, respectively [29, 30]. The metabolism of TG and TRLs has the involvement of lipoprotein lipase (LPL) which is capable of activating the hydrolysis of the TG component in the core of TRLs into fatty acids. As a result, residual VLDL-C and residual chylomicrons are formed, which contain less TG and more cholesterol than normal TRLs [29, 31]. A portion of VLDL-C residues and residual chylomicrons are captured in the liver and neutralized by hepatic bile. The remainder is metabolized again by LPL or hepatic lipase enzymes, forming cholesterol-rich LDL-C [29, 30]. The residual LDL-C, VLDL-C, and residual chylomicrons are all cholesterol-rich lipoproteins and are classified as non-HDL [29, 32]. As with LDL-C, residual VLDL-C and chyplomicron molecules can be engulfed by macrophages in the vascular wall, which contributes to vascular inflammation and progression of atheromal. However, unlike LDL-C, the residual VLDL-C and chylomicron molecules do not require oxidation when participating in the process of atherosclerosis [29, 30]. Many factors impact the metabolism of TG and TRLs, with LPL playing a major role. The activity of the LPL enzyme has a direct effect on the concentration of TG and TRLs in the blood; for example, increasing LPL activity lowers TG and TRL concentrations while increasing VLDL-C molecules and residual chylomicrons, and vice versa (**Figure 1**).

The reduction in TG and TRLs metabolism leads to less cholesterol-rich lipoprotein concentrations and is expected to reduce the risk of atherosclerosis. However, intensive genetic and molecular biology studies of TG, TRLs and LPL all showed conflicting results. The first observational studies in the field of genetics related to TG, TRLs and LPL found that mutations that decrease TRLs metabolism were associated with atherosclerosis and coronary artery disease, whereas mutations TRLs metabolism enhancer had the opposite effect. Several mutations directly in the LPL enzyme associated with CVD risk have been observed including Gly188Glu, Asp91Asn and Asn291Ser substitution mutations. In which, the Gly188Glu substitution mutation in LPL can increase the risk of coronary heart disease 5 times higher than those without the mutation [33]. ApoC-II and ApoA-V loss-of-function mutations, both have been conveyed to increase blood TG, increase the risk of myocardial infarction and coronary artery disease, while mutations in the APOC3 gene - the gene that codes for Apo C-III - such as the RX 9 mutation and some other rare mutations give the opposite result [29, 34]. Most recently, ANGPTL4 mutations have appeared to reduce TG levels and reduced the risk of coronary artery disease. When conducting whole-chromosome studies on single-nucleotide polymorphisms (SNPs), susceptibility loci in the genomic regions encoding ApoC-III, ApoA-V, ANGPTL3, and ANGPTL4 were revealed to be associated with ASCVD, which lays the foundation for gene therapy to improve CV risk. In addition, there are

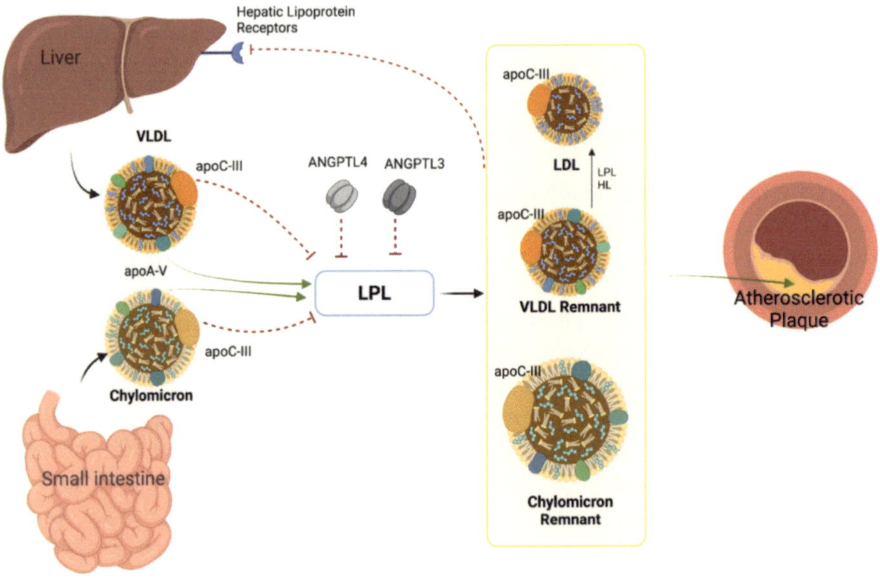

Figure 1.
The center role of LDL-C and TRLs in the formation of atherosclerotic plaque. ANGPTL = angiopoietin like protein, HL = hepatic lipase, LPL = lipoprotein lipase.

many other genetic studies with similar results regarding the role of TG in vascular events [29].

Due to the inverse correlation of HDL-C and TG, most of the previous epidemiological studies intimated the association between increased TG and atherosclerosis, which was explained by the lowering effect of HDL-C. However, there are studies that refute this view and provide strong evidence that TG is an independent factor affecting the risk of CV events. Furthermore, there appears to be a positive correlation between serum TG levels and mortality risk, even when adjusted for HDL-C and other factors [29].

With a few other CVD not caused by atherosclerosis, TG also showed a similar association. One study found that increase levels of TG and residual cholesterol molecules (total cholesterol minus LDL-C and HDL-C) were risks of aortic stenosis [35].

3.2.1 Treatment of hypertriglyceridemia

Because of the harmful effects of TG on the cardiovascular system, strategies to control TG levels were rapidly investigated to contribute to the control of CV risk in general population. Several epidemiological studies have indicated a reduction in the risk of CV events in subjects regularly consuming fish or foods rich in omega-3 fatty acid (EPA), which has been proved to reduce TG level [36–38]. However, studies testing natural EPA in subjects with ASCVD or heart failure or at high CV risk such as the ORIGIN study and most recently the STRENGTH study have showed no beneficial effect [39, 40]. Similarly, most trials of TG-lowering therapies have failed to improve CV risk. Until 2019, the REDUCE IT trial – a multicenter, double-blind, randomized, placebo-controlled study – was performed in statin-treated diabetic patients with CVD or other CV risk factors having TG levels between 135 and 499 mg/dl (1.52 to 5.63 mmol/L) and blood LDL-C levels between 41 and 100 mg/dl (1.06 to 2.59). mmol/L). There were one group treated with icosapent ethyl - a synthetic derivative of EPA with TG-lowering effects - and a placebo group. The results concluded that in patients with elevated TG, the use of icosapent ethyl reduced significantly CV events [41]. In addition to TG-reducing effect, the CV benefits of icosapent ethyl are also attributed to its effects on the main mechanisms underlying the progression of atherosclerosis, such as reduced inflammation and anti-oxidation, which stabilize and even regress atherosclerotic plaques [42]. Up to now, icosapent ethyl is considered a potential drug to help eliminate the residual CV risk caused by hypertriglyceridemia (**Figure 2**).

Research on the effects of fibrates which is a potent TG-lowering agent on CVD was also conducted quite early. In 1975, clofibrate in combination with niacin showed no significant benefit in reducing the risk of CVD [43]. However, VA-HIT study compared the gemfibrozil-treated group with the placebo group in patients with blood HDL-C levels <40 mg/dL and blood LDL-C levels <140 mg/dL showed effects on lipid parameters: HDL-C levels increased by 6%, total cholesterol decreased by 4% and TG decreased by 31% compared to the placebo group. In addition, VA-HIT also uncovered that gemfibrozil reduced the risk of mortality from major vascular events such as coronary artery disease, myocardial infarction, and stroke by 24% [44]. However, in 2010, ACCORD trial on combination of fenofibrate and statin in type 2 diabetes showed no favorable results [45]. A multicenter meta-analysis examinining data from 18 studies of fibrates during 1950–2010 to further assess their impact on CVD revealed fibrates decreased the risk of major CV events by 10% and coronary events by 13% but did not lower the overall risk of stroke or mortality rate [46]. With these results, there is practically no clear evidence that fibrates are beneficial in improving the risk of CVD or vascular events.

Novel therapies of hypertriglyceridemia are being applied to achieve maximum efficacy while minimizing undesirable side effects. For example, AKCEA-APOCIII-LRx is targeted on inhibiting the synthesis of Apo C-III by hindering the mRNA that translates it. In healthy volunteers, clinical trials of the treatment revealed a reduction in the risk of CV events in the treated group, as well as acceptable tolerability [47].

Residual lipoprotein cholesterol (RLP-C) which has close relation with TG level has also recently been demonstrated to be a residual CV risk factor even in those

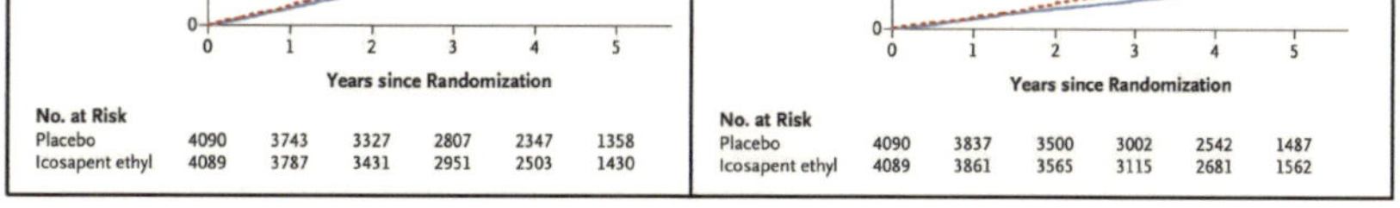

Figure 2.
(A) The Kaplan–Meier event curves for the primary end point of CV events without death. There was a statistically significant difference in primary CV events in the icosapent ethyl group (17.2%) compared with the placebo group (22%), corresponding to an absolute between-group difference of 4.8 percentage points, hazard ratio, 0.75 (95% CI, 0.68–0.83) P < 0.001, NNT = 21 over a median follow-up of 4.9 years. (B) The Kaplan–Meier event curves for the secondary end point of CV events without death. There was a statistically significant difference in secondary CV events in the icosapent ethyl group (17.2%) compared with the placebo group (22%), corresponding to an absolute between-group difference of 3.6 percentage points, hazard ratio, 0.74 (95% CI, 0.65–0.83) P < 0.001, NNT = 28 over a median follow-up of 4.9 years. NNT = number needed to treat, Cl = confidence interval. Reproduced with permission from Deepak L. Bhatt, M.D., 2019 [41].

with good LDL-C control. Elevated blood levels of RLP-C have been proved to predict coronary and other CV events [35, 48]. This is a new direction that need investigating in order to enhance the accuracy of assessing residual CV risk. In addition, more RLP-C intervention trials are required to demonstate the effect in CVD prophylaxis.

3.3 Low HDL-C

Research on the role of TG and TRLs in atherosclerotic disease are progressively providing conclusive evidence while trials to raise blood HDL-C levels have so far failed to show significant clinical benefit. This augments the possibility that the previously established causal link between higher HDL-C and a lower risk of vascular events is attributable to a comparable reduction in TG as HDL-C rises. The function of HDL-C in atherosclerosis-related CVD is still debatable nowadays.

There are several factors that contribute to HDL-C to protect blood vessels from atherosclerosis. The HDL-C molecule is responsible for cholesterol transfer from organs and peripheral blood vessels to the liver for biliary elimination. HDL-C also diminishes immune cell adherence and increases vasodilating process as well as inhibits platelet aggregation via prostacyclin. Prostacyclin modulation, in turn, aids in the breakdown of fibrin and thrombolysis in couple with decreasing inflammatory mediators and restoring vascular endothelial cell function. In addition, HDL-C is an inherent antioxidant involved in the preservation of blood vessels from oxidative damage [8, 49].

It is evident that HDL-C can prevent blood vessels from atherosclerosis. However, the role of HDL-C in lowering the overall risk of cardiovascular disease remains unknown. While epidemiological studies linked HDL-C to a lower risk of atherosclerotic CV events [50, 51], genetic study found that HDL-C had no effect on CV event risk [52, 53]. Indeed, when delving into a few gene mutations related to Scavenger receptor class B type 1 (SR-BI) and Cholesteryl ester transfer protein (CEPT) receptors - two components involved in HDL-C metabolism, these ones affect CV events differently. The pathway of HDL-C metabolism in the human body has the participation of SR-BI and CEPT receptors. When these two factors lose their function, the concentration of HDL-C in the blood will increase [54–56]. Studies in individuals with anomalies in the gene that cause loss of SR-BI receptor function have showed an increase in HDL-C levels but also an increased risk of CV events [55]. Nevertheless, studies of mutations that reduce function of CEPT showed irrelevant outcome. With the Ile405Val substitution alteration on CEPT, it is concluded that there was a decrease in CEPT activity and an increase in HDL-C regarding gender, but further an increased risk of ischemic heart disease in women but not in men [56]. Despite that, studies with other gene mutations such as TaqIB, I405V and -629C > A have clarified a reduced risk of coronary heart disease [57]. In 2009, a genetic study in different loci of the gene coding for CEPT, gave an explaination for this heterogeneity. There was an inverse association between HDL-C and the risk of cardiovascular events as a result of mutations; however, there are other alterations that do not demonstrate this correlation [8]. With achievements in functional decoding of HDL-C in terms of genes, researchers and clinical practitioners would assume the role of HDL-C in ASCVD will soon be clarified and become a state-of-art implement to assist in the treatment, prognosis, and prevention of CVD.

Since the role of HDL-C is uncertain, the use of the HDL-C measurement in clinical practice has been limited up until present. Due to the extreme prior belief that HDL-C is a favorable factor for lowering CVD risk, HDL-C was added to

SCORE – the CV risk assessment model – to create SCORE – HDL-C in European Society of Cardiology recommendations for the treatment of dyslipidemia [58, 59]. A study published in 2015 evaluated the predictive capacity of two models, SCORE - HDL-C and SCORE, and found that while the SCORE - HDL-C did not enhance CV mortality prognosis, it did lower the sensitivity of finding persons at high risk of CVD in the population [60].

3.3.1 Treatment of low HDL-C

Niacin is a medication that raises HDL-C levels and has been examined extensively in clinical studies. Its efficacy in controlling dyslipidemia and lowering the risk of cardiovascular disease is not well established. In a 1975 study comparing the CV merits of niacin, clofibrate, and placebo, treatment with a high dose of 3000 mg/day of moderate-release niacin resulted in a 14% reduction in coronary mortality, and 26% of stroke death [43]. When the research was expanded to include additional possible medicines in the treatment of dyslipidemia, such as estrogens, clofibrate, dextrothyroxine sodium, and niacin, and compared to lactose as a placebo, niacin was found to be encouraging reducing mortality [66]. However, in the AIM-HIGH and HPS2-THRIVE studies, the effects of niacin were only significant on lipid parameters without effect on CV outcomes [61, 62].

CEPT inhibitors came later than niacin and fibrates in terms of development and application. ILLUMINATE, dal-OUTCOMES, ACCELERATE, and REVIEW are among the most notable CEPT inhibitor trials to date. Nonetheless, the results of this medication were similarly unsuccessful due to inconsistencies in genetic research of CEPT. With the exception of the 2017 anacetrapid REVIEW study, which described a reduction in coronary events [63], the majority of the remaining studies suggested that CEPT inhibitors did not improve CVD risk but increased rates of CV mortality or adverse events such as increased CRP levels or increased systolic blood pressure [64–66]. Thus, clinical application studies of drugs that increase HDL-C have not yet provided evidence that HDL-C is beneficial in CVD.

In addition to the genetic aspect mentioned above, another hypothesis about HDL-C levels has been expanded to explicate the incompatible results of studies on HDL-C. When examining at HDL-C levels and mortality in the study population, several studies found a U-shaped relationship between HDL-C levels and overall mortality rates. This is understandable since extremely low or high HDL-C levels increase population mortality [67–69]. In fact, prior HDL-C studies neglected this aspect, requiring more study to more correctly assess HDL- C involvement in ASCVD.

Based on the available evidence, it can be stated that HDL-C modification in clinical practice is currently restricted. Not all HDL-C-increasing medications yield the same outcomes. To better understand the significance of HDL-C, these items must be considered to a greater extent: the threshold concentration of plasma HDL-C and the genetic aspect. It is indeed questionable if increasing HDL-C can assist reducing CV risk.

3.4 Lipoprotein (a)

Lp(a) is made up of an LDL-C molecule covalently bound to an apolipoprotein (a) that is homologous to the coagulation factor plasminogen. It also includes an apolipoprotein B100 as it contains LDL-C. Therefore, Lp(a) has both atherogenic and thrombolytic properties [70, 71]. The ability of Lp(a) to permeate the artery wall has been demonstrated [72]. Lp(a) has been showed to increase thrombus development, inflammatory response, and foam cell production in both laboratory and animal investigations [73].

Many studies prove that Lp(a) is a factor affecting the morbidity and mortality of CVD [74, 75]. The INTERHEART study proclaimed that Lp(a) levels >50 mg/dL increased the risk of myocardial ischemia [76]. The effect of Lp(a) on CV risk was independent of other risk factors, including LDL-C levels [77, 78]. Thus, elevation of blood Lp(a) levels confers a residual CV risk in dyslipidemia, which is similar to the role of TG mentioned above. A large study of LPA genetic variants also showed an independent role for Lp(a) in relation to coronary events, despite low LDL-C levels with statin therapy [79]. To specify the role of Lp(a) in reducing the risk of CVD, a study compared blood levels of Lp(a) with the risk of CVD and LDL-C levels with CVD risk, the results showed that the clinical benefit of lowering Lp(a) was directly proportional to the reduction of Lp(a) levels. Specifically, a 101.5 mg/dL reduction in Lp(a) resulted in a clinically significant reduction in CVD risk similar to a 38.67 mg/dL reduction in LDL-C [80].

Among the factors affecting Lp(a) levels, PCSK9 is one that has been observed in clinical trials to reduce Lp(a) concentration [78]. The role of proprotein convertase subtilisin/kexin type 9 (PCSK9) in influencing Lp(a) levels was also confirmed in a survey of PCSK9 functional-affecting mutants, which explicated that overexpressed function mutations of PCSK9 increased the CV risk while the PCSK9 R46L mutation reduced its function, showing a reduced risk of aortic stenosis and myocardial infarction [81]. The reduction in CV risk is proportional to the level of Lp(a) in the blood as mentioned above. Therefore, PCSK9 inhibitors are a potential agent for reducing the incidence of vascular events through its effect on Lp(a).

3.4.1 Treatment of high lipoprotein (a)

The cornerstone of current potential drug development is the new evidence on the benefits of Lp(a) reduction on the risk of CV events and mortality. Only in the last three years have trials of drugs that reduce Lp(a), such as alirocumab and evolocumab, been conducted. ODYSSEY OUTCOMES was a large trial of alirocumab, the results of which showed that alirocumab reduced the total number of CV events and CV mortality in patients diagnosed with acute coronary syndrome (ACS) [81]. In 2020, the data from the ODYSSEY OUTCOMES trial were reanalyzed to determine the effect of baseline Lp(a) levels and the trend of alirocumab-induced change on Lp(a) and LDL-C, results showed that each 5 mg/dL reduction in Lp(a) was predictive of a 2.5% reduction in CV events. Therefore, Lp(a) should now be considered a therapeutic target, especially after ACS [82]. There was a tremendous advantage when comparing alirocumab or evolocumab with placebo or ezetimibe plus a statin in another trial; however, the benefit difference between the two groups was not significant when comparing the two groups utilizing the combination of ezetimibe and statin [83].

Currently, new therapies that selectively target Lp(a) are being developed. The APO(a)-LRx study is currently ongoing, but preliminary findings indicate that APO(a)-LRx has the potential to reduce Lp(a) levels and their effects by up to 80%, potentially lowering CV risk [84]. In addition, testing a monoclonal antibody that reduces blood Lp(a) levels has demonstrated promising in vitro data [85]. The results of these trials are eagerly awaited.

To date, more persuasive evidence has exhibited that TG and Lp(a) are independent CV risk factors, even with LDL-C, and should be considered as new therapeutic targets in the management of CVD. Meanwhile, the importance of HDL-C has decreased compared to the previous era. However, in-depth studies analyzing genes and blood HDL-C levels are two hypotheses that need to be further studied to clarify the role of HDL-C.

4. Situations for considering residual cardiovascular risk factor intervention

4.1 After achieving LDL-C target

Based on the close association between hypercholesterolemia, especially LDL-C, with the incidence and mortality of ASCVD, the current treatment guidelines mainly focus on on lowering LDL-C levels [9, 11]. However, numerous clinical trials of statins, non-statin LDL-C lowering agents, and combination therapy have shown that the risk of ASCVD persists despite positive LDL-C reduction [14, 86, 87]. Accumulating evidence from epidemiological and genetic studies, as well as randomized clinical trials, suggests that TRLs [29, 41, 88], Lp(a) [77, 79, 82], inflammatory phenomenon [89–91] and thrombosis risk [92–95] are associated with risk of ASCVD in individuals with active LDL-C control and interventions to these factors yield promising results promise in improving the incidence of CV events [96].

Non-HDL-C dyslipidemia plays an important role in the residual risk of CVD. Recent recommendations for the quantification of atherogenic lipoproteins in addition to LDL-C for lipid-lowering strategies have been published [97].

4.2 Post-acute coronary syndrome

Advances in the treatment of ACS over the past few decades have improved the clinical outcomes of CV patients [98, 99]. Despite this, a substantial proportion of individuals continue to experience CV events, even when they are actively treated according to current guidelines [100]. This residual risk may be due to inflammation [90, 101, 102], thrombotic risk [93, 103] and metabolic causes such as TG [88, 104], Lp(a) [82, 105] and with or without HDL-C but has not been effectively addressed by current recommended approaches and is influenced by comorbidities [76, 102].

TG, Lp(a) have been shown to be independent risk factors affecting the risk of major CV events, some studies in subjects with a history of ACS also showed a similar correlation. Furthermore, the data to date suggest that TG and Lp(a) levels are positively correlated with the risk of ASCVD. Therefore, these two factors should be considered as new therapeutic targets to reduce residual CV risk [82, 88, 104, 105].

4.3 Diabetes mellitus

Insulin resistance and type 2 diabetes mellitus are associated with increased production of TRLs, such as VLDL-C and chylomicrons, as well as smaller and denser LDL-C particles (sdLDL-C), which makes LDL-C particles more compressed and therefore more prone to induce atherosclerosis. ApoB-100, the primary lipoproteins in VLDL-C, IDL-C, and sdLDL-C, as well as ApoB-48, the major lipoproteins in chylomicrons, have a significant risk of causing atherosclerosis. Despite effective LDL-C control with statin treatment, severe vascular events such as myocardial infarction, stroke, stable angina, and other vascular events, along with mortality from CV causes, occur substantially more frequently in diabetic patients. This has been shown to be related to TG [88, 104] because hyperglycemia is prevalent in those with type 2 diabetes mellitus [106]. Therefore, elevated TG is an important residual CV risk factor that should be considered in the treatment of diabetes.

In recent years, LDL-C-lowering treatments and other risk factor control strategies have significantly reduced the incidence of CVD, but in patients with type 2 diabetes there is still continue to increase the risk of ASCVD. Based on the evidence to date, it is suggested that non-LDL-C is a necessary therapeutic target in the prevention of CV events, especially in the TRLs group, in the setting of type 2 diabetes [107]. Furthermore, numerous studies suggest that low HDL-C levels and high TG, particularly TRLs, predict the risk of ASCVD in diabetes 2 which explains how low HDL-C levels impact cholesterol conversion from intravascular atherosclerotic plaque via CETP in TG metabolism. The consequence of all lipid abnormalities in type 2 diabetes is an increased risk of ASCVD. There is strong evidence, both genetic and clinical, that reducing residual TRLs and TG is likely to reduce the risk of CVD in CKD. diabetic patients with 2-insulin resistance [88, 104, 107]. Interventions on ApoC3, ANGPTL3, and ANGTL4 factors are being examined as potential TG- and TRL-lowering treatments and risk reductions in CVD, according to preclinical and human genetic research.

5. Conclusion

Based on the current evidence, the importance of residual CV risk factors in dyslipidemia are undoubtfully obvious. Since the complexity of the pathogenesis of atherosclerosis related to dyslipidemia, the recent interventional studies have shown controversial results. Therefore, identification and treatment of these risk factors is critical to optimizing treatment, particularly in subjects with recurrent vascular events, despite optimal treatment of traditional CV risk factors. In clinical practice, adequate attention should be paid when screening and managing residual CV risk factors in dyslipidemia in individualized approach. The ongoing trials will give more answers to elucidate this important clinical area.

Author details

Van Si Nguyen[1*], Xuan Truong Tran[2], Thanh Duy Vo[1] and Quang Truong Le[1]

1 Faculty of Medicine, Department of Internal Medicine, University of Medicine and Pharmacy, Ho Chi Minh City, Vietnam

2 Faculty of Medicine, Department of Internal Medicine, Pham Ngoc Thach Unversity of Medicine, Ho Chi Minh City, Vietnam

*Address all correspondence to: si.nguyen@ump.edu.vn

IntechOpen

© 2021 The Author(s). Licensee IntechOpen. This chapter is distributed under the terms of the Creative Commons Attribution License (http://creativecommons.org/licenses/by/3.0), which permits unrestricted use, distribution, and reproduction in any medium, provided the original work is properly cited. CC BY

References

[1] D. K. Arnett et al., 2019 ACC/AHA Guideline on the Primary Prevention of Cardiovascular Disease: A Report of the American College of Cardiology/ American Heart Association Task Force on Clinical Practice Guidelines, vol. 140, no. 11. 2019.

[2] "Heart-Healthy Living | NHLBI, NIH." https://www.nhlbi.nih.gov/ health-topics/heart-healthy-living (accessed Jun. 26, 2021).

[3] H. Kesteloot, "Prevention of cardiovascular disease," Tijdschr. Geneeskd., vol. 34, no. 10, pp. 627-630, 1978, doi: 10.1016/s0749-0690 (02)00015-0.

[4] S. M. Grundy et al., "WRITING COMMITTEE MEMBERS CHOLESTEROL CLINICAL PRACTICE GUIDELINES 2018 AHA/ACC/ AACVPR/AAPA/ABC/ACPM/ADA/ AGS/APhA/ASPC/NLA/PCNA Guideline on the Management of Blood Cholesterol Circulation," Circulation, vol. 139, pp. 1082-1143, 2018, doi: 10.1161/CIR.0000000000000625.

[5] R. Ferrari et al., "Current practice in identifying and treating cardiovascular risk, with a focus on residual risk associated with atherogenic dyslipidaemia," Eur. Hear. Journal, Suppl., vol. 18, pp. C2–C12, 2016, doi: 10.1093/eurheartj/suw009.

[6] J.-C. Fruchart et al., "Residual macrovascular risk in 2013: what have we learned? CARDIO VASCULAR DIABETOLOGY," 2014. doi: 10.1186/1475-2840-13-26.

[7] P. M. Ridker, "Clinician's Guide to Reducing Inflammation to Reduce Atherothrombotic Risk: JACC Review Topic of the Week," J. Am. Coll. Cardiol., vol. 72, no. 25, pp. 3320-3331, 2018, doi: 10.1016/j.jacc.2018.06.082.

[8] A. Hernández-Mijares et al., "Residual cardiovascular risk of lipid origin. Components and pathophysiological aspects," Clin. e Investig. en Arterioscler., vol. 31, no. 2, pp. 75-88, 2019, doi: 10.1016/j. arteri.2018.06.007.

[9] F. Mach et al., "2019 ESC/EAS Guidelines for the management of dyslipidaemias: Lipid modification to reduce cardiovascular risk," Eur. Heart J., vol. 41, no. 1, pp. 111-188, 2020, doi: 10.1093/eurheartj/ehz455.

[10] Ž. Reiner, "Managing the residual cardiovascular disease risk associated with HDL-cholesterol and triglycerides in statin-treated patients: A clinical update," Nutr. Metab. Cardiovasc. Dis., vol. 23, no. 9, pp. 799-807, 2013, doi: 10.1016/j.numecd.2013.05.002.

[11] S. M. Grundy et al., "2018 AHA/ ACC/AACVPR/AAPA/ABC/ACPM/ ADA/AGS/APhA/ASPC/NLA/PCNA Guideline on the Management of Blood Cholesterol: A Report of the American College of Cardiology/American Heart Association Task Force on Clinical Practice Guidelines," J. Am. Coll. Cardiol., vol. 73, no. 24, pp. e285–e350, 2019, doi: 10.1016/j.jacc.2018.11.003.

[12] J. L. Goldstein and M. S. Brown, "A century of cholesterol and coronaries: From plaques to genes to statins," Cell, vol. 161, no. 1, pp. 161-172, 2015, doi: 10.1016/j.cell.2015.01.036.

[13] B. A. Ference et al., "Low-density lipoproteins cause atherosclerotic cardiovascular disease. 1. Evidence from genetic, epidemiologic, and clinical studies. A consensus statement from the European Atherosclerosis Society Consensus Panel," Eur. Heart J., vol. 38, pp. 2459-2472, 2017, doi: 10.1093/ eurheartj/ehx144.

[14] C. Baigent et al., "Efficacy and safety of more intensive lowering of

LDL cholesterol: A meta-analysis of data from 170 000 participants in 26 randomised trials," Lancet, vol. 376, no. 9753, pp. 1670-1681, 2010, doi: 10.1016/S0140-6736(10)61350-5.

[15] U. K. Sampson, S. Fazio, and M. F. Linton, "Residual Cardiovascular Risk Despite Optimal LDL-Cholesterol Reduction with Statins: The Evidence, Etiology, and Therapeutic Challenges," Curr Atheroscler Rep, vol. 14, no. 1, pp. 1-10, 2012, doi: 10.1007/s11883-011-0219-7.

[16] C. P. Cannon et al., "Intensive versus Moderate Lipid Lowering with Statins after Acute Coronary Syndromes," N. Engl. J. Med., vol. 350, no. 15, pp. 1495-1504, Apr. 2004, doi: 10.1056/nejmoa040583.

[17] S. Sitia et al., "From endothelial dysfunction to atherosclerosis," Autoimmun. Rev., vol. 9, no. 12, pp. 830-834, 2010, doi: 10.1016/j.autrev.2010.07.016.

[18] M. Gliozzi et al., "Molecular Sciences Modulation of Nitric Oxide Synthases by Oxidized LDLs: Role in Vascular Inflammation and Atherosclerosis Development," 2019, doi: 10.3390/ijms20133294.

[19] J. Borén and K. J. Williams, "The central role of arterial retention of cholesterolrich apolipoprotein-B-containing lipoproteins in the pathogenesis of atherosclerosis: A triumph of simplicity," Curr. Opin. Lipidol., vol. 27, no. 5, pp. 473-483, 2016, doi: 10.1097/MOL.0000000000000330.

[20] I. Tabas, K. J. Williams, and J. Borén, "Subendothelial lipoprotein retention as the initiating process in atherosclerosis: Update and therapeutic implications," Circulation, vol. 116, no. 16, pp. 1832-1844, 2007, doi: 10.1161/CIRCULATIONAHA.106.676890.

[21] W. Liu, Y. Yin, Z. Zhou, M. He, and Y. Dai, "OxLDL-induced IL-1beta secretion promoting foam cells formation was mainly via CD36 mediated ROS production leading to NLRP3 inflammasome activation," Inflamm. Res., vol. 63, no. 1, pp. 33-43, 2014, doi: 10.1007/s00011-013-0667-3.

[22] E. Mammen, "Fibrinogen Abnormalities," Semin. Thromb. Hemost., vol. 9, no. 01, pp. 1-9, 1983, doi: 10.1055/s-2007-1004999.

[23] K. J. Moore, F. J. Sheedy, and E. A. Fisher, "Macrophages in atherosclerosis: A dynamic balance," Nat. Rev. Immunol., vol. 13, no. 10, pp. 709-721, 2013, doi: 10.1038/nri3520.

[24] A. Hultgårdh-Nilsson and M. Durbeej, "Role of the extracellular matrix and its receptors in smooth muscle cell function: Implications in vascular development and disease," Curr. Opin. Lipidol., vol. 18, no. 5, pp. 540-545, 2007, doi: 10.1097/MOL.0b013e3282ef77e9.

[25] Y. Kiyan, S. Tkachuk, D. Hilfiker-Kleiner, H. Haller, B. Fuhrman, and I. Dumler, "OxLDL induces inflammatory responses in vascular smooth muscle cells via urokinase receptor association with CD36 and TLR4," J. Mol. Cell. Cardiol., vol. 66, pp. 72-82, 2014, doi: 10.1016/j.yjmcc.2013.11.005.

[26] S. Vainio and E. Ikonen, "Macrophage cholesterol transport: a critical player in foam cell formation," 2009, doi: 10.1080/07853890310008198.

[27] M. M. Birck et al., "Endothelial cell death and intimal foam cell accumulation in the coronary artery of infected hypercholesterolemic minipigs," J. Cardiovasc. Transl. Res., vol. 6, no. 4, pp. 579-587, 2013, doi: 10.1007/s12265-013-9463-2.

[28] P. Libby, "Triglycerides on the rise: Should we swap seats on the seesaw?," Eur. Heart J., vol. 36, no. 13, pp. 774-776, 2015, doi: 10.1093/eurheartj/ehu500.

[29] M. Budoff, T. T. and H. W. G. of the E. S. Project, and and B. I. National Heart, Lung, "Triglycerides and Triglyceride-Rich Lipoproteins in the Causal Pathway of Cardiovascular Disease," Am. J. Cardiol., no. Cv, 2016, doi: 10.1016/j.amjcard.2016.04.004.

[30] S. A. Khetarpal and D. J. Rader, "Triglyceride-rich lipoproteins and coronary artery disease risk: New insights from human genetics," Arterioscler. Thromb. Vasc. Biol., vol. 35, no. 2, pp. e3–e9, 2015, doi: 10.1161/ATVBAHA.114.305172.

[31] H. Wang and R. H. Eckel, "Lipoprotein lipase: From gene to obesity," Am. J. Physiol. Endocrinol. Metab., vol. 297, no. 2, 2009, doi: 10.1152/ajpendo.90920.2008.

[32] "National Lipid Association recommendations for patient-centered management of dyslipidemia: Part 1 - executive summary | Elsevier Enhanced Reader." https://reader.elsevier.com/reader/sd/pii/S1933287414002748?token=67624B2012C13ABF4CA0F3EBA7A9423397ECD58FA715B75F15FFC4A6BF7758BD3BBCB8CE5D71F961F21F18C5ACB44458&originRegion=us-east-1&originCreation=20210630050921 (accessed Jun. 30, 2021).

[33] "24.Lipoprotein Lipase Mutations, Plasma Lipids and Lipoproteins, and Risk of Ischemic Heart Disease _ Enhanced Reader.pdf."

[34] C. J et al., "Loss-of-Function Mutations in APOC3, Triglycerides, and Coronary Disease," N. Engl. J. Med., vol. 371, no. 1, pp. 22-31, 2014, doi: 10.1056/nejmoa1307095.

[35] M. Kaltoft, A. Langsted, and B. G. Nordestgaard, "Triglycerides and remnant cholesterol associated with risk of aortic valve stenosis: Mendelian randomization in the Copenhagen General Population Study," Eur. Heart J., vol. 41, no. 24, pp. 2288-2299, 2020, doi: 10.1093/eurheartj/ehaa172.

[36] Allison A Brown and Frank B Hu, "Dietary modulation of endothelial function: implications for cardiovascular disease," 2001. [Online]. Available: https://academic.oup.com/ajcn/article/73/4/673/4737337.

[37] F. B. Hu et al., "Fish and Omega-3 Fatty Acid Intake and Risk of Coronary Heart Disease in Women," 2002. [Online]. Available: https://jamanetwork.com/.

[38] F. B. Hu, E. Cho, K. M. Rexrode, C. M. Albert, and J. E. Manson, "Fish and Long-Chain-3 Fatty Acid Intake and Risk of Coronary Heart Disease and Total Mortality in Diabetic Women," Circulation, vol. 107, pp. 1852-1857, 2003, doi: 10.1161/01.CIR.0000062644.42133.5F.

[39] "n–3 Fatty Acids and Cardiovascular Outcomes in Patients with Dysglycemia," N. Engl. J. Med., vol. 367, no. 4, pp. 309-318, 2012, doi: 10.1056/nejmoa1203859.

[40] S. J. Nicholls et al., "Effect of High-Dose Omega-3 Fatty Acids vs Corn Oil on Major Adverse Cardiovascular Events in Patients at High Cardiovascular Risk: The STRENGTH Randomized Clinical Trial," JAMA - J. Am. Med. Assoc., vol. 324, no. 22, pp. 2268-2280, 2020, doi: 10.1001/jama.2020.22258.

[41] D. L. Bhatt et al., "Cardiovascular Risk Reduction with Icosapent Ethyl for Hypertriglyceridemia," N. Engl. J. Med., vol. 380, no. 1, pp. 11-22, 2019, doi: 10.1056/nejmoa1812792.

[42] M. J. Budoff et al., "Effect of icosapent ethyl on progression of coronary atherosclerosis in patients with elevated triglycerides on statin therapy: final results of the EVAPORATE trial," 2020, doi: 10.1093/eurheartj/ehaa750.

[43] J. Stamler, "Clofibrate and Niacin in Coronary Heart Disease," JAMA J. Am. Med. Assoc., vol. 231, no. 4, pp. 360-381, 1975, doi: 10.1001/jama.1975.03240160024021.

[44] H. B. Rubinsv et al., "Gemfibrozil for the Secondary Prevention of Coronary Heart Disease in Men with Low Levels of High-Density Lipoprotein Cholesterol," J. Cardiopulm. Rehabil., vol. 20, no. 1, p. 66, 2000, doi: 10.1097/00008483-200001000-00015.

[45] B. Marshall et al., "Effects of Combination Lipid Therapy in Type 2 Diabetes Mellitus," pp. 1563-1574, 2010.

[46] M. Jun et al., "Effects of fibrates on cardiovascular outcomes: a systematic review and meta-analysis," Lancet, vol. 375, no. 9729, pp. 1875-1884, 2010, doi: 10.1016/S0140-6736(10)60656-3.

[47] V. J. Alexander et al., "N-acetyl galactosamine-conjugated antisense drug to APOC3 mRNA, triglycerides and atherogenic lipoprotein levels," Eur. Heart J., vol. 40, no. 33, pp. 2785-2796, 2019, doi: 10.1093/eurheartj/ehz209.

[48] P. H. Joshi et al., "Remnant Lipoprotein Cholesterol and Incident Coronary Heart Disease: The Jackson Heart and Framingham Offspring Cohort Studies," J. Am. Heart Assoc., vol. 5, no. 5, 2016, doi: 10.1161/JAHA.115.002765.

[49] S. Bandeali and J. Farmer, "High-density lipoprotein and atherosclerosis: The role of antioxidant activity," Curr. Atheroscler. Rep., vol. 14, no. 2, pp. 101-107, 2012, doi: 10.1007/s11883-012-0235-2.

[50] D. J. Gordon et al., "High-density lipoprotein cholesterol and cardiovascular disease. Four prospective American studies," Circulation, vol. 79, no. 1, pp. 8-15, 1989, doi: 10.1161/01.CIR.79.1.8.

[51] G. L. Moneta, "Major Lipids, Apolipoproteins, and Risk of Vascular Disease," Yearb. Vasc. Surg., vol. 2010, no. 18, pp. 42-44, 2010, doi: 10.1016/s0749-4041(10)79320-9.

[52] B. F. Voight et al., "Plasma HDL cholesterol and risk of myocardial infarction: A mendelian randomisation study," Lancet, vol. 380, no. 9841, pp. 572-580, 2012, doi: 10.1016/S0140-6736(12)60312-2.

[53] R. Frikke-Schmidt et al., "Association of Loss-of-Function Mutations in the ABCA1 Gene With High-Density," JAMA, vol. 299, no. 21, pp. 2524-2532, 2008.

[54] D. Rhainds and L. Brissette, "The role of scavenger receptor class B type I (SR-BI) in lipid trafficking: Defining the rules for lipid traders," Int. J. Biochem. Cell Biol., vol. 36, no. 1, pp. 39-77, 2004, doi: 10.1016/S1357-2725(03)00173-0.

[55] P. Zanoni et al., "Rare variant in scavenger receptor BI raises HDL cholesterol and increases risk of coronary heart disease," 2016. [Online]. Available: http://science.sciencemag.org/.

[56] B. Agerholm-Larsen, B. G. Nordestgaard, R. Steffensen, G. Jensen, and A. Tybjærg-Hansen, "Elevated HDL cholesterol is a risk factor for ischemic heart disease in white women when caused by a common mutation in the cholesteryl ester transfer protein gene," Circulation, vol. 101, no. 16, pp. 1907-1912, 2000, doi: 10.1161/01.CIR.101.16.1907.

[57] A. Thompson et al., "Association of cholesteryl ester transfer protein genotypes with CETP mass and activity, lipid levels, and coronary risk," JAMA - J. Am. Med. Assoc., vol. 299, no. 23, pp. 2777-2788, 2008, doi: 10.1001/jama.299.23.2777.

[58] Ž. Reiner et al., "ESC/EAS Guidelines for the management of

dyslipidaemias," Eur. Heart J., vol. 32, no. 14, pp. 1769-1818, 2011, doi: 10.1093/eurheartj/ehr158.

[59] J. Perk et al., "European Guidelines on cardiovascular diseaseprevention in clinical practice (version 2012): The Fifth Joint Task Force of the European Society of Cardiologyand Other Societies on Cardiovascular Disease Prevention in ClinicalPractice (constituted by representatives of nine societiesand by invited experts)," vol. 1, no. 5, 2012, doi: 10.1093/eurheartj/ehs092.

[60] M. B. Mortensen, S. Afzal, B. G. Nordestgaard, and E. Falk, "The high-density lipoprotein-adjusted SCORE model worsens SCORE-based risk classification in a contemporary population of 30 824 Europeans: The Copenhagen General Population Study," Eur. Heart J., vol. 36, no. 36, pp. 2446-2453, 2015, doi: 10.1093/eurheartj/ehv251.

[61] H. et. al Hampel, "Niacin in Patients with Low HDL Cholesterol Levels Receiving Intensive Statin Therapy," N. Engl. J. Med., pp. 687-696, 2011.

[62] M. J. Landray et al., "Effects of Extended-Release Niacin with Laropiprant in High-Risk Patients," N. Engl. J. Med., vol. 371, no. 3, pp. 203-212, 2014, doi: 10.1056/nejmoa1300955.

[63] "Effects of Anacetrapib in Patients with Atherosclerotic Vascular Disease," N. Engl. J. Med., vol. 377, no. 13, pp. 1217-1227, 2017, doi: 10.1056/nejmoa1706444.

[64] P. J. Barter, M. Caulfield, and M. Eriksson, "Effects of torcetrapib in patients at high risk for coronary events," J. Vasc. Surg., vol. 47, no. 4, p. 893, 2008, doi: 10.1016/j.jvs.2008.02.014.

[65] G. G. Schwartz et al., "Effects of Dalcetrapib in Patients with a Recent Acute Coronary Syndrome A bs t r ac t," N Engl J Med, vol. 367, pp. 2089-2099, 2012, doi: 10.1056/NEJMoa1206797.

[66] A. Lincoff, S. Nicholls, J. Riesmeyer, P. Barter, H. Brewer, and K. Fox, "Evacetrapib and Cardiovascular Outcomes in High-Risk Vascular Disease," 2017. doi: 10.1016/j.jvs.2017.08.007.

[67] C. M. Madsen and B. G. Nordestgaard, "Is it time for new thinking about high-density lipoprotein?," Arterioscler. Thromb. Vasc. Biol., vol. 38, no. 3, pp. 484-486, 2018, doi: 10.1161/ATVBAHA.118.310727.

[68] C. M. Madsen, A. Varbo, and B. G. Nordestgaard, "Extreme high high-density lipoprotein cholesterol is paradoxically associated with high mortality inmen and women: Two prospective cohort studies," Eur. Heart J., vol. 38, no. 32, pp. 2478-2486, 2017, doi: 10.1093/eurheartj/ehx163.

[69] M. Hamer, G. O'Donovan, and E. Stamatakis, "High-density lipoprotein cholesterol and mortality too much of a good thing?," Arterioscler. Thromb. Vasc. Biol., vol. 38, no. 3, pp. 669-672, 2018, doi: 10.1161/ATVBAHA.117.310587.

[70] R. C. Maranhão, P. O. Carvalho, C. Cassaro Strunz, and F. Pileggi, "Lipoprotein (a): Structure, Pathophysiology and Clinical Implications," 2013, doi: 10.5935/abc.20140101.

[71] E. Steyrer et al., "The role of lecithin: Cholesterol acyltransferase for lipoprotein (a) assembly. Structural integrity of low density lipoproteins is a prerequisite for Lp(a) formation in human plasma," J. Clin. Invest., vol. 94, no. 6, pp. 2330-2340, 1994, doi: 10.1172/JCI117598.

[72] M. B. Boffa, S. M. Marcovina, and M. L. Koschinsky, "Lipoprotein(a) as a risk factor for atherosclerosis and

thrombosis: Mechanistic insights from animal models," Clin. Biochem., vol. 37, no. 5, pp. 333-343, 2004, doi: 10.1016/j.clinbiochem.2003.12.007.

[73] M. Poon, X. Zhang, K. Dunsky, M. B. Taubman, and P. C. Harpel, "Apolipoprotein(a) is a human vascular endothelial cell agonist: Studies on the induction in endothelial cells of monocyte chemotactic factor activity," Clin. Genet., vol. 52, no. 5, pp. 308-313, 1997, doi: 10.1111/j.1399-0004.1997.tb04348.x.

[74] U. Kassner, T. Schlabs, A. Rosada, and E. Steinhagen-Thiessen, "Lipoprotein(a) - An independent causal risk factor for cardiovascular disease and current therapeutic options," Atheroscler. Suppl., vol. 18, pp. 263-267, 2015, doi: 10.1016/j.atherosclerosissup.2015.02.039.

[75] S. Erqou et al., "Lipoprotein(a) Concentration and the Risk of Coronary Heart Disease, Stroke, and Nonvascular Mortality," Jama-Journal Am. Med. Assoc., vol. 302, no. 4, pp. 412-423, 2009, [Online]. Available: http://jama.jamanetwork.com/.

[76] M. Mcqueen et al., "Lipoprotein (a) Levels and the Risk of Myocardial Infarction Among Seven Ethnic Groups," vol. 8, no. 905.

[77] A. V. Khera et al., "Lipoprotein(a) concentrations, rosuvastatin therapy, and residual vascular risk: An analysis from the JUPITER trial (justification for the use of statins in prevention: An intervention trial evaluating rosuvastatin)," Circulation, vol. 129, no. 6, pp. 635-642, 2014, doi: 10.1161/CIRCULATIONAHA.113.004406.

[78] M. L. O'Donoghue et al., "Lipoprotein(a), PCSK9 inhibition, and cardiovascular risk insights from the FOURIER trial," Circulation, vol. 139, no. 12, pp. 1483-1492, 2019, doi: 10.1161/CIRCULATIONAHA.118.037184.

[79] W. Q. Wei et al., "LPA variants are associated with residual cardiovascular risk in patients receiving statins," Circulation, vol. 138, no. 17, pp. 1839-1849, 2018, doi: 10.1161/CIRCULATIONAHA.117.031356.

[80] S. Burgess et al., "Association of LPA variants with risk of coronary disease and the implications for lipoprotein(a)-lowering therapies: A mendelian randomization analysis," JAMA Cardiol., vol. 3, no. 7, pp. 619-627, 2018, doi: 10.1001/jamacardio.2018.1470.

[81] A. Langsted, B. G. Nordestgaard, M. Benn, A. Tybjaerg-Hansen, P. R. Kamstrup, and G. Hospital, "PCSK9 R46L Loss-of-Function Mutation Reduces Lipoprotein(a), LDL Cholesterol, and Risk of Aortic Valve Stenosis and The Copenhagen General Population Study (A," J Clin Endocrinol Metab, vol. 101, pp. 3281-3287, 2016, doi: 10.1210/jc.2016-1206.

[82] M. Szarek et al., "Lipoprotein(a) lowering by alirocumabreduces the total burden of cardiovascularevents independent of low-densitylipo protein cholesterol lowering: ODYSSEYOUTCOMES trial," Eur. Heart J., vol. 41, pp. 4245-4255, 2020, doi: 10.1093/eurheartj/ehaa842.

[83] A. F. Schmidt et al., "PCSK9 monoclonal antibodies for the primary and secondary prevention of cardiovascular disease," Cochrane Database Syst. Rev., vol. 2020, no. 12, 2020, doi: 10.1002/14651858.CD011748.pub3.

[84] S. Tsimikas et al., "Lipoprotein(a) Reduction in Persons with Cardiovascular Disease," N. Engl. J. Med., vol. 382, no. 3, pp. 244-255, 2020, doi: 10.1056/nejmoa1905239.

[85] N. J. Viney et al., "Antisense oligonucleotides targeting apolipoprotein(a) in people with raised lipoprotein(a): two randomised,

double-blind, placebo-controlled, dose-ranging trials," Lancet, vol. 388, no. 10057, pp. 2239-2253, 2016, doi: 10.1016/S0140-6736(16)31009-1.

[86] C. P. Cannon et al., "Ezetimibe Added to Statin Therapy after Acute Coronary Syndromes," N. Engl. J. Med., vol. 372, no. 25, pp. 2387-2397, 2015, doi: 10.1056/nejmoa1410489.

[87] M. S. Sabatine et al., "Evolocumab and Clinical Outcomes in Patients with Cardiovascular Disease," N. Engl. J. Med., vol. 376, no. 18, pp. 1713-1722, 2017, doi: 10.1056/nejmoa1615664.

[88] G. A. Nichols, S. Philip, K. Reynolds, C. B. Granowitz, and S. Fazio, "Increased Cardiovascular Risk in Hypertriglyceridemic Patients With Statin-Controlled LDL Cholesterol," J Clin Endocrinol Metab, vol. 103, pp. 3019-3027, 2018, doi: 10.1210/jc.2018-00470.

[89] W. Koenig, "High-sensitivity C-reactive protein and atherosclerotic disease: From improved risk prediction to risk-guided therapy," Int. J. Cardiol., vol. 168, no. 6, pp. 5126-5134, 2013, doi: 10.1016/j.ijcard.2013.07.113.

[90] E. A. Bohula et al., "Achievement of dual low-density lipoprotein cholesterol and high-sensitivity c-reactive protein targets more frequent with the addition of ezetimibe to simvastatin and associated with better outcomes in IMPROVE-IT," Circulation, vol. 132, no. 13, pp. 1224-1233, 2015, doi: 10.1161/CIRCULATIONAHA.115.018381.

[91] P. M. Ridker et al., "Antiinflammatory Therapy with Canakinumab for Atherosclerotic Disease," N. Engl. J. Med., vol. 377, no. 12, pp. 1119-1131, 2017, doi: 10.1056/nejmoa1707914.

[92] R. Collins et al., "Aspirin in the primary and secondary prevention of vascular disease: collaborative meta-analysis of individual participant data from randomised trials," Lancet, vol. 373, no. 9678, pp. 1849-1860, 2009, doi: 10.1016/S0140-6736(09)60503-1.

[93] G. Gallone et al., "Medical Therapy for Long-Term Prevention of Atherothrombosis Following an Acute Coronary Syndrome: JACC State-of-the-Art Review," J. Am. Coll. Cardiol., vol. 72, no. 23, pp. 2886-2903, 2018, doi: 10.1016/j.jacc.2018.09.052.

[94] J. W. Eikelboom et al., "Rivaroxaban with or without Aspirin in Stable Cardiovascular Disease," N. Engl. J. Med., vol. 377, no. 14, pp. 1319-1330, 2017, doi: 10.1056/nejmoa1709118.

[95] S. S. Anand et al., "Rivaroxaban with or without aspirin in patients with stable peripheral or carotid artery disease: an international, randomised, double-blind, placebo-controlled trial," Lancet, vol. 391, no. 10117, pp. 219-229, 2018, doi: 10.1016/S0140-6736(17)32409-1.

[96] R. C. Hoogeveen and C. M. Ballantyne, "Residual Cardiovascular Risk at Low LDL: Remnants, Lipoprotein(a), and Inflammation," Clin. Chem., vol. 67, no. 1, pp. 143-153, 2021, doi: 10.1093/clinchem/hvaa252.

[97] M. R. Langlois et al., "Quantifying atherogenic lipoproteins for lipid-lowering strategies: Consensus-based recommendations from EAS and EFLM," Clin. Chem. Lab. Med., vol. 58, no. 4, pp. 496-517, 2020, doi: 10.1515/cclm-2019-1253.

[98] F. Schiele et al., "The FAST-MI 2005-2010-2015 registries in the light of the COMPASS trial: The COMPASS criteria applied to a post-MI population," Int. J. Cardiol., vol. 278, no. xxxx, pp. 7-13, 2019, doi: 10.1016/j.ijcard.2018.11.138.

[99] D. D. McManus, J. Gore, J. Yarzebski, F. Spencer, D. Lessard, and

R. J. Goldberg, "Recent trends in the incidence, treatment, and outcomes of patients with STEMI and NSTEMI," Am. J. Med., vol. 124, no. 1, pp. 40-47, 2011, doi: 10.1016/j.amjmed.2010.07.023.

[100] M. Hall et al., "Association of clinical factors and therapeutic strategies with improvements in survival following Non-ST-elevation myocardial infarction, 2003-2013," JAMA - J. Am. Med. Assoc., vol. 316, no. 10, pp. 1073-1082, 2016, doi: 10.1001/jama.2016.10766.

[101] P. M. Ridker et al., "Relationship of C-reactive protein reduction to cardiovascular event reduction following treatment with canakinumab: a secondary analysis from the CANTOS randomised controlled trial," Lancet, vol. 391, no. 10118, pp. 319-328, 2018, doi: 10.1016/S0140-6736(17)32814-3.

[102] P. Mani et al., "Association of Initial and Serial C-Reactive Protein Levels With Adverse Cardiovascular Events and Death After Acute Coronary Syndrome A Secondary Analysis of the VISTA-16 Trial," 2019, doi: 10.1001/jamacardio.2019.0179.

[103] J. L. Mega et al., "Rivaroxaban in Patients with a Recent Acute Coronary Syndrome," n engl j med, vol. 366, 2012, doi: 10.1056/NEJMoa1112277.

[104] G. A. Nichols, S. Philip PharmD, K. Reynolds, C. B. Granowitz, S. Fazio, and C. A. Gregory Nichols, "Increased residual cardiovascular risk in patients with diabetes and high versus normal triglycerides despite statin-controlled LDL cholesterol," 2018, doi: 10.1111/dom.13537.

[105] M. Szarek et al., "Alirocumab Reduces Total Nonfatal Cardiovascular and Fatal Events: The ODYSSEY OUTCOMES Trial," J. Am. Coll. Cardiol., vol. 73, no. 4, pp. 387-396, 2019, doi: 10.1016/j.jacc.2018.10.039.

[106] H. Ghandehari, S. Kamal-Bahl, and N. D. Wong, "Prevalence and extent of dyslipidemia and recommended lipid levels in US adults with and without cardiovascular comorbidities: The National Health and Nutrition Examination Survey 2003-2004," Am. Heart J., vol. 156, no. 1, pp. 112-119, 2008, doi: 10.1016/j.ahj.2008.03.005.

[107] S. Dash and L. A. Leiter, "Residual cardiovascular risk among people with diabetes," Diabetes, Obes. Metab., vol. 21, no. S1, pp. 28-38, Apr. 2019, doi: 10.1111/dom.13646.

Chapter 10

Experimental Model of Cardiotoxicity

Oytun Erbaş, İlknur Altuntaş, Özge Çağlar, Elif Özyilmaz, Ece Sari, İlayda Üzümcü and Kaan Erbakan

Abstract

The occurrence of heart electrophysiology dysfunction or/and muscle damage is referred to as cardiotoxicity. The heart weakens and becomes less efficient at pumping and hence circulating blood. Cardiomyopathy can be caused by a variety of factors, including viral infections, diseases such as diabetes, ischemia, hypertension, obesity, radiation therapy, antipsychotic drugs, cytotoxic drugs, most notably chemotherapeutic agents; antitumor antibiotics, monoclonal antibodies, tyrosine kinase inhibitors, platinum-based compounds, microtubule inhibitors, vinca alkaloids, antimetabolites, proteasome inhibitors, topoisomerase inhibitors, alkylating agents, corticosteroids. This chapter focuses on the mechanisms of cardiotoxicity, animal models and transgenic methods used in studies, and the effects of therapeutic agents on cardiotoxicity.

Keywords: cardiotoxicity, cardiomyopathy, chemotherapeutics, diabetes, ischemia, radiation therapy, toxicants, transgenic animal models

1. Introduction

Globally, heart disease is responsible for a third of all deaths [1]. Cardiotoxicity occurs when the heart, in whole or in part, is damaged as a result of factors such as obesity, chemotherapy (CT), alcohol exposure, anorexia, neurosis, unconscious drug use, occupational and environmental heavy metal exposure [2–4].

Toxicants impair pumping efficiency by reducing the number of active myocytes, cause oxidative damage and lipid peroxidation, which results in cell swelling, altered Ca^{2+} homeostasis, and irreversible myocyte injury, alter aerobic metabolism, myocardial conduction, cell membrane function, directly damaged myocardium, and induce vascular changes [5]. They also cause QT interval prolongation and ionic channel blockage, which can lead to syncope and ventricular fibrillation. The heart weakens and becomes less efficient at pumping and thus circulating blood. Because of the high energy demands of the heart, it is susceptible to toxins that interfere with oxygen availability, carbohydrate metabolism, and oxidative phosphorylation [6, 7].

Cardiotoxicity is characterized by cardiac dysfunctions, arrhythmia (changes in heart rhythm), hypotension, tachypnea, edema, heart muscle damage (cardiomyopathy), changes in transmission pathways, and toxic effects on the heart [3]. Cardiotoxicity includes changes in resting cardiac measurements as well as dynamic functional evaluations of the cardiovascular (CV) systems [3, 5, 6]. The formation of oxygen free radicals and calcium overload in myocytes, a deficiency of antioxidant systems such as catalase and superoxide dismutase, and a possible immunological reaction triggered by the drug are the main pathophysiological processes of cardiotoxicity [8]. Acute or subacute heart damage includes changes in the ventricular repolarization phase, the duration of the QT interval, arrhythmias, ischemia, acute heart failure (HF), and myocarditis-pericarditis-like syndrome. As a result of chronic (early/late) conditions, patients may have symptoms such as left ventricular (LV) dysfunction, systolic/diastolic impotence, and cardiac death [9, 10].

Cardiotoxicity is a well-known side effect of many cytotoxic drugs that can result in long-term morbidity.

2. Chemotherapy-induced cardiotoxicity (CIC)

The development of cancer screening methods, early diagnosis, and the widespread use of adjuvant chemotherapy can result in a significantly higher positive response rate in cancer treatment. Cancer drugs destroy cancerous cells in a variety of ways. These actions usually result in cell death (cytotoxicity), but they can also prevent the cell from growing without killing it (cytostatic action) [11].

Chemotherapeutics have a variety of modes of action, including alkylation of DNA, disruption of DNA and RNA synthesis by intercalating between base pairs, inhibition of DNA polymerase, stimulation of apoptosis, inhibition of DNA topoisomerase II, and preventing mitosis via altering tubulin polymerization. With this higher positive response, however, the number of people exposed to chemotherapy's early and late cardiac side effects emerges [12]. A wide range of adverse effects of chemotherapy and radiation on cardiac structure, hemostasis and thrombosis, cardiac dysfunctions and arrhythmias, and toxic effects on the heart have been well-documented [1, 13].

Side effects are common among cytotoxic drugs, notably chemotherapeutic agents; antitumor antibiotics, monoclonal antibodies, tyrosine kinase inhibitors, platinum-based compounds, microtubule inhibitors, vinca alkaloids, antimetabolites, proteasome inhibitors, topoisomerase inhibitors, alkylating agents, corticosteroids, and other drugs. They have the potential to cause long-term morbidity. They are linked to irreversible dilated cardiomyopathy and dose-dependent cardiotoxicity [14, 15].

Anthracyclines, a class of antibiotics derived from Streptomyces spp, have been used to treat a variety of cancers over the last 50 years, including lymphoma, leukemia, bladder cancer, breast cancer, and other metastatic cancers [16, 17]. Cardiotoxicity is a growing concern in clinical oncology due to the increasing use of anthracyclines, the introduction of new antitumor agents with potentially cardiotoxic properties, and the use of combined treatments that may have adverse effects on the heart [18, 19].

Anthracyclines catalyze intracellular oxygen radicals via enzymatic reactions in mitochondria, as well as non-enzymatic iron-mediated free radical reactions which damage DNA. They induce apoptosis in vascular cells and cardiomyocytes by activating caspases and degrading internucleosomal DNA [20]. When compared to other tissues, cardiomyocytes have a 35–40% larger amount of mitochondria. Cardiomyocytes use 90% of the ATP produced by mitochondria [21]. Due to bio-energetic failure, genotoxic stress, and oxidative stress, adenosine monophosphate-activated protein kinase (AMPK) signaling is suppressed during treatment, resulting in increased energy stress and hypertrophy [21]. Serum troponin levels in anthracycline-treated patients are also observed to be higher, indicating cell death [22, 23].

Daunorubicin, doxorubicin, epirubicin, idarubicin, mitoxantrone, and valrubicin are some of the most commonly used anthracyclines [17]. These drugs have similar effects on cardiotoxicity [24–26]. Following the existence of targeted therapy, doxorubicin is still widely used in cancer treatment today [10, 27]. However, anthracycline's medical use is limited due to dose-dependent and cumulative cardiotoxicity. The clinical efficacy of this drug is restricted due to its side effects, particularly cardiotoxicity when doses exceed 400–700 mg/m^2 for adults and 300 mg/m^2 for children [6, 7, 28]. Doxorubicin cardiomyopathy is more likely at 400 mg/m^2 (5%), at 550 mg/m^2 (26%), and at 700 mg/m^2, where the risk is as high as 48% [14].

A primary cause of doxorubicin-induced cardiomyocyte damage is assumed to be ROS (reactive oxygen species) generation and lipid peroxidation by inhibition of mitochondrial membrane potential and mitochondrial permeability transition pore [29]. To interfere with DNA replication, doxorubicin inhibits DNA topoisomerase 2-beta (Top2β) whereas a doxorubicin-Top2β DNA complex prevents the repair of damaged DNA and leads to cell death [27, 30, 31]. Doxorubicin also affects adrenergic function and adenylate cyclase inhibition of sarcoplasmic reticulum Ca^{2+} release, inhibits Ca^{2+}-ATPase activities causing diastolic dysfunction, reduces expression of cardiac-specific genes and down-regulates expression of a variety of cardiac muscle-specific proteins including mitochondrial proteins, contractile proteins, sarcoplasmic reticulum proteins [29]. Treatment with doxorubicin induces the immune system to generate a variety of inflammatory mediators (IL-1, IL-6, IL-7, TNF receptor 2, vascular endothelial growth factor/VEGF, matrix metalloproteinases/MMP2); natural killer cells stop functioning, cytotoxic T lymphocytes responses are triggered, and macrophage differentiation is inhibited [32, 33]. Doxorubicin cardiomyopathy increases oxidative stress, which is connected to an increase in Toll-like receptors 2, induces nuclear factor kappa B (NF-κB), and finally leads to apoptosis [34]. There is also an increase in the level of tumor necrosis factor (TNF-α) due to the toll-like receptor 4 [35].

The human epidermal growth factor receptor 2 (ERBB2) is a transmembrane tyrosine kinase receptor that plays in a variety of cellular processes, including cell survival in normal healthy tissue [36]. As a humanized monoclonal antibody, trastuzumab targets ERBB2 on the surface of tumor cells that overexpress ERBB2 [37]. Trastuzumab-induced cardiac damage was detected in metastatic breast cancer trials for the first time. It is the most common chemotherapeutic agent related to left ventricular dysfunction [38]. Bevacizumab is a humanized monoclonal antibody that inhibits vascular endothelial growth factor (VEGF) activity in patients with metastatic colorectal cancer, non-small cell lung cancer, and breast cancer. Although, congestive heart failure (CHF) has been reported in a study, its overall incidence and relative risk are still unknown [39].

Tyrosine kinase (TK) inhibitors (TKI) are molecules designed to target TKs that are overexpressed in cancer cells, but they also inhibit normal variants of tyrosine kinases in non-cancerous cells, which can cause severe side effects such as left ventricular failure [40].

Imatinib is an ATP-competitive small-molecule ABL kinase inhibitor that was developed primarily for the treatment of malignancies such as chronic myeloid leukemia (CML) [41, 42]. It has been shown that imatinib leads to significant mitochondrial damage, including loss of membrane potential, the release of cytochrome C, and markedly reduced energy production with significant declines in ATP concentration, in studies on cultured cardiomyocytes [43, 44]. Other tyrosine-kinase inhibitors such as dasatinib, nilotinib, sunitinib, sorafenib, and lapatinib have been related to drug-induced cardiotoxicity, although the true extent of the damage remains unknown. The literature mentions only a few cases of asymptomatic QT prolongation, pericardial effusion, acute coronary syndromes [45].

Anticancer drugs based on platinum bind to DNA, causing it to crosslink. End result: cancer cells die through apoptosis because of the crosslinks, which interfere with DNA repair and synthesis in the cancer cells. Cisplatin, carboplatin, and oxaliplatin, platinum-based compounds with severe nephrotoxic, neurotoxic, and ototoxic properties, are frequently used in the treatment of human neoplasms [46, 47]. Vascular toxicity, hypertension, dyslipidemia, early atherosclerosis, and coronary artery disease are the most serious late effects of cisplatin-based chemotherapy in patients [48].

Taxanes (paclitaxel, docetaxel, cabazitaxel, Nab-paclitaxel) are microtubule inhibitors (MIT) or mitotic inhibitors that play an important role in mitosis and have lower cardiotoxicity than anthracyclines. Vinca alkaloids such as vinblastine, vincristine, liposomal vincristine, and vinorelbine are also mitotic inhibitors that are used to treat a variety of cancers such as breast, lung, myelomas, lymphomas, and leukemia. As a result, several trials have been conducted to evaluate their use in combination with anthracyclines [49–52].

Antimetabolites such as 5-fluorouracil (5-FU), capecitabine, azacitidine, cytarabine, gemcitabine, methotrexate, hydroxyurea, and pentostatin which are commonly used to treat leukemia, ovarian, breast, gastrointestinal, and other solid tumors, damage proliferating cells during the S phase of mitosis by substituting the normal DNA/RNA building blocks [53]. Endothelial injury followed by thrombosis; energy depletion and myocardial ischemia; coronary arterial spasm following myocardial ischemia; and decreased ability of red blood cells to transfer oxygen leading to myocardial ischemia are all associated with antimetabolite toxicity [54, 55].

Proteasome inhibitors (PI), which primarily function as immunosuppressants and inhibit bone resorption, such as bortezomib, carfilzomib, and ixazomib, are a promising new class of drugs for the treatment of multiple myeloma, and they are also being studied for other types of cancer [56]. As non-proliferative cells with increased proteasome activity, cardiomyocytes are particularly sensitive to proteasome inhibition.

DNA topoisomerases (type I and type II) are the enzymes responsible for DNA unlinking, and play critical roles in a variety of biological processes involving DNA. Several topoisomerase I inhibitors (also known as camptothecins) include irinotecan, topotecan, and camptothecin, while topoisomerase II inhibitors (also known as epipodophyllotoxins) include etoposide, mitoxantrone, and teniposide [57]. Topoisomerase inhibitors cause the release of ROS, lead to DNA breaks and prevent ligase repair. The enzymes catalase (CAT), superoxide dismutase (SOD) and glutathione peroxidase (GSH-Px) are antioxidant enzymes in oxidative stress modulation, crucial for efficient removal of ROS. Cardiomyocytes are particularly vulnerable to damage because they have low levels of antioxidant enzymes required to detoxify ROS [58].

Cells are also prevented from reproducing by alkylating agents such as cisplatin, busulfan, mechlorethamine, temozolomide, dacarbazine, streptozocin, which damage their DNA [59].

Following are a few examples of *in vivo* models of chemotherapy-induced cardiotoxicity and protective agents based on the literature;

To explore cardiotoxic effects, animal models are being studied, and therapeutic approaches developed. Because considerable pharmacokinetic and pharmacodynamic data from studies examining the anticancer efficacy of drugs are available, rodents are an attractive model for studying cardiotoxicity.

In the initial periods of cardiotoxicity studies, rabbits were thought to be the standard model. In a study, scientists evaluated the protective effect of ICRF-187 (dexrazoxane, a drug used to prevent anthracycline-induced cardiotoxicity) in rabbits against chronic daunorubicin cardiotoxicity. For the experimental model, twenty-four male white rabbits were divided into four groups (group1; 25 mg ICRF-187/kg and 3.2 mg daunorubicin/kg, group2; daunorubicin (3.2mg/kg), group3;

ICRF-187 (25 mg/kg), group4; placebo). They treated animals six times at 3-week intervals over an 18-week period. Significantly different cardiotoxic effects were observed in animals treated only with daunorubicin and those treated only with daunorubicin + ICRF-187. Anthracycline cardiotoxicity was significantly reduced by pretreatment with ICRF-187 [60].

In another study, Zhang et al. divided 50 male Sprague-Dawley rats into three groups for a 15-day experiment: control (saline), doxorubicin (3 mg/kg), and doxorubicin+oxymatrine (12.5, 25, and 50 mg/kg) to detect oxymatrine's protective effects on cardiovascular diseases. Specifically, they found that oxymatrine pre-treatment protected against doxorubicin-induced cardiotoxicity in rats' hearts by inhibiting the apoptotic pathway [61].

Zilinyi et al. investigated metformin's (anti-diabetic drug) protective role and its effect on autophagy in doxorubicin-induced cardiotoxicity. In the first group of four Sprague-Dawley rats, doxorubicin (3 mg/kg every second day) was administered intraperitoneally, metformin (250 mg/kg/day) was administered via gavage, and the third group received doxorubicin + metformin, while the fourth group was a control group for two weeks. Doxorubicin-treated myocytes were significantly thinner than those in the control group. Myocyte diameters in the doxorubicin + metformin group were nearly identical to those in the control group. According to the histopathological examination of heart tissue samples, metformin normalized autophagy [62].

In a doxorubicin-induced cardiomyopathy model, Erbaş and his colleagues described the therapeutic effects of liraglutide (LIR), oxytocin, and granulocyte colony-stimulating factor. Four groups of 32 rats were given, respectively, group I; placebo 0.9% NaCl saline solution at a dose of 1 ml/kg/day i.p. (doxorubicin + saline), group II; 1.8 mg/kg/day of liraglutide i.p. (doxorubicin + LIR), group III; 160 μg/kg/day oxytocin i.p. (doxorubicin + OX), group IV; 100 μg/kg/day filgrastim i.p. (doxorubicin + G-CSF (Granulocyte colony-stimulating factor)). It was revealed through the study's findings inflammatory activity and improved tissue integrity were found to be decreased in response to oxytocin treatment. Besides, LIR reduces levels of proinflammatory cytokines, lipid peroxidation products, troponin T, pro-BNP levels, and CASPASE-3 in doxorubicin-treated rats [63].

Arsenic trioxide and imatinib mesilate cardiotoxicity were examined in male Wistar rats. In the experiment, for ten days, arsenic trioxide (5 mg/kg) and imatinib mesilate (30 mg/kg) was given intraperitoneally and orally, respectively. As a result, the cardiac tissue of the combination-treated group showed fibroblastic proliferation, myocardial disorganization, and myocardial necrosis [64].

According to a study by Saleh et al., tadalafil (Tad) might protect against cardiac and vascular damage caused by the chemotherapy drug cisplatin (CDDP). Seventy-two male albino rats were divided into four groups: the control group, the CDDP (4 mg/kg) i.p. group, the Tad (0.4 mg/kg BW Tad i.p. daily) group, and the Tad +CDDP (0.4 mg/kg BW Tad i.p. + 4 mg/kg BW CDDP i.p) group. In the heart homogenate sample from CDDP treated rats, Tad was able to reduce blood pressure, heart rate, and levels of cardiac troponin, malondialdehyde (MDA), while increasing levels of reduced glutathione (GSH) and nitric oxide (NO) [65].

3. Radiation therapy-induced cardiotoxicity

Cardiotoxicity caused by radiation therapy (RT) is not only seen in adults, but also in children. High radiation exposure, being female, higher anthracycline cumulative dose, trisomy 21, and race are all risk factors for cardiotoxicity in children [66]. Since the early 1900s, ionizing radiation therapy has been utilized to treat cancer [67]. Along with medical advancements, the role of imaging modalities in the administration of the treatment process has gradually increased, in addition to surgical and systematic treatment [68, 69]. Considering the significance of these procedures in the treatment process and in enhancing survival, heart problems from radiotherapy remain a risk [69]. Radiation-induced heart disease (RIHD) is an important cause of long-term non-cancer death after thoracic irradiation [70]. Studies have shown that people who live at least 5 years after diagnosis have a high rate of cardiovascular death [71]. Studies have shown that significant cardiovascular events usually occur within 10–15 years [72]. Lung cancer, mediastinal lymphoma, and breast cancer are cancers that are proximal to the heart and have the highest prevalence of RT, which means they have a significant risk of cardiotoxicity [73]. When Saika et al. looked at breast cancer radiotherapy treatment and heart failure risk, they discovered that women who had RT for breast cancer had a 10 times higher risk of heart failure than the control group, regardless of age or cancer type [74]. Cardiotoxicity from RT causes a worsening of cardiac function in a variety of illnesses, including cardiomyopathy, pericardial injury, coronary artery disease, and heart disease [75, 76].

The effects of factors such as the total radiation volume applied to the patient, the patient's age, the radiation exposure process, and the simultaneous use of cardiotoxic chemotherapeutic drugs such as anthracyclines are seen in radiation-induced heart diseases [1, 4]. Symptoms of these diseases include pericardial and myocardial fibrosis, rhythm disorders, conduction abnormalities, atherosclerosis, and heart valve injuries. Although, cardiac issues do not manifest themselves until later in life in people, evidence of cardiac toxicity can be found after 10–15 years of follow-up [1, 77]. It has been stated in the literature that RT may have detrimental effects on several important tissues in the heart [68]. In studies, it has been explained that the basis of the mechanism of cardiac damage caused by RT is related to microvascular changes and inflammation that causes longer-term fibrotic changes [1, 68, 78].

Following are a few examples of *in vivo* models of radiation-induced cardiotoxicity and protective agents based on the literature;

In the studies carried out so far, models have been created with different animals to create experimental animal models of cardiotoxicity. Some of these models are Male Albino rats [79, 80], Male Sprague-Dawley rats [63], Albino Wistar rats [81], male C57/BL6 mice [82].

Mezzaroma et al. used three-month-old C57BL/6J male mice in their study, and 12 of them were irradiated with a single 20 Gray (Gy) dose of radiation therapy, while the other six underwent sham-irradiation. They found that when compared to sham non-irradiated mice, radiation therapy-treated mice exhibited a 2-fold higher rate of myocardial interstitial fibrosis after six months [83].

Using Mast cell-deficient rats (Ws/Ws) and mast cell–competent littermate controls (+/+), researchers exposed the rats for six months to 18 Gy localized single-dose irradiation to investigate cardiac function. They found that mast cell–deficient rats had a higher upward/leftward shift in the left ventricular (LV) diastolic pressure-volume relationship, a decrease in vivo LV diastolic area, and a greater rise in the thickness of the LV posterior wall [84].

Dreyfuss et al. in their study aimed to develop a new mouse model to investigate the pathophysiological mechanism of RT-induced cardiotoxicity and to detect clinically targetable biomarkers of cardiac damage. They used 9–11 weeks of female C57BL/6 mice to form the model. Single radiation doses of 20, 40 or 60 Gy were given to the selected mice, with or without the adjacent lung tissue, using conformal radiation therapy to the cardiac apex. When the results were analyzed, perivascular fibrosis was seen 8 and 24 weeks after RT. The developed model can be utilized to incorporate radiomic and biochemical markers of cardiotoxicity to guide early treatment intervention and human translation studies [85].

In another study, Ibrahim et al. aimed to detect cardiac magnetic resonance (CMR) imaging markers of early RT-induced cardiac dysfunction. In the study, the effect of CMR on global and regional cardiac function and myocardial T1/T2 values at 2-time points after RT with the use of CMR in a localized cardiac RT rat model was investigated. Rats that received 24 Gy radiation, whole-heart radiation were compared to sham-treated rats. They concluded that MRI regional myocardial strain is sensitive imaging diagnostic for detecting RT-induced subclinical cardiac damage before global cardiac function was compromised [86].

4. Ischemic cardiomyopathy

Ischemia is another of the most typical cardiotoxic effects [87]. This term comes from the Greek language (isch means restriction and haema means blood) and refers to a situation where there is an imbalance between the demand for blood and the supply in the tissue [88]. Cardiomyocytes, unlike other tissue cells, do not store energy in the form of glycogen, hence the relationship between myocardial oxygen use and the amount of oxygen given to the myocardial cells is extremely delicate. Cardiovascular problems are further increased by myocardial ischemia [89]. Stress, aging, alcohol consumption, and poor nutrition are all risk factors [90]. 5-fluorouracil (5-FU), cisplatin, and capecitabine are the most common chemotherapeutic agents that cause cardiac ischemia as a cardiotoxic side effect [88, 91, 92]. Isoproterenol (ISP) is another drug that is commonly used to treat bradycardia and heart block, but it can cause myocardial ischemia [92]. 5-FU is a common anticancer drug that can cause cardiotoxicity and is related to myocardial ischemia. In this case, the potential mechanism that occurs in myocardial ischemia is indirectly induced coronary vasospasm. Coronary vasospasm may be caused by the synthesis of vasoactive compounds, intimal hyperplasia which results in hyperactive coronary arteries, or it can be myocardial cell damage that occurs as an autoimmune reaction in individuals who are susceptible to 5-FU. Eskilsson et al. investigated verapamil to see if it could protect against 5-FU-induced cardiac ischemia, but the results were not significant [88]. Capecitabine, another agent that is used in chemotherapy, is the oral prodrug of 5-FU. In other words, it is the inactive form of 5-FU, which is activated by thymidine phosphorylase in tumor cells. It is used for its advantages compared to 5-FU. However, capecitabine cardiotoxicity is also known to be reported in the literature [92]. In a case of cardiac ischemia associated with capecitabine-induced cardiotoxicity, acute onset of severe anterior chest pain is observed. The development of chest pain and ischemic changes on ECG is no more observed after capecitabine is ceased [93].

Isoproterenol (ISP) is a medication used to treat conditions such as bradycardia, Torsades de pointes (TdP), and heart block. However, ISP also generates free radicals, which cause oxidative stress. Underlying molecular mechanisms in ISP-induced cardiotoxicity include oxidative stress, the renin-angiotensin system (RAS), apoptosis, and DNA damage. All of these causes cell death and, as a result, cardiac injury, including ischemia [90].

Cisplatin is an antineoplastic drug based on platinum. It is used to treat tumors of the lung, ovary, sarcoma, and lymphoma. The most common cardiotoxic complications caused by cisplatin are thromboembolic events, including myocardial ischemia and infarction [94]. Depolarization of the mitochondrial membrane due to structural abnormalities is one of the mechanisms involved in cisplatin-induced myocardial dysfunction. Furthermore, the endoplasmic reticulum stress response is activated, and apoptosis and caspase-3 activity are increased in cardiomyocytes [95].

Arsenic trioxide (As_2O_3) is an anticancer agent used in patients with acute promyelocytic leukemia. Arsenic is a chemical element that can be consumed or absorbed through the environment, such as through water and air. Arsenic-related cardiopathological consequences include heart failure and arrhythmia. Caspase activation, mitochondrial disruption, and the pk53 and MAPK signaling pathways all contribute to apoptosis in arsenic cardiotoxicity [96].

Following are a few examples of *in vivo* models of ischemic cardiomyopathy and protective agents based on the literature;

Paclitaxel, a taxoloid drug, is a cardiotoxicity-inducing drug that causes ischemia, with mechanisms including oxidative stress and apoptosis [97]. Studies on mice have shown that L-glutamine protects against the cardiotoxicity of the anticancer drug cantharidin, which is similar to ischemia in its mechanism of action [98]. ISP is used in protective drug research to create acute or progressive cardiotoxicity in animal models. Curcumin, quercetin, coriander, Momordica, and Withania somnifera are plant-based agents that have been shown to reduce myocardial ischemia in ISP models [90]. The extract of the Spondias mombin plant was used as a treatment in an ISP model on rats. The findings strongly imply that the plant could be used as a cardioprotective treatment. Spondias mombin improves the contractility of the ISP model rat hearts, which are unable to pump blood due to ischemia [99]. Another ISP model investigation was conducted by Jain et al., and ferulic acid was found to be a cardioprotective agent for ISP-induced cardiotoxicity [100]. Pituitrin, like ISP, induces myocardial ischemia. Another rat model for cardiotoxicity is being investigated, and a flavonoid named latifolin derived from Lignum dalbergiae odoriferae was shown to protect against acute myocardial ischemia induced by pituitrin and ISP [101]. Zhang et al. investigated latifolin's cardioprotective effects on doxorubicin-induced cardiotoxicity. They determined that latifolin protects against the cardiotoxic effects of doxorubicin [102].

5. Diabetic cardiomyopathy

Diabetes mellitus (DM) is a heterogeneous metabolic disease characterized by chronic hyperglycemia resulting from defects in insulin action, insulin secretion, or both. Although, some of the patients die from acute metabolic complications such as ketoacidosis, hyperosmolar hyperglycemic state, and hypoglycemia, the main problem is the increased morbidity and mortality resulting from long-term complications of diabetes. Morbidity and mortality are related to decreased life expectancy and decreased quality of life due to diabetes-related complications [103]. The main cause of morbidity and mortality in diabetic patients is cardiovascular complications [104].

40% of DM patients have heart failure and cardiotoxicity. The increase in the incidence of these conditions is because insulin resistance is a risk factor [105]. Insulin desensitization greatly diminishes the important effects of insulin on heart tissue. It is expressed on many cell surfaces, including cardiomyocytes, where insulin receptor, ligand binding, and insulin receptor substrates (IRS) 1 and 2 are taken up. In addition to IRS1 and IRS2, regulation of the PI3K/Akt pathway is also important in the ERK and MAP kinase cascade. They provide control of metabolism and cell survival. One of the Akt isoforms, AKT1 is involved in the survival of cardiomyocytes; AKT2 is required for the modulation of genes involved in cardiac metabolism. AKT2 promotes glucose uptake through mobilization and fusion of GLU4-containing vesicles to the plasma membrane. Short-term activation of AKT shows cardioprotective effects, can increase glycolysis, and decrease oxidative phosphorylation. The long-term activity of AKT1 in the adult heart is associated with a higher risk of cardiac complications and reduced mitochondrial function [106].

Following insulin stimulation, AKT1 phosphorylates and blocks FOXO1 nuclear translocation, inhibiting the expression of proapoptotic proteins belonging to the Bcl-2 family. FOXO1 has emerged as one of the key players in chronic metabolic diseases, promoting hyperglycemia and glucose intolerance [107]. In physiological conditions, pro-survival stimuli were induced by insulin-suppressing FOXO1 activity via the PI3K/AKT1 pathway. Following stress stimuli, FOXO1 translocates in the nucleus and causes negative feedback on the insulin pathway via a JNK-dependent mechanism that greatly reduces IRS-1 activity [108].

The heart of healthy people without DM obtains 60–90% of its energy from free fatty acids (FFA) oxidation and the rest from lactate and glucose [109]. In patients with DM, glucose uptake is greatly reduced, FFA uptake is increased, and the metabolic balance shifts to lipid oxidation. Increased FFA oxidation is complicated by lipotoxicity and high levels of triglyceride synthesis causing myocyte apoptosis. Additionally, in the diabetic heart, increased lipid oxidation increases mitochondrial dissociation and oxidative stress, which can lead to decreased myocardial energy production and myocardial contractile dysfunction [110]. Hyperglycemia is an important component in diabetes-associated cardiotoxicity because glucotoxicity leads to cardiac dysfunction by inducing oxidative stress and producing enhanced glycation end products. In addition, hyperglycemia may activate the renin-angiotensin-aldosterone system (RAAS) and cause an increase in cell necrosis and fibrosis [111]. Another important component is the inflammation that occurs in diabetes. Expression of inflammatory cytokines such as tissue necrosis factor-alpha (TNF-α) and interleukin-6 (IL-6) is increased in the myocardium associated with myocardial contractile dysfunction [112]. In a study by Stentz et al., it was reported that acute hyperglycemic crises such as diabetic ketoacidosis (DKA) and hyperosmolar hyperglycemic syndrome (HHS) are associated with the inflammatory state and independently cause changes in proinflammatory cytokines, oxidative stress, and cardiovascular markers [113].

Increased leukocytes in the myocardium also contribute to the relationship between diabetes and cardiotoxicity. Pathological stresses such as hyperglycemia, hyperlipidemia, high RAAS, and advanced glycation end products (AGEs) stimulate the secretion of proinflammatory molecules, adhesion molecules, and danger-associated molecular patterns (DAMPs) from leukocytes. In addition, these triggers induce ROS-mediated endothelial dysfunction, which also causes cardiac remodeling. Secreted proinflammatory cytokines bind to receptors such as TLR4-MyD88 complex, the receptor for AGEs (RAGE), and IL-1R and initiate intracellular signaling pathways. These pathways activate NF-kB, resulting in transcriptional upregulation of inflammatory cytokines and NLRP3 inflammasome. NF-kB activation and increased oxidative stress mature IL-1B and IL-18 with induction of pyroptosis. At the same time, stressed and damaged cardiomyocytes contribute to inflammatory cascades by releasing pro-inflammatory cytokines and DAMPs. The chronic inflammatory cytokine-induced intracellular response causes pathological cardiac remodeling and cardiac dysfunction [114].

In summary, it involves complex and multifactorial mechanisms such as hyperglycemia, hyperinsulinemia, insulin resistance, increased free fatty acids, microvascular damage and inflammatory cytokines, changes cellular metabolic pathways in cardiomyocytes and contributes to cardiotoxicity by impairing heart function.

Following are a few examples of *in vivo* models of diabetic cardiomyopathy and protective agents based on the literature;

Rodent models of type 1 and type 2 diabetes share many features with human diabetic cardiomyopathy and have greatly advanced our understanding of the underlying pathology of diabetic cardiomyopathy. Each model has certain limitations, and there is no perfect model that fully phenotypes the human condition. Genetic heterogeneity and lifestyle differences among people make it difficult to produce a suitable model. Some studies with these models are given below.

In one study, empagliflozin treatment was applied to investigate the cardiac metabolic profile of Zucker diabetic fatty rats, which is an early-stage DMT2 model. This treatment activated the cardioprotective master regulator of cellular energy homeostasis, AMP-activated protein kinase, and decreased IL-6 and cardiac mRNA levels while increasing autophagy at the cardiac level. In addition, it reduced cardiac levels of the essential glucose mediators 2,3-bisphosphoglycerate and phosphoenolpyruvate, and regulated several amino acids important in the metabolic control of cardiac function, such as glutamic acid. Therefore, it has been proven that empagliflozin has a protective effect on the development of cardiometabolic diseases associated with cardiac bioenergetic dysregulation and cardiac lipidoma dysregulation [115].

In a study at the ERBAS Institute of Experimental Medicine, 12 rats were used to create a diabetic model after receiving an i.p injection of streptozocin. Rats were randomly assigned to one of two groups: the diabetes group, received 1 mL/kg saline, and the second one received 160 g/kg/day i.p oxytocin for 28 days. They found that oxytocin treatment reduced cardiac myocyte thicknesses significantly over a 4-week period. Besides, as plasma TGF-β levels increased in diabetic rats, oxytocin application significantly decreased plasma TGF-β levels [116].

In another study, rats with and without diabetes were used as models. The hearts of those predisposed to diabetes exhibited depressed contractility and ventricular relaxation at high filling pressures, and abnormalities in the contractile performance of these hearts were observed [117].

Diabetic patients suffer from dual stress on the heart: (1) diabetic cardiomyopathy caused by hyperglycemia and (2) cardiotoxicity caused by anti-diabetic drugs. The following drugs are used as a solution to cardiotoxicity [118].

Metformin (Met) is an oral biguanide antihyperglycemic drug commonly used in the treatment of type 2 diabetes. It activates AMPK and induces cardiac autophagy through the AMPK signaling pathway and improves cardiac functions. In other words, metformin activates AMP-activated protein kinases that play an important role in insulin signaling and fat and glucose metabolism [119]. Kobashigawa and colleagues demonstrated that the cardioprotective effect of metformin against DOX-induced toxicity is mediated through the upregulation of AMPK and its downstream target molecules [120]. However, treatment with high doses of metformin induces the same change in the AMPK pathway, but its protective effect is lost. The authors suggested that this may be due to the downregulation of the platelet-derived growth factor receptor. Moreover, silencing of adiponectin receptors suppressed AMPK activation and cell viability in metformin and DOX-treated cells [121]. In another study, metformin was able to activate AMPK, restore autophagy, and improve heart function [122].

Another drug, Pio, is hyperglycemic drug; it is FDA (Food and Drug Administration) approved and does not show liver toxicity, but cardiotoxicity. It stimulates the peroxisome proliferator-activated receptor (PPAR) γ, which controls the storage of fatty acids and glucose metabolism [123].

One study shows that curcumin has the potential to reverse cardiotoxicity caused by the anti-diabetic drugs Pio and Met. It confirms the generation of ROS in cardiomyoblasts upon treatment with anti-diabetic drugs that Pio is more toxic than Met. Curcumin significantly reduced the oxidative stress caused by anti-diabetic drugs and strengthened the built-in oxidative machinery. It also reduces mitochondrial changes and thus reduces apoptotic cell death of cardiomyoblasts *in vitro* [118].

6. Antipsychotic drug-induced cardiotoxicity

Antipsychotic drugs have been used to treat psychosis caused by a variety of disorders such as bipolar disorder, delirium, paranoia, schizophrenia, substance-induced psychosis, Tourette's syndrome, dementia, Huntington's disease, multiple sclerosis, and parkinsonism. They come in a variety of forms and affect dopamine, serotonin, and other receptors as well as physiological systems. This can cause a wide range of negative effects, such as palpitations, akathisia, dystonia, tardive dyskinesia, orthostatic hypotension, tachycardia, arrhythmias, and heart failure [124]. Antipsychotics are grouped into two types: first-generation (typical, conventional or neuroleptics) antipsychotics (FGAs) such as butyrophenones, chlorpromazine, haloperidol, phenothiazines, thioridazine, and thiothixene, and second-generation (atypical) antipsychotics (SGAs) such as aripiprazole, asenapine, brexpiprazole, clozapine, iloperidone, lurasidone, olanzapine, paliperidon, quetiapine, risperidone, ziprasidone. They can have a variety of effects on cardiovascular function, including direct effects such as blocking cardiac muscarinic receptors, blocking 1-adrenoceptors, blocking sodium, potassium, and calcium channels, and blocking calmodulin, causing QT prolongation as well as indirect effects such as blocking 2-adrenoceptors in the central nervous system (CNS). Antipsychotic drug-induced toxic cardiomyopathy has also frequently been linked to myocardial infarction [125, 126].

Clozapine, the only drug approved for resistant schizophrenia, comes with a warning for an increased risk of fatal myocarditis [124, 127].

Cyclic antidepressants, such as tricyclic and tetracyclic forms, were among the first antidepressants to be developed. TCAs (tricyclic antidepressants) inhibit norepinephrine and serotonin reuptake, leading to an overproduction of these neurotransmitters in the presynaptic cleft [128]. They also inhibit postsynaptic histamine, alpha-1 adrenergic, and muscarinic-acetylcholine receptors [129]. These tricyclic antidepressants were approved by the FDA for the treatment of depression and anxiety disorders: amitriptyline, amoxapine, desipramine, doxepin, Imipramine, nortriptyline, protriptyline, and trimipramine [130].

Most mortality from arrhythmias, hypotension, QTc prolongation, myocardial depression, and ventricular fibrillation is caused by cardiac toxicity, which is the most common side effect of TCAs. TCAs lengthen the cardiac action potential by inhibiting cardiac sodium channels and slowing phase 0 depolarization [131].

Amitriptyline (AMT) intoxication is the third most prevalent cause of mortality among prescription medication-related toxicities, after sedative-hypnotic drugs and analgesic drugs [132].

Following are a few examples of *in vivo* models of antipsychotic drug-induced cardiotoxicity and protective agents based on the literature;

In a study conducted at the ERBAS Institute of Experimental Medicine, they investigated and compared the electrophysiological, immunohistochemical, and biochemical effects of metoprolol, lipid emulsion, and $MgSO_4$ on AMT-induced cardiotoxicity. Thirty male Sprague-Dawley rats were used in the study. Five groups were given the following treatments: saline intraperitoneally (i.p.); AMT 100 mg/kg per os (p.o.) and saline i.p.; AMT 100 mg/kg p.o. and 5 mg/kg metoprolol i.p.; AMT 100 mg/kg p.o. and 20 ml/kg lipid emulsion. As a result of the study, the QT intervals were significantly prolonged in the AMT + saline group than in the other groups. The QT interval was significantly reduced in all the other groups when compared to the AMT + saline group. They reported that AMT has severe cardiotoxic effects and manifests with ECG abnormalities such as prolongation of QTc duration, which is crucial in cardiotoxicity. The study's findings also demonstrated that $MgSO_4$ was more potent than other treatments in AMT-toxic rats in terms of shortness of QTc prolongation and immunohistochemical/biochemical effects [133].

In their research, Erbas and his colleague examined the impact of metoprolol and diltiazem on ziprasidone-induced QTc prolongation. For the experiment, 24 rats were divided equally into four groups: I, control, II, 3 mg/kg ziprasidone and saline, III, 3 mg/kg ziprasidone and 1 mg/kg metoprolol, IV, and 3 mg/kg ziprasidone and 2 mg/kg diltiazem. As a result, they observed that rats treated solely with antipsychotic drugs developed ECG abnormalities. When the QTc intervals of the four groups were compared, the QTc of the second group (ziprasidone + saline) was significantly prolonged than that of the control group. Moreover, in the study, metoprolol and diltiazem were found to have a beneficial effect on a prolonged QT interval [134].

A study on clozapine-induced cardiotoxicity was conducted using young male Wistar rats that were given clozapine (10, 15, and 25 mg/kg/day, i.p.) for 21 days. Clozapine, particularly at relatively high doses, was found to have a clear cardiotoxic effect after haemodynamic and echocardiographic studies were performed to assess cardiac functions. An increase in the serum activity of CK-MB (creatine kinase-myocardial band) and LDH (lactate dehydrogenase), two markers of cardiotoxicity, supported these findings [135].

7. Transgenic methods in cardiotoxicity research

Cardiotoxicity develops later as a result of stress, chronic diseases, cancer therapies, and immunotherapies in general, but it can occur *in vivo* and *in vitro* if the necessary genetic facilities are available. Mimicking proteomic and genetic disorders, in particular, can cause cardiomyopathies, cardiac transmission problems, and a variety of heart diseases. These models are created using a variety of transgenic methods. The method to be used in a study also varies depending on the pathophysiological mechanisms being studied.

The main methods for creating transgenic models are TALEN (transcription activation-like effector nucleases), CRISPR/Cas9 (clustered regularly interspaced short palindromic repeats/CRISPR associated protein 9), sleeping beauty, piggyBac (PB), pronuclear microinjection (PMI), viral transgenesis, RNAi (RNA interference), and hiPSC (human induced pluripotent stem cells). Numerous studies are currently being conducted in which these methods are being used not only to create pathological models, but also to develop new treatment methods.

Following are a few examples of *in vivo* models of *transgenic methods* based on the literature;

Genetically modified cell lines are frequently used due to their ease of maintenance and manipulation. Unfortunately, cell culture results do not always accurately reflect human physiology.

hPSCs (human pluripotent stem cells) can be genetically reprogrammed and converted into iPSCs (induced pluripotent stem cells), which can then be used for functional analysis in a variety of studies. Isogenic hPSC lines derived from ZFNs (zinc-finger nucleases), TALENs, or CRISPR/Cas9 add to our understanding of a variety of cardiovascular diseases, particularly cardiomyopathies and electrophysiological disorders [136].

Disease models can be created in a matter of weeks using current gene-editing methods, including knock-in, knock-out or mutation of certain genes in experimental animals, such as rats. CRISPR/Cas9 systems have recently been used to edit DNA more efficiently based on direct injection of genome editing machines into single-celled mouse embryos. Various cardiovascular diseases have been studied in mammalian models, including but not limited to rats, rabbits, and pigs, to date. Even in zebrafish models alone, various cardiac development, cardiac regeneration, vascular development, and hereditary cardiomyopathy were studied. In addition to single-cell embryo studies, it has been demonstrated that somatic *in vivo* genome editing studies in adult animals using CRISPR/Cas9 delivery via viral vectors and lipid nanoparticles are possible. Adenovirus and adeno-associated viruses (AAVs) are viral vectors that can be used to efficiently present genetic material in adult animals [136].

Several transgenic models of inherited arrhythmias have been described. Long-QT syndrome (LQTS-1/2/3/8/15), Atrial fibrillation (AF), Brugada Syndrome, and Catecholaminergic polymorphic ventricular tachycardia (CPVT) are just a few of the inherited arrhythmias that have been created using the hPSC [137].

LQTS: Ion channel genes KCNQ1 and KCNH2 with dominant-negative mutations that cause LQTS Type 1 and 2, respectively, were successfully integrated into the AAVS1 locus, which is considered a safe haven using ZFN technology and created an LQTS model in a study on iPSC-CMs (iPSC-Cardiomyocytes). The potential duration of action in regulated iPSC-CMs was significantly longer than in control cells that were not regulated as characteristic phenotypes of the long-QT syndrome, according to patch-clamp results [138].

Dermal fibroblasts from two people in a family with LQTS-1 and two healthy people were infected with retroviral vectors encoding the human transcription factors OCT3/4, SOX2, KLF4, and c-MYC and converted into hPSCs in another study [139]. Another research examined the therapeutic potential of new IKs activators in LQTS using dermal fibroblasts differentiated into hPSCs [140].

To create the LQT15 model, an electrophysiological study mimicked mutations in CALM2 from the CALM1, CALM2, and CALM3 genes that encode Calmodulin, a Ca^{2+} sensor on hPSC [141].

Transgenic models are also frequently used in studies on other types of Long QT Syndrome [142–147].

Brugada Syndrome: a large class of arrhythmias caused by a mutation in SCN5A (sodium voltage-gated channel alpha subunit 5), a cardiac sodium channel gene. Brugada Syndrome, Bradycardia, Atrioventricular (AV) Blocks, and Ventricular Fibrillation are few examples (VF).

A scn5a+/− (heterozygous knock-out) transgenic rat model was created for therapeutic evaluation, and the Brugada Syndrome phenotype was mimicked in a study [148]. The models created in a study targeting the SCN5A gene demonstrate cardiac conduction slowdowns and ventricular tachycardia (VT) [149].

In an *in vitro* study, dermal fibroblasts from two patients with Brugada Syndrome and two healthy individuals were differentiated to iPSC-CMs using Sendai virus (SeV) [150].

CPVT: The mutation in the RYR2 gene, which encodes the cardiac ryanodine receptor and is associated with CPVT cases, is modeled on hiPSCs differentiated from dermal fibroblasts via retrovirus [151].

The main cardiomyopathies investigated by developing transgenic models are dilate cardiomyopathy (DCM), hypertrophic cardiomyopathy (HCM), and restrictive cardiomyopathy (RCM).

Dilate cardiomyopathy: A study focused on striated muscle alpha-tropomyosin (α-TM), an essential thin filament protein involved in the pathogenesis of both dilate and hypertrophic cardiomyopathy. The Glu54Lys mutation, one of two prominent mutations in this protein (Glu40Lys and Glu54Lys), was expressed in transgenic rats. In echocardiography examinations, the successful dilate cardiomyopathy phenotype was observed [152].

In an iPSC-based study, an iPSC-CMs model was created from dermal fibroblasts from patients in a DCM family with a spot mutation (R173W) on the gene encoding cardiac troponin T (cTnT), a sarcomric protein [153].

In a study targeting Leiomodin proteins, which play a vital role in muscle thin filament length, the Lmod2 mutation was modeled in rats using the piggyBac transposon. It has been demonstrated that these rats with ventricular arrhythmias and increased postnatal mortality have a typical DCM phenotype [154].

In a recent study, a knock-in mouse model was created in which endogenous genes were altered to include the deletion of three base pairs encoded in cardiac troponin T for K210 in dilate cardiomyopathy patients [155].

In a study focusing on the titin protein, preserved blood samples from three DCM patients with the dominant TTN mutation were reprogrammed, and high-quality iPSC clones were expanded, differentiated, and enriched by metabolic selection to create a culture with >% iPSC-CMs. To analyze the effects of titin mutation on sarcoma structure, the iPSC-CMs method was created [156].

Hypertrophic cardiomyopathy: A transgenic hypertrophic cardiomyopathy model based on the erasure of 468–527 amino acids, which is bridged by the addition of a point mutation (G1445A) and 9 nonmyosin amino acids (SerSerLeuProHisLeuLysLeu) resulting in Arg403Gln, was created in a study targeting two mutations in the myosin heavy chain gene. Transgenic sequences were shown to be extracted from prokaryotic vector sequences, purified on agarose gels, and injected into the pronuclei of fertilized rat eggs [157].

In a comparative study, two different mutations (R92Q and E163R) in the TNNT2 gene, which encodes cardiac troponin T, were used. Echocardiography showed left ventricular hypertrophy, increased contractility, and diastolic dysfunction in both models. These phenotypes, however, were found to be more pronounced in R92Q mice [158]. HCM rat models with these two mutations had previously been described [159, 160].

In a study on the actin protein, the molecular mechanisms of apical hypertrophic changes were tried to be clarified in rat models created by a mutation (E99K) in the cardiac actin gene (ACTC). The phenotypic investigation of the created models was carried out using echocardiography, electrocardiography, magnetic resonance imaging, and a conductance catheter [161].

In a study examining the central role of calcium-related disorders in the disease pathogenesis in HCM, the iPSC-CMs model was created using fibroblasts derived from HCM patients with the Arg663His mutation in the MYH7 gene, which encodes the heavy chain of myosin [162].

A recent study used transgenic mouse models with the cardiac troponin-I mutation ($cTnI^{Gly146}$) to try to demonstrate that the exosomally derived Y-RNA fragment could regress the HCM clinic [163].

Restrictive cardiomyopathy: Mogensen and colleagues first described six different TnI C-terminal mutations linked to restrictive cardiomyopathy (L144Q, R145W, A171T, K178E, D190G, and R192H) in 2003 [164, 165].

In a study in RCM examining troponin mutations, transgenic rat models were explained by focusing on $cTnI^{193His}$ (R193H) and R145W mutations [165].

Numerous transgenic methods from the past to the present have developed *in vivo* and *in vitro* models that are commonly utilized to describe the pathophysiology of the disease. Aside from these studies, which look at the phenotypic manifestations of disease molecular mechanisms, the fact that transgenic approaches give hope for the treatment of numerous diseases has sparked a lot of research. Transgenic methods have therapeutic potential, particularly for cardiotoxic conditions induced by proteomic and genetic disorders that cannot be treated with drugs.

Besides these, R14del mutation in the phospholamban gene (PLN) is another important cause of cardiomyopathy development. Correcting this mutation on induced cardiomyocytes (iCMs) using the TALEN vector method resulted in improved Ca^{2+} handling, hypertrophic phenotype regression, and homogeneous reticular distribution of phospholamban [166]. In another study using 3D human engineering heart tissue technology, the PLN R14del mutation disrupts cardiac contractility; however, the contractile function is restored in this model with TALEN-mediated genetic correction [167].

A study of the human embryo revealed that the heterozygous MYBPC3 mutation associated with HCM is corrected by an endogenous, germline-specific DNA repair response using the homology-directed repair (HDR) with CRISPR/Cas9, an up-to-date genome editing method [168].

Long QT syndrome is caused by three major mutations: KCNQ1 (LQT1), KCNH2 (LQT2), and SCN5A (LQT3) [169]. These mutations disrupt potassium flow or prolong inward storage flows, prolonging the potential duration of cardiac action and reducing repolarization reserve. According to a study that modeled the E637K mutation in KCNH2, potassium currents were also corrected to relatively close levels after transfection with an optimized siRNA targeted against the mutant potassium channel [170].

A study of CASQ2 knockout rat models reported that exogenous CASQ2 expression, provided via intraperitoneal adeno-associated virus serotype 9 (AAV9) vector, improves CPVT phenotype by correcting arrhythmogenic phenotype and ultrastructural abnormalities [171].

In addition to these models, studies on the therapeutic potentials of transgenic studies for heart failure (HF) have been conducted. An earlier study revealed that overexpression of SERCA2a in cells isolated from HF patients improved myocyte contractile function [172]. Furthermore, genetic therapies for Duchenne muscular dystrophy (DMD), which causes HF with cardiomyopathy, were emphasized. Previous research tried to improve dystrophin mutations using transgenic methods such as ZFN, TALEN, and meganucleases [173–177]. Even more recently, the CRISPR/Cas9 method was used with AAV to treat mice with dystrophin deficiency induced by a spontaneous mutation in the dystrophin gene [178]. The aim was to remove exon 23 from the dystrophin gene, provide partial functional dystrophin expression in skeletal myofibers and heart muscle, and increase muscle strength [179–181].

8. Conclusion

Cardiomyopathy is a serious disease in which the heart muscle becomes inflamed and does not work as well as it should. Although, that drug administration and radiation therapy for the disease have a higher positive response, the number of patients experiencing early and late cardiac side effects is growing. There are dozens of diseases related to cardiotoxicity described in the literature, each with dozens of distinct proteomic/genetic mechanisms. The difficulty in modeling and treating diseases stems from the fact that disease mechanisms emerge from a variety of causes that interact with one another in a complex structure. New therapeutic agents, advanced genetic editing technologies and the effective revelation of molecular mechanisms every day, however, are a beacon of hope for humanity to overcome these diseases.

Author details

Oytun Erbaş[1,2*], İlknur Altuntaş[1,2], Özge Çağlar[1,3], Elif Özyilmaz[4], Ece Sari[1], İlayda Üzümcü[1] and Kaan Erbakan[1]

1 ERBAS Institute of Experimental Medicine, USA, Turkey

2 CEPHALINK Institute, USA, EU

3 Faculty of Science, Department of Chemistry, Selçuk University, Konya, Turkey

4 Faculty of Science, Department of Biochemistry, Selçuk University, Konya, Turkey

*Address all correspondence to: oytunerbas@yahoo.com

IntechOpen

© 2022 The Author(s). Licensee IntechOpen. This chapter is distributed under the terms of the Creative Commons Attribution License (http://creativecommons.org/licenses/by/3.0), which permits unrestricted use, distribution, and reproduction in any medium, provided the original work is properly cited.

References

[1] Tapio S. Pathology and biology of radiation-induced cardiac disease. Journal of Radiation Research. 2016;**57**(5):439-448. DOI: 10.1093/jrr/rrw064. Epub 2016 Jul 15

[2] Georgiadis N, Tsarouhas K, Rezaee R, Nepka H, Kass GEN, Dorne JCM, et al. What is considered cardiotoxicity of anthracyclines in animal studies. Oncology Reports. 2020;**44**(3):798-818. DOI: 10.3892/or.2020.7688. Epub 2020 Jul 14. Erratum in: Oncol Rep. 2020;**44**(4): 1772

[3] Bidulescu DT, Alexandrescu SR. Cardiotoxicology. In: Nriagu JO, editor. Encyclopedia of Environmental Health: Elsevier; 2011. pp. 524-531. ISBN: 9780444522726

[4] Boerma M, Hauer-Jensen M. Preclinical research into basic mechanisms of radiation-induced heart disease. Cardiology Research and Practice. 2010;**2011**:858262

[5] Hoffman JW Jr, Gilbert TB, Poston RS, Silldorff EP. Myocardial reperfusion injury: etiology, mechanisms, and therapies. Journal of Extra Corporeal Technology. 2004 Dec;**36**(4):391-411

[6] Li DL, Hill JA. Cardiomyocyte autophagy and cancer chemotherapy. Journal of Molecular and Cellular Cardiology. 2014;**71**:54-61. DOI: 10.1016/j.yjmcc.2013.11.007. Epub 2013 Nov 14

[7] Sheppard RJ, Berger J, Sebag IA. Cardiotoxicity of cancer therapeutics: Current issues in screening, prevention, and therapy. Frontiers in Pharmacology. 2013;**4**:19. DOI: 10.3389/fphar.2013.00019

[8] Kaneko M, Matsumoto Y, Hayashi H, Kobayashi A, Yamazaki N. Oxygen free radicals and calcium homeostasis in the heart. Mol Cell Biochem. Jun 1994 15;**135**(1):99-108. doi: 10.1007/BF00925965. Molecular and Cellular Biochemistry. 1994;**139**(1): 91-100

[9] Antoniou CK, Dilaveris P, Manolakou P, Galanakos S, Magkas N, Gatzoulis K, et al. QT prolongation and malignant arrhythmia: How serious a problem? European Cardiology. 2017;**12**(2):112-120. DOI: 10.15420/ecr.2017:16:1

[10] Force T, Kolaja KL. Cardiotoxicity of kinase inhibitors: The prediction and translation of preclinical models to clinical outcomes. Nature Reviews. Drug Discovery. 2011;**10**(2):111-126. DOI: 10.1038/nrd3252

[11] Waldman AD, Fritz JM, Lenardo MJ. A guide to cancer immunotherapy: From T cell basic science to clinical practice. Nature Reviews. Immunology. 2020;**20**(11):651-668. DOI: 10.1038/s41577-020-0306-5. Epub 2020 May 20

[12] Lenneman CG, Sawyer DB. Cardio-oncology: An update on cardiotoxicity of cancer-related treatment. Circulation Research. 2016;**118**(6):1008-1020. DOI: 10.1161/CIRCRESAHA.115.303633

[13] Cardinale D, Sandri MT. Role of biomarkers in chemotherapy-induced cardiotoxicity. Progress in Cardiovascular Diseases. 2010;**53**(2):121-129. DOI: 10.1016/j.pcad.2010.04.002

[14] Swain SM, Whaley FS, Ewer MS. Congestive heart failure in patients treated with doxorubicin: A retrospective analysis of three trials. Cancer. 2003;**97**(11):2869-2879. DOI: 10.1002/cncr.11407

[15] Yeh ET, Tong AT, Lenihan DJ, Yusuf SW, Swafford J, Champion C, et al. Cardiovascular complications of cancer therapy: Diagnosis, pathogenesis, and management. Circulation. 2004;**109**(25):3122-3131. DOI: 10.1161/01.CIR.0000133187.74800.B9

[16] Geisberg CA, Sawyer DB. Mechanisms of anthracycline cardiotoxicity and strategies to decrease cardiac damage. Current Hypertension Reports. 2010;**12**(6):404-410. DOI: 10.1007/s11906-010-0146-y

[17] Venkatesh P, Kasi A. Anthracyclines. In: StatPearls [Internet]. Treasure Island (FL): StatPearls Publishing. p. 2021. Available from: https://www.ncbi.nlm.nih.gov/books/NBK538187/

[18] Barry E, Alvarez JA, Scully RE, Miller TL, Lipshultz SE. Anthracycline-induced cardiotoxicity: Course, pathophysiology, prevention and management. Expert Opinion on Pharmacotherapy. 2007;**8**(8):1039-1058. DOI: 10.1517/14656566.8.8.1039

[19] Jones RL, Ewer MS. Cardiac and cardiovascular toxicity of non-anthracycline anticancer drugs. Expert Review of Anticancer Therapy. 2006; **6**(9):1249-1269. DOI: 10.1586/14737140.6.9.1249

[20] Wang L, Ma W, Markovich R, Chen JW, Wang PH. Regulation of cardiomyocyte apoptotic signaling by insulin-like growth factor I. Circulation Research. 1998;**83**(5):516-522. DOI: 10.1161/01.res.83.5.516

[21] Goffart S, von Kleist-Retzow JC, Wiesner RJ. Regulation of mitochondrial proliferation in the heart: Power-plant failure contributes to cardiac failure in hypertrophy. Cardiovascular Research. 2004;**64**(2):198-207. DOI: 10.1016/j.cardiores.2004.06.030

[22] Lipshultz SE, Rifai N, Sallan SE, Lipsitz SR, Dalton V, Sacks DB, et al. Predictive value of cardiac troponin T in pediatric patients at risk for myocardial injury. Circulation. 1997;**96**(8):2641-2648. DOI: 10.1161/01.cir.96.8.2641

[23] Chen W, Liu I, Tomiyasu H, Lee J, Cheng C, Liao AT, et al. Imatinib enhances the anti-tumour effect of doxorubicin in canine B-cell lymphoma cell line. Veterinary Journal. 2019;**254**: 105398

[24] Piska K, Koczurkiewicz P, Bucki A, Wójcik-Pszczoła K, Kołaczkowski M, Pękala E. Metabolic carbonyl reduction of anthracyclines—Role in cardiotoxicity and cancer resistance. Reducing enzymes as putative targets for novel cardio-protective and chemosensitizing agents. Investigational New Drugs. 2017;**35**(3): 375-385. DOI: 10.1007/s10637-017-0443-2. Epub 2017 Mar 10

[25] Minotti G, Menna P, Salvatorelli E, Cairo G, Gianni L. Anthracyclines: Molecular advances and pharmacologic developments in antitumor activity and cardiotoxicity. Pharmacological Reviews. 2004;**56**(2):185-229. DOI: 10.1124/pr.56.2.6

[26] Simůnek T, Stérba M, Popelová O, Adamcová M, Hrdina R, Gersl V. Anthracycline-induced cardiotoxicity: Overview of studies examining the roles of oxidative stress and free cellular iron. Pharmacological Reports. 2009;**61**(1): 154-171. DOI: 10.1016/s1734-1140(09)70018-0

[27] Zhang S, Liu X, Bawa-Khalfe T, Lu LS, Lyu YL, Liu LF, et al. Identification of the molecular basis of doxorubicin-induced cardiotoxicity. Nature Medicine. 2012;**18**(11):1639-1642. DOI: 10.1038/nm.2919. Epub 2012 Oct 28

[28] Renu K, Abilash VG, Tirupathi Pichiah PB, Arunachalam S. Molecular mechanism of doxorubicin-induced cardiomyopathy —An update. European Journal of Pharmacology. 2018;**818**:241-253. DOI: 10.1016/j.ejphar.2017.10.043. Epub 2017 Oct 23

[29] Takemura G, Fujiwara H. Doxorubicin-induced cardiomyopathy from the cardiotoxic mechanisms to management. Progress in Cardiovascular Diseases. 2007;**49**(5):330-352. DOI: 10.1016/j.pcad.2006.10.002

[30] Capranico G, Tinelli S, Zunino F. Formation, resealing and persistence of DNA breaks produced by 4-demethoxy-daunorubicin in P388 leukemia cells. Chemico-Biological Interactions. 1989;**72**(1-2):113-123.DOI:10.1016/0009-2797(89)90022-7

[31] Lyu YL, Kerrigan JE, Lin CP, Azarova AM, Tsai YC, Ban Y, et al. Topoisomerase IIbeta mediated DNA double-strand breaks: Implications in doxorubicin cardiotoxicity and prevention by dexrazoxane. Cancer Research. 2007;**67**(18):8839-8846. DOI: 10.1158/0008-5472.CAN-07-1649

[32] Wu T, Qiao Q, Qin X, Zhang D, Zhang Z. Immunostimulatory cytokine and doxorubicin co-loaded nanovesicles for cancer immunochemotherapy. Nanomedicine. 2019;**18**:66-77. DOI: 10.1016/j.nano.2019.02.008. Epub 2019 Mar 2

[33] Holopainen T, Räsänen M, Anisimov A, Tuomainen T, Zheng W, Tvorogov D, et al. Endothelial Bmx tyrosine kinase activity is essential for myocardial hypertrophy and remodeling. Proceedings of the National Academy of Sciences of the United States of America. 2015;**112**(42):13063-13068. DOI: 10.1073/pnas.1517810112. Epub 2015 Oct 1

[34] Nijholt KT, Westenbrink BD, de Boer RA. Mitochondrial therapy for doxorubicin cardiomyopathy: Nuclear factor-κB to the rescue? Cardiovascular Research. 2020;**116**(6):1092-1094. DOI: 10.1093/cvr/cvz344

[35] Tacar O, Sriamornsak P, Dass CR. Doxorubicin: An update on anticancer molecular action, toxicity and novel drug delivery systems. The Journal of Pharmacy and Pharmacology. 2013;**65**(2):157-170. DOI: 10.1111/j.2042-7158.2012.01567.x. Epub 2012 Aug 2

[36] Carver JR. Management of trastuzumab-related cardiac dysfunction. Progress in Cardiovascular Diseases. 2010;**53**(2):130-139. DOI: 10.1016/j.pcad.2010.07.001

[37] Dean L, Kane M. Trastuzumab therapy and ERBB2 genotype. In: Pratt VM, Scott SA, Pirmohamed M, Esquivel B, Kane MS, Kattman BL, Malheiro AJ, editors. Medical Genetics Summaries [Internet]. Bethesda (MD): National Center for Biotechnology Information (US); 2012

[38] Witteles RM, Fowler MB, Telli ML. Chemotherapy-associated cardiotoxicity: How often does it really occur and how can it be prevented? Heart Failure Clinics. 2011;**7**(3):333-344. DOI: 10.1016/j.hfc.2011.03.005. Epub 2011 May 14

[39] Choueiri TK, Mayer EL, Je Y, Rosenberg JE, Nguyen PL, Azzi GR, et al. Congestive heart failure risk in patients with breast cancer treated with bevacizumab. Journal of Clinical Oncology. 2011;**29**(6):632-638. DOI: 10.1200/JCO.2010.31.9129. Epub 2011 Jan 4

[40] Chu TF, Rupnick MA, Kerkela R, Dallabrida SM, Zurakowski D, Nguyen L, et al. Cardiotoxicity associated with tyrosine kinase inhibitor sunitinib. Lancet. 2007;**370**(9604):2011-2019. DOI: 10.1016/S0140-6736(07)61865-0

[41] Tiribelli M, Medeot M. Cardiotoxicity of imatinib: At the heart of the problem. Leukemia Research. 2011;**35**(1):36-37. DOI: 10.1016/j.leukres.2010.09.021

[42] Garcia-Alvarez A, Garcia-Albeniz X, Esteve J, Rovira M, Bosch X. Cardiotoxicity of tyrosine-kinase-targeting drugs. Cardiovascular & Hematological Agents in Medicinal Chemistry. 2010;**8**(1):11-21. DOI: 10.2174/187152510790796192

[43] Dyck JR, Lopaschuk GD. AMPK alterations in cardiac physiology and pathology: Enemy or ally? The Journal of Physiology. 2006;**574**(Pt 1):95-112. DOI: 10.1113/jphysiol.2006.109389. Epub 2006 May 11

[44] Force T, Krause DS, Van Etten RA. Molecular mechanisms of cardiotoxicity of tyrosine kinase inhibition. Nature Reviews. Cancer. 2007;**7**(5):332-344. DOI: 10.1038/nrc2106

[45] Talpaz M, Shah NP, Kantarjian H, Donato N, Nicoll J, Paquette R, et al. Dasatinib in imatinib-resistant Philadelphia chromosome-positive leukemias. The New England Journal of Medicine. 2006;**354**(24):2531-2541. DOI: 10.1056/NEJMoa055229

[46] Dilruba S, Kalayda GV. Platinum-based drugs: Past, present and future. Cancer Chemotherapy and Pharmacology. 2016;**77**(6):1103-1124. DOI: 10.1007/s00280-016-2976-z. Epub 2016 Feb 17

[47] Bjerring AW, Fosså SD, Haugnes HS, Nome R, Stokke TM, Haugaa KH, et al. The cardiac impact of cisplatin-based chemotherapy in survivors of testicular cancer: A 30-year follow-up. European Heart Journal Cardiovascular Imaging. 2021;**22**(4):443-450. DOI: 10.1093/ehjci/jeaa289

[48] Demkow U, Stelmaszczyk-Emmel A. Cardiotoxicity of cisplatin-based chemotherapy in advanced non-small cell lung cancer patients. Respiratory Physiology & Neurobiology. 2013;**187**(1):64-67. DOI: 10.1016/j.resp.2013.03.013. Epub 2013 Mar 30

[49] Pai VB, Nahata MC. Cardiotoxicity of chemotherapeutic agents: Incidence, treatment and prevention. Drug Safety. 2000;**22**(4):263-302. DOI: 10.2165/00002018-200022040-00002

[50] Sledge GW, Neuberg D, Bernardo P, Ingle JN, Martino S, Rowinsky EK, et al. Phase III trial of doxorubicin, paclitaxel, and the combination of doxorubicin and paclitaxel as front-line chemotherapy for metastatic breast cancer: An intergroup trial (E1193). Journal of Clinical Oncology. 2003;**21**(4):588-592. DOI: 10.1200/JCO.2003.08.013

[51] Chatterjee K, Zhang J, Tao R, Honbo N, Karliner JS. Vincristine attenuates doxorubicin cardiotoxicity. Biochemical and Biophysical Research Communications. 2008;**373**(4):555-560. DOI: 10.1016/j.bbrc.2008.06.067. Epub 2008 Jun 30

[52] Gros R, Hugon V, Thouret JM, Peigne V. Coronary spasm after an injection of vincristine. Chemotherapy. 2017;**62**(3):169-171. DOI: 10.1159/000455224. Epub 2017 Feb 1

[53] Alter P, Herzum M, Soufi M, Schaefer JR, Maisch B. Cardiotoxicity of 5-fluorouracil. Cardiovascular & Hematological Agents in Medicinal Chemistry. 2006;**4**(1):1-5. DOI: 10.2174/187152506775268785

[54] Polk A, Vistisen K, Vaage-Nilsen M, Nielsen DL. A systematic review of the pathophysiology of 5-fluorouracil-induced cardiotoxicity. BMC Pharmacology and Toxicology. 2014;**15**:47. DOI: 10.1186/2050-6511-15-47

[55] Meyer CC, Calis KA, Burke LB, Walawander CA, Grasela TH. Symptomatic cardiotoxicity associated with 5-fluorouracil. Pharmacotherapy. 1997;**17**(4):729-736

[56] Fricker LD. Proteasome inhibitor drugs. Annual Review of Pharmacology and Toxicology. 2020;**60**:457-476. DOI: 10.1146/annurev-pharmtox-010919-023603. Epub 2019 Sep 3

[57] Delgado JL, Hsieh CM, Chan NL, Hiasa H. Topoisomerases as anticancer targets. Biochemical Journal. 2018;**475**(2):373-398. DOI: 10.1042/BCJ20160583

[58] Evison BJ, Sleebs BE, Watson KG, Phillips DR, Cutts SM. Mitoxantrone, more than just another topoisomerase II poison. Medicinal Research Reviews. 2016;**36**(2):248-299. DOI: 10.1002/med.21364. Epub 2015 Aug 19

[59] Jain D, Aronow W. Cardiotoxicity of cancer chemotherapy in clinical practice. Hospital Practice. 2019;**47**(1):6-15. DOI: 10.1080/21548331.2018.1530831. Epub 2018 ANTIPSYCHOTICMID: 30270693

[60] Herman EH, Ferrans VJ. Pretreatment with ICRF-187 provides long-lasting protection against chronic daunorubicin cardiotoxicity in rabbits. Cancer Chemotherapy and Pharmacology. 1986;**16**(2):102-106. DOI: 10.1007/BF00256157

[61] Zhang YY, Yi M, Huang YP. Oxymatrine ameliorates doxorubicin-induced cardiotoxicity in rats. Cellular Physiology and Biochemistry. 2017;**43**(2):626-635. DOI: 10.1159/000480471. Epub 2017 Sep 21

[62] Zilinyi R, Czompa A, Czegledi A, Gajtko A, Pituk D, Lekli I, et al. The cardioprotective effect of metformin in doxorubicin-induced cardiotoxicity: The role of autophagy. Molecules. 2018;**23**(5):1184. DOI: 10.3390/molecules23051184

[63] Taşkıran E, Erdoğan MA, Yiğittürk G, Erbaş O. Therapeutic effects of liraglutide, oxytocin and granulocyte colony-stimulating factor in doxorubicin-induced cardiomyopathy model: An experimental animal study. Cardiovascular Toxicology. 2019; **19**(6):510-517. DOI: 10.1007/s12012-019-09524-x

[64] Saad SY, Alkharfy KM, Arafah MM. Cardiotoxic effects of arsenic trioxide/imatinib mesilate combination in rats. The Journal of Pharmacy and Pharmacology. 2006;**58**(4):567-573. DOI: 10.1211/jpp.58.4.0017

[65] Saleh RM, Awadin WF, El-Shafei RA, Elseady YY, Wehaish FE, Elshal MF. Cardioprotective role of tadalafil against cisplatin-induced cardiovascular damage in rats. European Journal of Pharmacology. 2015;**765**:574-581. DOI: 10.1016/j.ejphar.2015.09.015. Epub 2015 Sep 14

[66] Lipshultz SE, Sambatakos P, Maguire M, Karnik R, Ross SW, Franco VI, et al. Cardiotoxicity and cardioprotection in childhood cancer. Acta Haematologica. 2014;**132**(3-4): 391-399

[67] Gianfaldoni S, Gianfaldoni R, Wollina U, Lotti J, Tchernev G, Lotti T. An overview on radiotherapy: From its history to its current applications in dermatology. Open Access Macedonian Journal of Medical Sciences. 2017;**5**(4): 521-525

[68] Ell P, Martin JM, Cehic DA, Ngo DTM, Sverdlov AL. Cardiotoxicity of radiation therapy: Mechanisms, management, and mitigation. Current Treatment Options in Oncology. 2021;**22**(8):70

[69] Wei T, Cheng Y. The cardiac toxicity of radiotherapy—A review of characteristics, mechanisms, diagnosis, and prevention. International Journal of Radiation Biology. 2021;**97**:1-8

[70] Yi P, Li H, Fang Y, Su J, Xu C, Cao L, et al. Administration of trastuzumab with heart irradiation induced acute cardiotoxicity in mice. American Journal of Cancer Research. 2020;**10**(2):536-544

[71] Koczwara B, Meng R, Miller MD, Clark RA, Kaambwa B, Marin T, et al. Late mortality in people with cancer: A population-based Australian study. The Medical Journal of Australia. 2021;**214**(7):318-323. DOI: 10.5694/mja2.50879. Epub 2020 Dec 9

[72] Adams MJ, Hardenbergh PH, Constine LS, Lipshultz SE. Radiation-associated cardiovascular disease. Critical Reviews Oncology Hematologyl. 2003 Jan;**45**(1):55-75. DOI: 10.1016/s1040-8428(01)00227-x

[73] Ratosa I, Ivanetic PM. Cardiotoxicity of mediastinal radiotherapy. Reports of Practical Oncology and Radiotherapy. 2019;**24**(6):629-643. DOI: 10.1016/j.rpor.2019.09.002. Epub 2019 Oct 30

[74] Saiki H, Petersen IA, Scott CG, Bailey KR, Dunlay SM, Finley RR, et al. Risk of heart failure with preserved ejection fraction in older women after contemporary radiotherapy for breast cancer. Circulation. 2017;**135**(15): 1388-1396

[75] Frankart AJ, Nagarajan R, Pater L. The impact of proton therapy on cardiotoxicity following radiation treatment. Journal of Thrombosis and Thrombolysis. 2021;**51**(4):877-883

[76] Hoppe BS, Flampouri S, Su Z, Latif N, Dang NH, Lynch J, et al. Effective dose reduction to cardiac structures using protons compared with 3DCRT and IMRT in mediastinal Hodgkin lymphoma. International Journal of Radiation Oncology, Biology, Physics. 2012;**84**(2):449-455

[77] Giraud P, Cosset JM. Toxicité cardiaque de la radiothérapie: physiopathologie, données cliniques [Radiation toxicity to the heart: Physiopathology and clinical data]. Bulletin du Cancer. 2004;**91**(Suppl 3):147-153. French

[78] Yusuf SW, Venkatesulu BP, Mahadevan LS, Krishnan S. Radiation-induced cardiovascular disease: A clinical perspective. Frontiers in Cardiovascular Medicine. 2017;**4**:66

[79] Elkady AA, Mohamed ET. Possible role of Withania somnifera against gamma radiation induced cardiotoxicity in male albino rats. Pakistan Journal of Zoology. 2016;**48**(2):539-545

[80] Mohamed ET, Elkady AA, Mohamed S, Said E, Kiki E. Protective effect of Symplocos racemosa Roxb against gamma radiation induced cardiotoxicity in male albino rats. Pakistan Journal of Zoology. 2016;**48**(6):1831-1837

[81] Mansour HH, Eid M, El-Arnaouty MB. Effect of silver nanoparticles synthesized by gamma radiation on the cytotoxicity of doxorubicin in human cancer cell lines and experimental animals. Human & Experimental Toxicology. 2018;**37**(1): 38-50

[82] EBCTCG (Early Breast Cancer Trialists' Collaborative Group), McGale P, Taylor C, Correa C, Cutter D, Duane F, et al. Effect of radiotherapy after mastectomy and axillary surgery on 10-year recurrence and 20-year breast cancer mortality: Meta-analysis of individual patient data for 8135 women in 22 randomised trials. Lancet. 2014;**383**(9935):2127-2135. DOI: 10.1016/S0140-6736(14)60488-8. Epub 2014 Mar 19. Erratum in: Lancet. 2014 Nov 22;384(9957):1848

[83] Mezzaroma E, Di X, Graves P, Toldo S, Van Tassell BW, Kannan H, et al. A mouse model of radiation-induced cardiomyopathy. International Journal of Cardiology. 2012;**156**(2):231-233. DOI: 10.1016/j.ijcard.2012.01.038. Epub 2012 Feb 16

[84] Boerma M, Wang J, Wondergem J, Joseph J, Qiu X, Kennedy RH, et al. Influence of mast cells on structural and functional manifestations of radiation-induced heart disease. Cancer Research. 2005;**65**(8):3100-3107. DOI: 10.1158/0008-5472.CAN-04-4333

[85] Dreyfuss AD, Goia D, Shoniyozov K, Shewale SV, Velalopoulou A, Mazzoni S, et al. A novel mouse model of radiation-induced cardiac injury reveals biological and radiological biomarkers of cardiac dysfunction with potential clinical relevance. Clinical Cancer Research. 2021;**27**(8):2266-2276. DOI: 10.1158/1078-0432.CCR-20-3882. Epub 2021 Feb 4

[86] Ibrahim EH, Baruah D, Croisille P, Stojanovska J, Rubenstein JC, Frei A, et al. Cardiac magnetic resonance for early detection of radiation therapy-induced cardiotoxicity in a small animal model.

JACC: CardioOncology. 2021;**3**(1):113-130. DOI: 10.1016/j.jaccao.2020.12.006. Epub 2021 Mar 16

[87] Frank A, Bonney M, Bonney S, Weitzel L, Koeppen M, Eckle T. Myocardial ischemia reperfusion injury: From basic science to clinical bedside. Seminars in Cardiothoracic and Vascular Anesthesia. 2012;**16**(3):123-132

[88] Eskilsson J, Albertsson M. Failure of preventing 5-fluorouracil cardiotoxicity by prophylactic treatment with verapamil. Acta Oncologica. 1990;**29**(8): 1001-1003

[89] Pagliaro BR, Cannata F, Stefanini GG, Bolognese L. Myocardial ischemia and coronary disease in heart failure. Heart Failure Reviews. 2020; **25**(1):53-65

[90] Allawadhi P, Khurana A, Sayed N, Kumari P, Godugu C. Isoproterenol-induced cardiac ischemia and fibrosis: Plant-based approaches for intervention. Phytotherapy Research. 2018;**32**(10): 1908-1932

[91] Oun R, Rowan E. Cisplatin induced arrhythmia; electrolyte imbalance or disturbance of the SA node? European Journal of Pharmacology. 2017;**811**: 125-128

[92] Tunio MA, Hashmi A, Shoaib M. Capecitabine induced cardiotoxicity: A case report and review of literature. Pakistan Journal of Pharmaceutical Sciences. 2012;**25**(1):277-281

[93] McGoldrick TA, Jodrell D, Clive S. Capecitabine (oral 5-fluorouracil pro-drug) treatment for colorectal carcinoma causing ischaemic chest pain. BML Case Reports. 2009;**2009**:bcr07.2008.0449

[94] Bursac D. Myocardial ischemia during combined chemotherapy with etoposide and cisplatin for non-small lung cancer. Oncology & Cancer Case Reports. 2018;**4**:141

[95] Varga ZV, Ferdinandy P, Liaudet L, Pacher P. Drug-induced mitochondrial dysfunction and cardiotoxicity. American Journal of Physiology. Heart and Circulatory Physiology. 2015;**309**(9):H1453-H1467

[96] Alamolhodaei NS, Shirani K, Karimi G. Arsenic cardiotoxicity: An overview. Environmental Toxicology and Pharmacology. 2015;**40**(3):1005-1014

[97] Lamberti M, Giovane G, Garzillo EM, Avino F, Feola A, Porto S, et al. Animal models in studies of cardiotoxicity side effects from antiblastic drugs in patients and occupational exposed workers. BioMed Research International. 2014;**2014**:240642

[98] Shao H, Dong L, Feng Y, Wang C, Tong H. The protective effect of L-glutamine against acute cantharidin-induced cardiotoxicity in the mice. BMC Pharmacology and Toxicology. 2020;**21**(1):71

[99] Akinmoladun AC, Obuotor EM, Barthwal MK, Dikshit M, Farombi EO. Ramipril-like activity of Spondias mombin linn against no-flow ischemia and isoproterenol-induced cardiotoxicity in rat heart. Cardiovascular Toxicology. 2010;**10**(4):295-305

[100] Jain PG, Mahajan UB, Shinde SD, Surana SJ. Cardioprotective role of FA against isoproterenol induced cardiac toxicity. Molecular Biology Reports. 2018;**45**(5):1357-1365

[101] Li XL, Chen LY, Guan ZY, Luo Y, Cui YR, Liu RH, et al. Effect of neoflavonoid latifolin isolated from Dalbergia odorifera on acute myocardial ischemia in rats and its mechanism of Nrf2 signaling pathway. Zhongguo Zhong Yao Za Zhi. 2017;**42**(20):3974-3982. Chinese. DOI: 10.19540/j.cnki.cjcmm.20170907.009

[102] Zhang N, Shou B, Chen L, Lai X, Luo Y, Meng X, et al. Cardioprotective

effects of latifolin against doxorubicin-induced cardiotoxicity by macrophage polarization in mice. Journal of Cardiovascular Pharmacology. 2020;**75**(6):564-572

[103] Tuomi T, Santoro N, Caprio S, Cai M, Weng J, Groop L. The many faces of diabetes: A disease with increasing heterogeneity. Lancet. 2014;**383**(9922): 1084-1094

[104] Seferović PM, Petrie MC, Filippatos GS, Anker SD, Rosano G, Bauersachs J, et al. Type 2 diabetes mellitus and heart failure: A position statement from the Heart Failure Association of the European Society of Cardiology. European Journal of Heart Failure. 2018;**20**(5):853-872

[105] Tromp J, Voors AA, Sharma A, Ferreira JP, Ouwerkerk W, Hillege HL, et al. Distinct pathological pathways in patients with heart failure and diabetes. JACC: Heart Failure. 2020;**8**:234-242

[106] DeBosch B, Sambandam N, Weinheimer C, Courtois M, Muslin AJ. Akt2 regulates cardiac metabolism and cardiomyocyte survival. The Journal of Biological Chemistry. 2006;**281**(43):32841-32851

[107] Riehle C, Abel ED. Insulin signaling and heart failure. Circulation Research. 2016;**118**(7):1151-1169

[108] Eijkelenboom A, Burgering BM. FOXOs: Signalling integrators for homeostasis maintenance. Nature Reviews. Molecular Cell Biology. 2013;**14**(2):83-97

[109] Stanley WC, Chandler MP. Energy metabolism in the normal and failing heart: Potential for therapeutic interventions. Heart Failure Reviews. 2002;**7**:115-130

[110] Aneja A, Tang WH, Bansilal S, Garcia MJ, Farkouh ME. Diabetic cardiomyopathy: Insights into pathogenesis, diagnostic challenges, and therapeutic options. The American Journal of Medicine. 2008;**121**(9):748-757

[111] Schilling JD, Mann DL. Diabetic cardiomyopathy: Bench to bedside. Heart Failure Clinics. 2012;**8**(4):619-631

[112] Westermann D, Van Linthout S, Dhayat S, Dhayat N, Schmidt A, Noutsias M, et al. Tumor necrosis factor-alpha antagonism protects from myocardial inflammation and fibrosis in experimental diabetic cardiomyopathy. Basic Research in Cardiology. 2007;**102**(6):500-507. DOI: 10.1007/s00395-007-0673-0. Epub 2007 Oct 5

[113] Stentz FB, Umpierrez GE, Cuervo R, Kitabchi AE. Proinflammatory cytokines, markers of cardiovascular risks, oxidative stress, and lipid peroxidation in patients with hyperglycemic crises. Diabetes. 2004;**53**(8):2079-2086

[114] Kaur N, Guan Y, Raja R, Ruiz-Velasco A, Liu W. Mechanisms and therapeutic prospects of diabetic cardiomyopathy through the inflammatory response. Frontiers in Physiology. 2021;**21**(12):694864

[115] Aragón-Herrera A, Feijóo-Bandín S, Otero Santiago M, Barral L, Campos-Toimil M, Gil-Longo J, et al. Empagliflozin reduces the levels of CD36 and cardiotoxic lipids while improving autophagy in the hearts of Zucker diabetic fatty rats. Biochemical Pharmacology. 2019;**170**:113677

[116] Çavuşoğlu T, Çiftçi ÖD, Çağıltay E, Meral A, Kızıloğlu İ, Gurgul S, et al. Histological and biochemical examination of the effect of oxytocin on diabetic cardiomyopathy rat model. Dicle Medical Journal. 2017;**44**(2):135-143

[117] Broderick TL, Hutchison AK. Cardiac dysfunction in the euglycemic diabetic-prone BB Wor rat. Metabolism. 2004;**53**(11):1391-1394

[118] Jain A, Rani V. Curcumin-mediated effects on anti-diabetic drug-induced cardiotoxicity. 3 Biotech. 2018;**8**(9):399

[119] Hostalek U, Gwilt M, Hildemann S. Therapeutic use of metformin in prediabetes and diabetes prevention. Drugs. 2015;**75**(10):1071-1094

[120] Kobashigawa LC, Xu YC, Padbury JF, Tseng YT, Yano N. Metformin protects cardiomyocyte from doxorubicin induced cytotoxicity through an AMP-activated protein kinase dependent signaling pathway: An in vitro study. PLoS ONE. 2014;**9**(8):e104888

[121] Asensio-López MC, Lax A, Pascual-Figal DA, Valdés M, Sánchez-Más J. Metformin protects against doxorubicin-induced cardio-toxicity: Involvement of the adiponectin cardiac system. Free Radical Biology & Medicine. 2011;**51**(10):1861-1871

[122] Rena G, Hardie DG, Pearson ER. The mechanisms of action of metformin. Diabetologia. 2017;**60**(9):1577-1585. DOI: 10.1007/s00125-017-4342-z. Epub 2017 Aug 3

[123] Smith U. Pioglitazone: Mechanism of action. International Journal of Clinical Practice. Supplement. 2001;**121**:13-18

[124] Khasawneh FT, Shankar GS. Minimizing cardiovascular adverse effects of atypical antipsychotic drugs in patients with schizophrenia. Cardiology Research and Practice. 2014;**2014**:273060. DOI: 10.1155/2014/273060. Epub 2014 Feb 4

[125] Buckley NA, Sanders P. Cardiovascular adverse effects of antipsychotic drugs. Drug Safety. 2000;**23**(3):215-228. DOI: 10.2165/00002018-200023030-00004

[126] Harrigan EP, Miceli JJ, Anziano R, Watsky E, Reeves KR, Cutler NR, et al. A randomized evaluation of the effects of six antipsychotic agents on QTc, in the absence and presence of metabolic inhibition. Journal of Clinical Psychopharmacology. 2004;**24**(1):62-69. DOI: 10.1097/01.jcp.0000104913.75206.62

[127] Kilian JG, Kerr K, Lawrence C, Celermajer DS. Myocarditis and cardiomyopathy associated with clozapine. Lancet. 1999;**354**(9193): 1841-1845. DOI: 10.1016/s0140-6736(99)10385-4

[128] Schneider J, Patterson M, Jimenez XF. Beyond depression: Other uses for tricyclic antidepressants. Cleveland Clinic Journal of Medicine. 2019;**86**(12):807-814. DOI: 10.3949/ccjm.86a.19005

[129] Obata H. Analgesic mechanisms of antidepressants for neuropathic pain. International Journal of Molecular Sciences. 2017;**18**(11):2483. DOI: 10.3390/ijms18112483

[130] Moraczewski J, Aedma KK. Tricyclic Antidepressants. In: StatPearls [Internet]. Treasure Island (FL): StatPearls Publishing. p. 2021. Available from: https://www.ncbi.nlm.nih.gov/books/NBK557791/

[131] Foianini A, Joseph Wiegand T, Benowitz N. What is the role of lidocaine or phenytoin in tricyclic antidepressant-induced cardiotoxicity? Clinical Toxicology (Philadelphia, Pa.). 2010;**48**(4):325-330. DOI: 10.3109/15563650.2010.487050

[132] Bateman DN, Chick J, Good AM, Kelly CA, Masterton G. Are selective serotonin re-uptake inhibitors associated with an increased risk of self-harm by antidepressant overdose? European Jouirnal of Clinical Pharmacology. 2004;**60**(3):221-224. DOI: 10.1007/s00228-004-0748-x

[133] Bora S, Erdoğan MA, Yiğittürk G, Erbaş O, Parlak İ. The effects of lipid emulsion, magnesium sulphate and metoprolol in amitriptyline-induced cardiovascular toxicity in rats.

Cardiovascular Toxicology. 2018;**18**(6): 547-556. DOI: 10.1007/s12012-018-9466-y

[134] Erbas O, Yilmaz M. Metoprolol and diltiazem ameliorate ziprasidone-induced prolonged corrected QT interval in rats. Toxicology and Industrial Health. 2015;**31**(12):1152-1157. DOI: 10.1177/0748233713487249. Epub 2013 Apr 26

[135] Abdel-Wahab BA, Metwally ME. Clozapine-induced cardiotoxicity in rats: Involvement of tumour necrosis factor alpha, NF-κβ and caspase-3. Toxicology Reports. 2014;**1**:1213-1223. DOI: 10.1016/j.toxrep.2014.11.012

[136] Chadwick AC, Musunuru K. Genome editing for the study of cardiovascular diseases. Current Cardiology Reports. 2017;**19**(3):22. DOI: 10.1007/s11886-017-0830-5

[137] Christidi E, Huang HM, Brunham LR. CRISPR/Cas9-mediated genome editing in human stem cell-derived cardiomyocytes: Applications for cardiovascular disease modelling and cardiotoxicity screening. Drug Discovery Today: Technologies. 2018;**28**:13-21. DOI: 10.1016/j.ddtec.2018.06.002. Epub 2018 Jun 25

[138] Wang Y, Liang P, Lan F, Wu H, Lisowski L, Gu M, et al. Genome editing of isogenic human induced pluripotent stem cells recapitulates long QT phenotype for drug testing. Journal of the American College of Cardiology. 2014;**64**(5):451-459. DOI: 10.1016/j.jacc.2014.04.057

[139] Moretti A, Bellin M, Welling A, Jung CB, Lam JT, Bott-Flügel L, et al. Patient-specific induced pluripotent stem-cell models for long-QT syndrome. The New England Journal of Medicine. 2010;**363**(15):1397-1409. DOI: 10.1056/NEJMoa0908679. Epub 2010 Jul 21

[140] Ma D, Wei H, Lu J, Huang D, Liu Z, Loh LJ, et al. Characterization of a novel KCNQ1 mutation for type 1 long QT syndrome and assessment of the therapeutic potential of a novel IKs activator using patient-specific induced pluripotent stem cell-derived cardiomyocytes. Stem Cell Research & Therapy. 2015;**6**(1):39. DOI: 10.1186/s13287-015-0027-z

[141] Yamamoto Y, Makiyama T, Harita T, Sasaki K, Wuriyanghai Y, Hayano M, et al. Allele-specific ablation rescues electrophysiological abnormalities in a human iPS cell model of long-QT syndrome with a CALM2 mutation. Human Molecular Genetics. 2017;**26**(9):1670-1677. DOI: 10.1093/hmg/ddx073

[142] Matsa E, Rajamohan D, Dick E, Young L, Mellor I, Staniforth A, et al. Drug evaluation in cardiomyocytes derived from human induced pluripotent stem cells carrying a long QT syndrome type 2 mutation. European Heart Journal. 2011;**32**(8):952-962. DOI: 10.1093/eurheartj/ehr073. Epub 2011 Mar 2

[143] Bellin M, Casini S, Davis RP, D'Aniello C, Haas J, Ward-van Oostwaard D, et al. Isogenic human pluripotent stem cell pairs reveal the role of a KCNH2 mutation in long-QT syndrome. The EMBO Journal. 2013;**32**(24):3161-3175. DOI: 10.1038/emboj.2013.240. Epub 2013 Nov 8

[144] Mehta A, Sequiera GL, Ramachandra CJ, Sudibyo Y, Chung Y, Sheng J, et al. Re-trafficking of hERG reverses long QT syndrome 2 phenotype in human iPS-derived cardiomyocytes. Cardiovascular Research. 2014;**102**(3): 497-506. DOI: 10.1093/cvr/cvu060. Epub 2014 Mar 12

[145] Terrenoire C, Wang K, Tung KW, Chung WK, Pass RH, Lu JT, et al. Induced pluripotent stem cells used to reveal drug actions in a long QT syndrome family with complex genetics.

The Journal of General Physiology. 2013;**141**(1):61-72. DOI: 10.1085/jgp.201210899

[146] Spencer CI, Baba S, Nakamura K, Hua EA, Sears MA, Fu CC, et al. Calcium transients closely reflect prolonged action potentials in iPSC models of inherited cardiac arrhythmia. Stem Cell Reports. 2014;**3**(2):269-281. DOI: 10.1016/j.stemcr.2014.06.003. Epub 2014 Jul 4

[147] Limpitikul WB, Dick IE, Tester DJ, Boczek NJ, Limphong P, Yang W, et al. A precision medicine approach to the rescue of function on malignant calmodulinopathic long-QT syndrome. Circulation Research. 2017;**120**(1):39-48. DOI: 10.1161/CIRCRESAHA.116.309283. Epub 2016 Oct 20

[148] Stokoe KS, Balasubramaniam R, Goddard CA, Colledge WH, Grace AA, Huang CL. Effects of flecainide and quinidine on arrhythmogenic properties of Scn5a+/− murine hearts modelling the Brugada syndrome. The Journal of Physiology. 2007;**581**(Pt 1):255-275. DOI: 10.1113/jphysiol.2007.128785. Epub 2007 Feb 15

[149] Papadatos GA, Wallerstein PM, Head CE, Ratcliff R, Brady PA, Benndorf K, et al. Slowed conduction and ventricular tachycardia after targeted disruption of the cardiac sodium channel gene Scn5a. Proceedings of the National Academy of Sciences of the United States of America. 2002;**99**(9):6210-6215. DOI: 10.1073/pnas.082121299. Epub 2002 Apr 23

[150] Liang P, Sallam K, Wu H, Li Y, Itzhaki I, Garg P, et al. Patient-specific and genome-edited induced pluripotent stem cell-derived cardiomyocytes elucidate single-cell phenotype of Brugada Syndrome. Journal of the American College of Cardiology. 2016;**68**(19):2086-2096. DOI: 10.1016/j.jacc.2016.07.779

[151] Itzhaki I, Maizels L, Huber I, Gepstein A, Arbel G, Caspi O, et al. Modeling of catecholaminergic polymorphic ventricular tachycardia with patient-specific human-induced pluripotent stem cells. Journal of the American College of Cardiology. 2012;**60**(11):990-1000. DOI: 10.1016/j.jacc.2012.02.066. Epub 2012 Jun 27

[152] Rajan S, Ahmed RP, Jagatheesan G, Petrashevskaya N, Boivin GP, Urboniene D, et al. Dilated cardiomyopathy mutant tropomyosin mice develop cardiac dysfunction with significantly decreased fractional shortening and myofilament calcium sensitivity. Circulation Research. 2007;**101**(2):205-214. DOI: 10.1161/CIRCRESAHA.107.148379. Epub 2007 Jun 7. Erratum in: Circ Res. 2007 Sep 14;101(6):e80

[153] Sun N, Yazawa M, Liu J, Han L, Sanchez-Freire V, Abilez OJ, et al. Patient-specific induced pluripotent stem cells as a model for familial dilated cardiomyopathy. Science Translational Medicine. 2012;**4**(130):130ra47. DOI: 10.1126/scitranslmed.3003552

[154] Li S, Mo K, Tian H, Chu C, Sun S, Tian L, et al. Lmod2 piggyBac mutant mice exhibit dilated cardiomyopathy. Cell & Bioscience. 2016;**6**:38. DOI: 10.1186/s13578-016-0101-y

[155] Du CK, Morimoto S, Nishii K, Minakami R, Ohta M, Tadano N, et al. Knock-in mouse model of dilated cardiomyopathy caused by troponin mutation. Circulation Research. 2007;**101**(2):185-194. DOI: 10.1161/CIRCRESAHA.106.146670. Epub 2007 Jun 7

[156] Hinson JT, Chopra A, Nafissi N, Polacheck WJ, Benson CC, Swist S, et al. HEART DISEASE. Titin mutations in iPS cells define sarcomere insufficiency as a cause of dilated cardiomyopathy. Science. 2015;**349**(6251):982-986. DOI: 10.1126/science.aaa5458

[157] Vikstrom KL, Factor SM, Leinwand LA. Mice expressing mutant myosin heavy chains are a model for familial hypertrophic cardiomyopathy. Molecular Medicine. 1996;**2**(5):556-567

[158] Ferrantini C, Coppini R, Pioner JM, Gentile F, Tosi B, Mazzoni L, et al. Pathogenesis of hypertrophic cardiomyopathy is mutation rather than disease specific: A comparison of the cardiac troponin T E163R and R92Q mouse models. Journal of the American Heart Association. 2017;**6**(7):e005407. DOI: 10.1161/JAHA.116.005407

[159] Tardiff JC, Hewett TE, Palmer BM, Olsson C, Factor SM, Moore RL, et al. Cardiac troponin T mutations result in allele-specific phenotypes in a mouse model for hypertrophic cardiomyopathy. The Journal of Clinical Investigation. 1999;**104**(4):469-481. DOI: 10.1172/JCI6067

[160] Moore RK, Abdullah S, Tardiff JC. Allosteric effects of cardiac troponin TNT1 mutations on actomyosin binding: A novel pathogenic mechanism for hypertrophic cardiomyopathy. Archives of Biochemistry and Biophysics. 2014;**552-553**:21-28. DOI: 10.1016/j.abb.2014.01.016. Epub 2014 Jan 28

[161] Song W, Dyer E, Stuckey DJ, Copeland O, Leung MC, Bayliss C, et al. Molecular mechanism of the E99K mutation in cardiac actin (ACTC Gene) that causes apical hypertrophy in man and mouse. The Journal of Biological Chemistry. 2011;**286**(31):27582-27593. DOI: 10.1074/jbc.M111.252320. Epub 2011 May 26

[162] Lan F, Lee AS, Liang P, Sanchez-Freire V, Nguyen PK, Wang L, et al. Abnormal calcium handling properties underlie familial hypertrophic cardiomyopathy pathology in patient-specific induced pluripotent stem cells. Cell Stem Cell. 2013;**12**(1):101-113. DOI: 10.1016/j.stem.2012.10.010

[163] Huang F, Na N, Ijichi T, Wu X, Miyamoto K, Ciullo A, et al. Exosomally derived Y RNA fragment alleviates hypertrophic cardiomyopathy in transgenic mice. Molecular Therapy—Nucleic Acids. 2021;**24**:951-960. DOI: 10.1016/j.omtn.2021.04.014

[164] Mogensen J, Kubo T, Duque M, Uribe W, Shaw A, Murphy R, et al. Idiopathic restrictive cardiomyopathy is part of the clinical expression of cardiac troponin I mutations. Journal of Clinical Investigation. 2003;**111**(2):209-216. DOI: 10.1172/JCI16336. Erratum in: The Journal of Clinical Investigation 2003 Mar;111(6):925

[165] Liu X, Zhang L, Pacciulli D, Zhao J, Nan C, Shen W, et al. Restrictive cardiomyopathy caused by troponin mutations: Application of disease animal models in translational studies. Frontiers in Physiology. 2016;**7**:629. DOI: 10.3389/fphys.2016.00629

[166] Karakikes I, Stillitano F, Nonnenmacher M, Tzimas C, Sanoudou D, Termglinchan V, et al. Correction of human phospholamban R14del mutation associated with cardiomyopathy using targeted nucleases and combination therapy. Nature Communications. 2015;**6**:6955. DOI: 10.1038/ncomms7955

[167] Stillitano F, Turnbull IC, Karakikes I, Nonnenmacher M, Backeris P, Hulot JS, et al. Genomic correction of familial cardiomyopathy in human engineered cardiac tissues. European Heart Journal. 2016;**37**(43):3282-3284. DOI: 10.1093/eurheartj/ehw307. Epub 2016 Jul 22

[168] Ma H, Marti-Gutierrez N, Park SW, Wu J, Lee Y, Suzuki K, et al. Correction of a pathogenic gene mutation in human embryos. Nature. 2017;**548**(7668):413-419. DOI: 10.1038/nature23305. Epub 2017 Aug 2

[169] Mizusawa Y, Horie M, Wilde AA. Genetic and clinical advances in congenital long QT syndrome. Circulation Journal. 2014;**78**(12): 2827-2833. DOI: 10.1253/circj.cj-14-0905. Epub 2014 Oct 1

[170] Lu X, Yang X, Huang X, Huang C, Sun HH, Jin L, et al. RNA interference targeting E637K mutation rescues hERG channel currents and restores its kinetic properties. Heart Rhythm. 2013;**10**(1):128-136. DOI: 10.1016/j.hrthm.2012.09.124. Epub 2012 Sep 26

[171] Denegri M, Avelino-Cruz JE, Boncompagni S, De Simone SA, Auricchio A, Villani L, et al. Viral gene transfer rescues arrhythmogenic phenotype and ultrastructural abnormalities in adult calsequestrin-null mice with inherited arrhythmias. Circulation Research. 2012;**110**(5):663-668. DOI: 10.1161/CIRCRESAHA.111.263939. Epub 2012 Jan 31

[172] del MonteF HSE, Schmidt U, Matsui T, Kang ZB, Dec GW, Gwathmey JK, et al. Restoration of contractile function in isolated cardiomyocytes from failing human hearts by gene transfer of SERCA2a. Circulation. 1999;**100**(23):2308-2311. DOI: 10.1161/01.cir.100.23.2308

[173] Chapdelaine P, Pichavant C, Rousseau J, Pâques F, Tremblay JP. Meganucleases can restore the reading frame of a mutated dystrophin. Gene Therapy. 2010;**17**(7):846-858. DOI: 10.1038/gt.2010.26. Epub 2010 Apr 15

[174] Ousterout DG, Perez-Pinera P, Thakore PI, Kabadi AM, Brown MT, Qin X, et al. Reading frame correction by targeted genome editing restores dystrophin expression in cells from Duchenne muscular dystrophy patients. Molecular Therapy. 2013;**21**(9):1718-1726. DOI: 10.1038/mt.2013.111, . Epub 2013 Jun 4. Erratum in: Mol Ther. 2013 Nov;21(11):2130

[175] Ousterout DG, Kabadi AM, Thakore PI, Perez-Pinera P, Brown MT, Majoros WH, et al. Correction of dystrophin expression in cells from Duchenne muscular dystrophy patients through genomic excision of exon 51 by zinc finger nucleases. Molecular Therapy. 2015;**23**(3):523-532. DOI: 10.1038/mt.2014.234. Epub 2014 Dec 10

[176] Popplewell L, Koo T, Leclerc X, Duclert A, Mamchaoui K, Gouble A, et al. Gene correction of a duchenne muscular dystrophy mutation by meganuclease-enhanced exon knock-in. Human Gene Therapy. 2013;**24**(7): 692-701. DOI: 10.1089/hum.2013.081

[177] Cordova G, Negroni E, Cabello-Verrugio C, Mouly V, Trollet C. Combined therapies for duchenne muscular dystrophy to optimize treatment efficacy. Frontiers in Genetics. 2018;**9**:114. DOI: 10.3389/fgene.2018.00114

[178] Nance ME, Duan D. Perspective on adeno-associated virus capsid modification for duchenne muscular dystrophy gene therapy. Human Gene Therapy. 2015;**26**(12):786-800. DOI: 10.1089/hum.2015.107. Epub 2015 Oct 15

[179] Nelson CE, Hakim CH, Ousterout DG, Thakore PI, Moreb EA, Castellanos Rivera RM, et al. In vivo genome editing improves muscle function in a mouse model of Duchenne muscular dystrophy. Science. 2016;**351**(6271):403-407. DOI: 10.1126/science.aad5143. Epub 2015 Dec 31

[180] Wang JZ, Wu P, Shi ZM, Xu YL, Liu ZJ. The AAV-mediated and RNA-guided CRISPR/Cas9 system for gene therapy of DMD and BMD. Brain & Development. 2017;**39**(7):547-556. DOI: 10.1016/j.braindev.2017.03.024. Epub 2017 Apr 5

[181] Zhu P, Wu F, Mosenson J, Zhang H, He TC, Wu WS. CRISPR/Cas9-mediated genome editing corrects dystrophin mutation in skeletal muscle stem cells in a mouse model of muscle dystrophy. Molecular Therapy—Nucleic Acids. 2017;7:31-41. DOI: 10.1016/j.omtn.2017.02.007. Epub 2017 Feb 28